THE WRITINGS OF ANNA FREUD

Volume V

RESEARCH AT THE HAMPSTEAD CHILD-THERAPY CLINIC AND OTHER PAPERS

1956-1965

THE WRITINGS OF ANNA FREUD
VOLUME V

RESEARCH
AT THE HAMPSTEAD
CHILD-THERAPY
CLINIC AND
OTHER PAPERS
1956-1965

INTERNATIONAL UNIVERSITIES PRESS, INC.

NEW YORK

Manufactured in the United States of America

Editor's Note

ORGANIZATION OF VOLUME V

The grouping of papers contained in this volume is based on the same principles used in Volume IV:*

1. according to the audience to which they were addressed,
2. in chronological sequence in each section.

However, Volume V, covering the period 1956-1965, differs in some respects from Volume IV. This difference is a reflection of the author's extension of her activities from working in private practice on her own to studies with a group of co-workers in a clinic setting which provided unique opportunities for systematic psychoanalytic research.

Thus, the items contained in Part I represent a new category: they are not papers written for publication but

---

* For details, see Vol. IV, *Indications for Child Analysis and Other Papers*, pp. vi-ix.

are communications addressed to a very specific "audience": fund-granting foundations. They describe the author's plans for projects as well as her methodological thinking.

Being of intrinsic interest to all those engaged in psychoanalytic research, the outlines included in Part I also provide important background information for an understanding of the author's subsequent work. They document the initial steps leading to the development of important new clinical tools (e.g., the Developmental Profile) and new conceptualizations (e.g., the concept of Developmental Lines, which, incidentally, appeared in print for the first time in a paper addressed to nursery school educators [see ch. 19]).

It should also be stressed that the author's contributions resulting from this period of work are contained not only in this volume but in her major publication, *Normality and Pathology in Childhood* (Volume VI). For this reason Volume V is, in terms of content, much more closely connected with Volume VI than with Volume IV.

The author's extension of activities to systematic research carried out by a team is also reflected in the greater number of items contained in Part IV, miscellaneous brief writings, half of which introduce work carried out at the Hampstead Child-Therapy Clinic.

Another extension of the author's activities has resulted in the enlargement of Part III, papers addressed to nonanalytic audiences. During the springs of 1963 and 1964 she was a member of the Yale Law School faculty. Evidence of this new interest is found in chs. 26 and 27.

Finally, ch. 38 has been placed in a category by itself,

Part V, because it is essentially a personal biographical document.

As was stressed in the Editor's note to Volume IV, the classification of papers according to the audience to which they were addressed does not imply that the contribution of individual papers is confined to that particular area. Even the personal biographical account contains ideas and suggestions applicable to present-day psychoanalytic training and education.

Contents

ix

Part II

Part III

Part IV

Part I

The items included in this section are with minor exceptions taken from applications to various fund-granting and supporting foundations. They represent outlines of research projects as first formulated by the author. In many instances they are presented in the form required by the specific foundation to which they were addressed. It should be stressed that they are not papers written for publication. They are nevertheless published here because they reflect the author's thinking about and planning for the research work carried out at the Hampstead Child-Therapy Clinic. The author's outlines included here as well as the papers by her colleagues listed in the Appendix bear witness to the Hampstead Clinic's specific approach to clinical facts and the pursuit of them to their theoretical implications.

Editor's note

1

The Hampstead
Child-Therapy Course
and Clinic
(1957)

DEVELOPMENT OF ACTIVITIES

As is expressed in our name, our organization serves several purposes which we separate into training, therapy, and research.

Training

We began as the Hampstead Child-Therapy Course in 1947 as a training scheme to equip graduate students of

From applications to the Psychoanalytic Research and Development Fund, New York, January 23, 1957; the Grant Foundation, New York, July 29, 1957; and the Taconic Foundation, New York, May 2, 1960.

psychology (or other disciplines dealing with human behavior) for analytic therapy with difficult children. The personal analyses of students, theoretical and technical lectures, and supervision of students' clinical work are carried out by a panel of analysts who are members of the British Psycho-Analytical Society.

Therapy

In 1951, a treatment center was added to the existing training scheme.[1] This treatment center began to function on January 1, 1952, under the name of Hampstead Child-Therapy Clinic. The Clinic is staffed by child analysts, by qualified analytic child therapists who have completed our own training course, and by senior students who are still in training with us.

Research

While engaged in teaching and therapy, we developed gradually a number of special interests and studies based on our case material. We appointed a number of our own qualified students as research assistants and asked for help and cooperation from the analysts on our panel.

DESCRIPTION OF UNITS (SERVICES) AND THEIR ACTIVITIES

Services

A MEDICAL-PSYCHOLOGICAL SERVICE FOR INFANTS

In this Well-Baby Clinic, our pediatrician, Dr. Josefine Stross, who was trained in both medicine and psycho-

[1] Supported by the Field Foundation.

analysis, sees approximately sixty mothers and their infants at regular intervals to guide them through the hazards of the first two years of life. Apart from the valuable help given to the mothers, she and her two assistants have developed a special interest in the general aspects of such preventive work. They try to determine the extent to which, and also the limits within which, such guidance serves to relieve important tensions that arise between mother and child at this early age; how far inexperienced mothers can be induced to cope efficiently with the problems arising around the child's sleeping and feeding attitudes, the processes of weaning and toilet training, and the repercussions of these bodily experiences on the infant's mind. The first interactions between the child's innate nature and the environmental influences can be traced at this time of life. Thus, while applying knowledge and serving the mothers, the Well-Baby Clinic becomes secondarily the source of much valuable observational material.

THE EDUCATIONAL UNIT

The nursery school, under the direction of Mrs. M. Friedman, is intended primarily for a small group of normal children from three to five years of age, but is sometimes attended by children who are in treatment at the Clinic. In addition, two groups of younger children (under three years of age) attend regularly once a week with their mothers.

While being used on occasion as an observational center for diagnostic purposes, our nursery school has set itself the further aim to explore how far children can be helped through the more common difficulties by educational measures based on analytic understanding. This leads to lively discussions among the staff concerning the relative merits of educational handling on the one hand and child analysis on the other hand.

In addition to the nursery school, the educational unit consists of other services:

(a) remedial teaching is given to a number of children who are in treatment in the Clinic;

(b) individual educational sessions are held with older children who are too disturbed for group activities and for some reason not suitable for treatment.

A NURSERY GROUP FOR BLIND CHILDREN, COMBINED WITH A SMALL ADVISORY SERVICE FOR THE MOTHERS OF BLIND BABIES

This special unit, of which Dorothy Burlingham is in charge, with Mrs. A. Curzon as head teacher, serves a small number of children. Our motive in setting up this venture was the following: while many mothers of normal infants may dispense with the services of a guiding clinic and find their own practical solutions, we find that no mother is normally equipped for the task of raising a child with a severe physical handicap such as blindness, deafness or deformity. Usually, much advice on physical matters is given to the mothers, but no consistent psychological guidance. The facts are that many of these physically handicapped children acquire secondary severe mental disturbances.

After analyzing several mentally disturbed handicapped children, we have approached this field from the specific aspect of the upbringing of the blind. While giving active help to the mothers and the children, we try to trace in the

cases under our observation not only the mental consequences of the primary physical defect, but also the consequences of the additional severe shocks administered to
such children from birth onward by such factors as the
mother's depression, her emotional difficulty in accepting
and loving a damaged child; by the repeated hospitalizations with separation from the mother; by many frightening
medical procedures carried out with complete disregard for
the child's (and the mother's) emotions and anxieties, etc.
—all these leading to secondary but major emotional disorders, many of which, we feel, could be prevented.

The Clinic as a Center for Training, Therapy, Research, and Preventive Work

While all other schemes and projects of our organization
work with comparative independence of each other, the
Clinic serves, and is used, by all departments. The Diagnostic Service of the Clinic is at the disposal of all other
services and governs the entry into the nursery school and
nursery group for the blind. All research projects depend on
the Clinic for their case material.

The fourfold orientation of the Clinic toward training,
therapy, research, and prevention is reflected in the selection of cases for analytic treatment, which fall, roughly, into
four categories:

(a) children with typical infantile neuroses, suitable for
treatment by students as part of their clinical training under the supervision of senior analysts or child
therapists;

(b) children with gross but incipient disturbances, needing treatment to prevent the development of severe abnormality;

(c) severely ill children sent to us for intensive therapy by other clinics where analytic treatment is not available;

(d) cases serving our specific research projects such as adolescents, handicapped, blind, orphaned children, child heroes, mother-child couples.[2]

[2]For a more detailed description of the Hampstead Child-Therapy Clinic, see Sandler (1965).

2

Research Projects of the Hampstead Child-Therapy Clinic

(1957–1960)

THE QUESTION OF PLANNED RESEARCH IN ANALYSIS

Analysts have often been reproached for taking no interest in planned research and the methods serving it; of making their discoveries haphazardly and incidentally; of not choos-

Based, in part, on a paper entitled "Clinical Studies in Psychoanalysis," which was published in *Proceedings of the Royal Society of Medicine*, 51:938-942, 1958, and also in *The Psychoanalytic Study of the Child*, 14:122-131, 1959. Other parts are selected from applications to the Psychoanalytic Research and Development Fund, New York, January 23, 1957, and the Grant Foundation, New York, July 29, 1957. The last section on "Research into the Prevention of Mental Illness" is taken from an application to the Taconic Foundation, New York, May 2, 1960.

ing their material according to plan; of working as individuals and not in teams; and of allowing their case material to drift out of sight without follow-up. All these failings exist, or have existed, but have to be attributed to the conditions of the past, when psychoanalysis was wholly a matter of private practice and hedged in by the difficulties and restrictions imposed by the circumstances of the latter. It was these conditions which permitted no planned selection of cases, imposed limits on the undistorted publication of material, and made the follow-ups dependent on the goodwill of the former patients. That a steady accumulation of findings was possible even under these conditions, unfavorable as they now seem, was due only to the lucky chance that in psychoanalysis the method of therapy is identical with the method of inquiry. This rare combination allowed for no routine work in analysis and conferred the potential of a research case on every patient who entered psychoanalysis for his private therapeutic purposes.

Conditions changed in this respect when psychoanalysts began to make contacts with established research centers and when the first psychoanalytic clinics were established. Examples of new research activities were reported in the literature. Interestingly enough, the earliest undertakings of this nature did not confine themselves to the field of psychoanalysis proper but explored the borderlines, on the one hand, between psychoanalysis and organic medicine, on the other hand, between psychoanalysis and academic genetic psychology. In both instances, extraneous research techniques were either added to the analytic method or substituted for it for purposes of exactness. It remained an open and debated question whether research could also be planned to take place within analysis itself, on topics of purely analytic interest, carried out by analysts who employ the analytic method only, without sacrificing any part of it. It is this latter question which the workers in the Hampstead Child-Therapy Clinic have set out to answer in the affirmative. It is still too early to report on the results of the research projects which are in progress; this will have to wait until the investigations are further advanced, or concluded, and brought into publishable form.[1] The present intention is only to use these activities as examples and illustrations of the possibility of research within the analytic field. At the same time the question is being raised which devices may be used legitimately in an analytic clinic to operate research projects. Two such devices will be discussed: (1) the pooling of clinical material among a group of analytic workers; (2) the planned selection of cases; the contention being that the consistent employment of both, singly or in combination with each other, improves the conditions for fact finding to a considerable degree and opens up new opportunities for evaluating, comparing, and verifying data. Pooling of material and planned case selection are also used to counteract disadvantages for research which are inherent in analytic work, such as the comparative absence of specialization and the impossibility of setting up experiments. Thus, the projects of the Clinic can be shown to have a double motivation. On the one hand, they are aimed at increasing knowledge of mental processes and contents, and the techniques of handling them in therapy; on the other hand, at eliminating or decreasing some of the most common handi-

---

[1] [Since this was written many of these investigations have been published. A list of all the publications resulting from the research projects outlined in this chapter as well as the next ones is appended at the end of Part I.—*Editor's note*.]

caps under which analysts labor when they work privately, unaided, and in isolation.

THE ABSENCE OF SPECIALIZATION IN ANALYSIS
REMEDY BY POOLING MATERIAL

A definite and directed search for material runs counter to the analytic technique according to which the analyst's attention should be free-floating and receptive to all the vagaries of the patients' associations and attitudes. Therefore, specialization, with its inevitable centering of attention on selected topics, is not encouraged in analytic training and practice, essential as it may be for research purposes in other branches of work. With exceptions, it remains rare for an analyst to treat simultaneously more than two or three cases of the same type and diagnosis, apart, of course, from the broader divisions into adult analysis, child analysis, the analysis of delinquents or psychotics.

The remedy in clinic practice is a simple one. Instead of one analyst treating eight to ten cases of similar type simultaneously, eight to ten such patients are distributed among an equal number of analysts, their clinical material being shared by means of weekly and bimonthly reports and compared weekly in a discussion group. This method intensifies typical features in contrast to individual ones and helps to minimize any subjective elements introduced into objective material by the persons, or variations of technique, of the individual analysts.

So far two projects of the Clinic have been based on this principle.

An Inquiry into the Analytic Treatment of Adolescents

CONTENT AND AIM OF PROJECT

There is among analysts a fair amount of consensus regarding the nature and range of the conscious and unconscious conflicts which underlie the neurotic or prepsychotic upheavals of adolescence. In spite of this knowledge the technical handling of adolescents in analysis has remained a problem since neither the technique of child analysis nor the technique for adults is wholly applicable. The technical tool of free association cannot be used in most cases; even common honesty, i.e., the sharing of conscious experience with the analyst, usually remains incomplete. Heightened defenses against irruptions from the unconscious render resistances impregnable in many cases. Transference tends to be acted out as it is in borderline and psychotic patients. Owing to these difficulties, adolescents break off treatment at unsuitable moments in far greater numbers than any other type of case. According to our experience, analytic patients who begin treatment in preadolescence invariably leave it when adolescence proper sets in, i.e., when the typical revolt against the parents as love objects is acted out with the analyst. When analysis begins in adolescence proper, the analyst has a better chance to complete treatment. It is the aim of this study to establish by common effort the most typical features of the adolescent process and to base the necessary variations and adaptations of technique on them.[2]

[2] For further details of this project see a preliminary report given by Ilse Hellman (1958).

An Inquiry into the Analysis of Borderline Cases (in Latency and Preadolescence)

CONTENT AND AIM OF STUDY

The material of these cases is reviewed and discussed especially from the aspect of (a) use of language and its distortion; (b) acting out of primitive impulses versus their verbalization; (c) the profusion of fantasy life and its defensive use; (d) comparison of ego functions and activities with those of normal or neurotic children; (e) the specific nature of the object ties and their transference. The study is aimed at providing material for improved differential diagnoses between the neurotic and borderline disturbances.

THE ABSENCE OF EXPERIMENTATION IN PSYCHOANALYSIS SUGGESTED USE OF EXPERIMENTAL SITUATIONS PROVIDED BY NATURE OR FATE

The analytic technique as such precludes the setting up of experiments, the only approximation to it being the establishment of the analytic setting itself which acts as an invitation to the patient to re-enact his neurosis under the eyes of the analyst and centered around his person. But this repetition of the neurotic process in the transference represents for the patient a new and complex life situation and offers no possibility for the artificial isolation of factors.

On the other hand, this embargo on experimentation, to which every analyst has resigned himself, can be compensated for by the selection for treatment of cases in which either nature or fate has caused either the elimination or the exaggeration of one specific innate or environmental factor. Two projects of the Clinic have been based on this principle.

Inquiry into the Development of Motherless Children

Method: Analysis in the latency period, preadolescence, or adolescence

Subject of this inquiry are children who have been separated from their mothers or families, either at birth or during the first two years of life: orphans, war children, and certain concentration-camp children from the European continent who grew up in England.

AIM OF STUDY

This inquiry is aimed at testing the hypothesis that continual absence of mothering from early life onward causes severe abnormality. The analytic study of these cases reveals

(a) the varying emotional reactions to the loss of the mother at different ages;

(b) the pathological consequences of this experience;

(c) the ways and means in which some children cope with the loss and succeed in building up comparatively normal personalities.

(d) On the other hand, the deviations in personality development in the absence of a stable mother relationship throw much light on, and emphasize by comparison, the part played normally by the mother image in the child's instinctual, emotional, and ego development.

Results are obtained especially by studying the transference reactions of these orphaned children which reveal

(a) the primitive character of their object ties to the adult;

(b) the substitute ties to individual contemporaries or a group;

(c) the search for a true mother relationship in adolescence before the step into adulthood can be made.

An Analytic Study of Children Who Are Blind from Birth

Method: Group work in preparation for child analysis; child analysis.

CONTENT OF STUDY

It is a common assumption that visual impressions play an integral part in the individual's early contact with the environment, i.e., in his object relations and the introjections and identifications built on them, as well as in the mental processes of memory, dream, and fantasy life. Much additional information about this topic can be gained where the role of imagery is isolated by its total absence from the personality.

Secondarily the same study is aimed at analytic insight into the compensatory processes to be found in the development of totally blind children and into the origin of certain attitudes and qualities of the blind such as the variations in their object ties, their use of language, their methods of recall, etc.

DIFFICULTIES OF STUDY

It is important not to overrate the isolation of factors which can be achieved in this manner. The analyst of the blind child has to work through a whole series of complicating secondary factors and disentangle their effect on the child's development from the effects proper of the blindness, quite apart from the frequency of a second, complicating defect. Such secondary factors are: (a) the impact on the child of the mother's depression and emotional upheaval consequent on the discovery of the child's defect; (b) the severe restriction of mobility which usually occurs in the second year of life to safeguard the blind child; (c) the repeated hospitalizations, surgical interventions with the eyes, and traumatic separations from the mother which are the rule with blind children under the management adopted and advocated at present.

Suggestions for Further Studies

It is suggested that parallel analytic studies could be undertaken of children who are born deaf, with a view toward establishing the deviations in the development of secondary process thinking, superego formation, and other mental processes normally built on auditory perception.

Other studies could concentrate on children who were born with a severe physical handicap. In the analyses of such children we could trace what happens to their development when the normally occurring fears of being mutilated and castrated are not fantasies but realities.

COMPARATIVE STUDIES BASED ON ANALYTIC TEAMWORK

Simultaneous Analysis of Mother and Child for the Purpose of Inquiring into the Interrelation between Neurotic or Psychotic Disorders of Mothers and Their Children

Method: Adult analysis, child analysis

Current analytic opinion ascribes almost every abnormality of a child to a latent or manifest abnormality of the mother, an assumption which needs further examination and validation. Detailed demonstration is also needed of the various ways in which the mother's unconscious mental life, her fantasy activity, her anxieties, her symptoms, etc., reach and affect the child's mental processes. We feel that interrelations of this nature can be uncovered best where mother and child are studied by means of the same analytic method, i.e., where the same depth of psychic material is reached in both partners. This cannot be accomplished if only one partner of the mother-child couple is analyzed, the other partner merely observed and interviewed. The method of choice is the simultaneous analysis of both partners.

PROCEDURE

The analyst of the mother and the analytic therapist of the child communicate weekly the material of their respective patients to a third, coordinating analyst for correlation and comparison. In some cases, no communication exists between the therapists themselves; in other selected cases, such communication is permitted for experimental purposes.

VERIFICATION STUDIES (COMPARISON OF OBSERVATIONAL WITH ANALYTIC DATA)

Comparison of Material Elicited in the Analyses of Older Children with Existing Observational Data Recorded in Their First Two Years of Life

When establishing the life history of a patient from his analytic material, every analyst would welcome confirmation of his reconstructions, at least so far as historical and environmental data are concerned. Ordinarily such confirmation from outside depends on chance. To counteract the lack of confrontation of external and internal reality, a longitudinal study has recently been set up in the United States (by Ernst Kris at the Child Study Center, Yale University) to collect all available observational data concerning the development of a given number of infants, to be held for comparison with the result of their analyses in later childhood.

The Hampstead Clinic has similar material at its disposal. In connection with a study on identical twins, a detailed observational record of a number of infants had been compiled by some of the Clinic workers during their war work in the Hampstead Nurseries. The present analyses of four of these children, now adolescents, offer constructive and revealing material concerning the processes of inner elaboration of external events, distortion of memories by developmental processes, the formation of cover memories.[3]

[3] For the results of this project see the preliminary report given by Dorothy Burlingham (1958).

Inquiry into the Difficulty of Diagnosis by Comparing the Impressions in the Diagnostic Interviews with the Material Elicited in the Course of Analysis[4]

A STUDY OF CHILD HEROES, CARRIED OUT WITH A COMBINATION OF METHODS

The case material of the Clinic contains predominantly instances of breakdowns, regressions, and malfunctions in ego and superego development. In contrast to these neurotic and borderline cases, it is of interest to inquire into the opposite phenomenon, i.e., children in whom qualities such as altruism, social responsibility, and the capacity for self-sacrifice develop abnormally early or to an abnormally high degree. Although these children are not to be found in clinics, they become conspicuous in society through the performance of heroic acts and are treated as child prodigies in the moral sense. After collecting reports of this kind, a study in three parts has been initiated in the Clinic, of which so far only Parts 1 and 2 have been completed.

Part 1 consists of a survey of thirty children (age range from four years to adolescence) who have performed *actual rescue acts,* saving the lives of other children from fire, water, or in traffic accidents. They were examined according to parental and family background, intelligence and manifest behavior, school performance, social adaptation, etc. Their developmental history was investigated so far as this is possible by methods of interviews and questionnaires. Rorschach tests were given.

[4] For the details of this project see the preliminary report by L. Frankl (1958). See also ch. 3 in this volume.

Part 2 consists of a parallel survey of *rescue fantasies and dreams* collected from sixty cases under analytic treatment at the Clinic. Since this material forms part of the children's analyses, it is possible to group these rescue fantasies according to their unconscious motivation, i.e., to characterize them according to their nature as impulsive manifestations, reaction formation built up in defense against hostile attitudes and death wishes, identifications with the protective father or mother, etc. None of the children studied in whom rescue fantasies are prominent had carried out actual rescue actions.

Part 3 will consist of the analysis of a small number of selected cases of actual child heroes. This will make it possible to determine the relationship between rescue fantasy and rescue action, to investigate whether the unconscious background of both manifestations is identical, and to provide material for a more intensive study of the early development of highly valued social attitudes, such as altruism, the capacity for sacrifice, taking responsibility for others at one's own expense, etc.

POOLING OF MATERIAL
A METHODOLOGICAL PROJECT

As mentioned before, the material of all cases under analytic treatment is made available to all other members of the Clinic by means of weekly and bimonthly summaries. This makes it common property so far as study and discussion are concerned; for all other purposes, especially for the purpose of publication, it remains the property of the analytic worker who carried out the treatment and should not be used or quoted without permission and acknowledgment.

Subject Index

To make the whole analytic material at the disposal of the Clinic more readily available for use by research workers, a plan has been devised to classify the data and to summarize them in the form of a subject index.[5] Work of this kind has so far not been done systematically by any analytic group. We find ourselves in a favorable position for attempting it since

(a) the members of our working group are in an unusually close cooperation with each other and thus can pool their material and share a common frame of reference;
(b) the material is systematically recorded in weekly notes and bimonthly reports; and
(c) the material is then categorized by the therapists under the direct supervision of a small group of senior people.

For the purpose of the Index the analytic material of each individual case is broken into its elements. Although certain categories such as environmental factors, personal history, manifest behavior on the one hand, and internal factors such as instinctual content, ego activities, object relationships, fantasies, anxieties, defenses, compromise formations, etc., on the other hand, are considered in each case, no rigid system of categories is adopted; they are revised and added to according to the material which the case presents.

We hope that the indexing of a relatively large number of cases will enable research workers to acquire an overall

[5] For details of this project see the preliminary report given by C. de Monchaux (1958).

picture of what the treatment of a particular child or series of children has revealed. It may also enable research workers to follow the analytic ramifications of a particular subject in a way which may lead to a better and clearer formulation of concepts. It may also become possible to trace certain associations within a given subject, for instance, whether a certain kind of analytic material is associated with certain reality factors, traumatic experiences, etc.

The Index may also pinpoint some important differences between child analysis and the analysis of adults. I name as an example two instances:

(a) the lesser role played in child analysis by *verbalization* as a vehicle for unconscious (preconscious) material, a fact which becomes very conspicuous in our summaries; and, in contrast to this,

(b) the more frequent occurrence in child analysis of direct, i.e., *unmodified expressions* of sexual and aggressive impulses during the analytic session. (The frequency of such instances can be gathered at a glance from the Index.)

APPLICATION OF FACTS
RESEARCH INTO THE PREVENTION OF
MENTAL ILLNESS

As analysts and child analysts we feel that we possess valuable knowledge concerning early childhood and personality development, and we should like to see this knowledge applied effectively in the field of mental hygiene, especially where the services for children are concerned. We feel convinced that many of the later psychological abnormalities can be prevented provided that the common developmental upsets and the problems of mental growth are handled correctly at their start in childhood; provided that the first signs of mental trouble are spotted, diagnosed, and dealt with before they have time to give rise to organized symptoms; and provided that, where illness makes it necessary, full clinical treatment is available in the initial stages rather than in the final stages of a specific disorder.

Under the title of "The Child Guidance Clinic as a Center of Prophylaxis and Enlightenment," I have recently tried to describe the preventive work which could be done in the community by organizations such as ours (see ch. 17 in this volume). In the same paper I made the point that the usefulness of any one clinic stands in direct proportion to the extent of knowledge on which its practical work is based. Guided by these ideas, I feel certain that any body of trained workers, such as ours, has a double duty: on the one hand, to apply existing knowledge about child development to the practical work with children; on the other hand, to work consistently toward an increase of knowledge by investigating problems which have been insufficiently studied so far.

Thus, it is the double aim of application of facts and further fact finding which underlies the range of our activities. Although, ostensibly, our therapeutic, educational, and guidance work is geared to the former, our research projects to the latter purpose, it can be shown easily that in essence all parts of the work serve both purposes, even if in varying proportions.

Up to now, preventive psychiatry, and above all child psychiatry, has been hampered in its efficiency because general interest focused on traditional types of psychopathology. As I have tried to show, I am convinced that the relevant factors in the causation of mental illness could be studied better if the *unusual* cases were better known. The unusual cases represent variations of the norm, caused either by nature or by fate which—almost like experiments set up in a laboratory—throw special light on specific innate or environmental factors, either by eliminating them or by overemphasizing their action. We have proved the value of such cases for the purpose of study in the analyses of blind, physically deformed, and orphaned children.

I feel that there is the possibility of improving on our results by initiating a scheme of "Research into the Prevention of Mental Illness by the Study of Nontypical Cases," i.e., a project which gives us freedom to accept for analytic investigation any case of a child, adolescent or parent which promises to yield additional insight into the intricacies of mental life.[6]

[6] Such a study would have to be continued for a number of years. I stress the importance of the time element, since every case, even if taken on for the purpose of scientific study, has to be brought to a satisfactory therapeutic conclusion, which, in psychoanalysis, takes considerable time.

3

Assessment of Pathology
in Childhood
Part I
(1962)

SPECIFIC AIMS

Our long-term aim is a new approach to the Assessment of Pathology in Childhood, with special regard to the Variations of Normality and the Imbalance of Lines of Development. It is the essence of this approach that developmental considerations take precedence over consideration of symptomatology and manifest abnormal behavior.

To work toward this aim we propose to use on the one hand the case material of the Hampstead Child-Therapy

From applications to the National Institute of Mental Health, Washington, D.C., 1962, 1964, and 1966 [1965].

Clinic and on the other hand the accumulated experience acquired by our staff in a variety of clinical research projects and services for children. We propose as an appropriate tool for assessment the setting up of Developmental Profiles for the detailed characterization of individual children, whether manifestly ill or healthy, such Profiles to be repeated at stated intervals and at various stages of the children's contact with our services or our clinical department, namely:

(1) at the stage of initial assessment, utilizing the findings of all personnel engaged in the diagnostic process;
(2) with children in need of therapy, at the end of psychoanalytic treatment, utilizing the findings of the child analyst or therapist who has carried out the analysis;
(3) at a period of two or three years after termination of treatment, utilizing the results of a follow-up procedure.

METHOD OF PROCEDURE

The method used for eliciting the material which is needed for these assessments is psychoanalytic observation and—in treatment—the psychoanalytic technique. The frame of reference for assessing the significance of the various elements elicited is the psychoanalytic theory. Evaluation of the material concerning its developmental significance is carried out in discussion between the various participants in the scheme, on the basis of their initial and diverse training and experience in the disciplines of normal and abnormal child development, education, psychology, psychiatry, and of their subsequent uniform training in the theory and practice of psychoanalysis.

A Developmental Profile to be used as the tool of assessment has been drafted provisionally (see below). It aims at covering all parts of the child's personality, thereby revealing where in the structure pathology is anchored or foreshadowed. The draft is tentative and open to revision and amplification in all directions. Its usefulness for purposes of assessment and categorization will have to be proved through application to a great variety of cases of all ages and stages of development.

Our method of procedure in collecting the material necessary for the Profiles will be a different one at each stage of the assessment.

Profile I

(set up at the stage of initial assessment)

All personnel engaged in the diagnostic process, i.e., psychiatrist, psychologist, and psychiatric social worker, record their observations and impressions immediately after the interviews with child and parent (or parents) and after the testing of the child. In these records raw material is kept apart from the conclusions drawn from it. The records are distributed among all participants in the diagnostic conference and read before the conference.

In the diagnostic conference itself, the psychiatrist in charge of the case presents the material in Profile form (see "Draft of Developmental Profile") and invites discussion, criticisms, and amendments which are contributed freely by all participants and the principal investigator. The need to fulfill the requirements of the Profile will show up eventual gaps and deficiencies in the diagnostic process. If the participants in the conference are not satisfied that all items of the Profile (or a sufficient number of them) are covered adequately, the case will be referred back for further diagnostic interviews, further tests, further reports, or, if necessary, a period of observational treatment. A second (or third) diagnostic conference on the same case will be called whenever the presenting psychiatrist judges that sufficient additional material has been collected.

Diagnostic conferences are minuted, the minutes containing the separate views expressed by different members of the group. The finished first Profile, amended by the psychiatrist in charge of the case on the basis of discussion, concludes the diagnostic process.

Profile II

(set up at the end of psychoanalytic treatment)

Our procedure concerning the collection of material elucidated during the treatment stage is very different from the one described for the diagnostic stage and has been worked out carefully over a number of years. Child analysts and child therapists prepare the material elucidated by them as follows:

A. RECORDING

(1) in short weekly reports, which contain raw material plus the main inferred analytic themes and the interpretations given to the child;

(2) in extensive bimonthly reports, expanding on the weekly reports and summarizing material;

(3) in informal presentations to the staff conferences of the whole Clinic, where the whole analytic procedure and validity of interpretations are put up for discussion;

(4) in a closing report which summarizes the therapeutic procedure and demonstrates the structure of the case.

B. ORGANIZING

The analytic data laid down in these four stages are, in addition, "indexed," i.e., they are subjected to a process of categorization which makes it possible to store them and to make them available for scientific discussion. Case material is broken up into items which are collected under analytically meaningful subject headings. Indexing is carried out by the analyst or therapist in charge of the case, under the supervision of a special Index Committee. The first indexing of a case is carried out after nine to twelve months of treatment; further indexings follow at yearly intervals.

C. UTILIZATION OF THE RECORDED AND ORGANIZED MATERIAL FOR THE SECOND PROFILE

The second Profile, which is the most extensive one, utilizes all the available sources of material described above for the validation or amendment of the initial diagnosis as well as for the assessment of treatment results.

Profile III

(set up two or three years after termination of treatment)

At present, several different follow-up procedures are being tried out in the attempt to assess which of them will yield the greatest number of relevant data for Profile III, which is meant to assess the permanence of treatment results or to show up pathology as merely temporarily removed.

The various follow-up procedures now in use are:

(a) follow-up of the case by the analyst or therapist formerly in charge of treatment or by a different analyst or therapist;
(b) follow-up through contact with the child only;
(c) follow-up by means of reports on the child's behavior, performance, etc., using parents, school, employers, etc.;
(d) a combination of (b) and (c);
(e) follow-up by means of a repetition of the initial diagnostic process (in cases where some form of pathology has returned).

DRAFT OF DEVELOPMENTAL PROFILE

The Profile for each case should be preceded by a description of the child, his family relationships, his history and, in case of disturbance, descriptive symptomatology. The Profile itself contains the internal picture of the child, including information about the structure of his personality; the dynamic interplay within the structure; the economic factors concerning drive activity; and (during and after treatment) the genetic findings. This picture is to be broken up into items as follows:

I. Drive Development based on the known sequences of phases

(a) Libido Development: here the essential point is to determine whether a child (above the age of four) has reached the appropriate phallic phase, including the oedipus complex; further, whether regression from this phase to earlier ones has taken place.

(b) Development of Aggression: to be scrutinized as above with special regard to the forms of aggression used, and the employment of aggression either toward the external world or internally within the personality.

II. Ego Development based on the age-adequate status and intactness of ego apparatus, functions, and defenses.

(a) Ego apparatus, normal or abnormal, as shown by psychological testing.

(b) Ego functions (memory, reality testing, integration, control of motility, speech, secondary rational thought processes) as established in diagnostic interviews, treatment material, follow-up material.

(c) Ego defenses against drive activity, characterized on the basis of their known chronology as age adequate, primitive, or advanced.

(d) Superego development, with special regard to moral dependence or independence of the significant love objects who have served as instigators and models for this division within the ego.

(e) Secondary interference of defense activity with the ego functions, as shown especially in the impact on the ego and superego of repression, regression, denial, etc.[1]

III. Lines of Development and Mastery of Tasks

While drive and ego development are regarded as separate entities for the purpose of analysis, their action has to be seen as combined in the *lines of development* which lead from an individual's state of infantile immaturity and de-

---

[1] For a more detailed description of the Developmental Profile, see Anna Freud (1962) and Volume VI, pp. 140-147.

pendence to the gradual mastery of his own body and its functions, to adaptation to reality, the object world and the wider social community, and to the building up of an inner organization. Whatever level has been reached by a given child in any of these respects represents the end point of a historical sequence which can be traced, reconstructed, scrutinized for defects, and in which ego as well as drive development have played their part. Under the influence of internal and external factors these lines of development may proceed at a fairly equal rate, i.e., harmoniously, or with wide divergences in speed, leading to the many existent imbalances, variations, and incongruities in personality development. (Examples are: excessive speech and thought development combined with infantilism of needs, fantasies, and wishes; achievement of object constancy combined with low frustration tolerance and primitive defense system; or complete dependence in feeding, defecation, etc., combined with fairly mature intellectual and moral standards.)

The status of these developmental lines is revealed clearly whenever a child is confronted with one of the many situations in life which pose for him a difficult problem of mastery. Although such tasks may seem simple and harmless when viewed externally, the demands made by them on the personality show up clearly when they are translated into psychological terms. Such translation is the indispensable prerequisite for assessing the meaning of successful mastery as well as for understanding failure and ascribing it correctly to the right sources in either the drives or the ego agencies.

Examples of such situations as they occur in the life of every child are the following:

separation from the mother;
birth of a sibling;
illness and surgical intervention;
hospitalization;
entry into nursery school;
school entry;
the step from the triangular oedipal situation into a community of peers;
the step from play to work;
tolerance for the new genital strivings in preadolescence and adolescence;
the step from the infantile objects within the family to new love objects outside the family.

For one particular life situation of this kind, namely, "Entry into Nursery School," the psychological significance has been worked out in detail, taking into account the demands on all parts of the personality (see ch. 19 in this volume).[2]

IV. Fixation Points and Regressions

So far as regression in childhood proceeds on the same lines as in adult psychopathology, the return to early fixation points as revealed in symptoms and abnormal behavior betray to the diagnostician the areas around which pathogenic conflicts have been centered, i.e., they provide genetic information.

On the other hand, it is important to recognize that infantile regression differs basically from regression in the adult; it does not always require fixation points and does

[2] For a more detailed description of the concept of Developmental Lines, see Anna Freud (1963a) and Volume VI, pp. 62-93.

not need to remain permanent. As "temporary regression" it takes place along the developmental lines, as part and parcel of infantile development, i.e., as an attempt at adaptation and ever-available response to frustration. Such temporary regressions may give rise to pathology, but the latter will be short-lived and reversible. For purposes of diagnosis and assessment the two types of regression (temporary or permanent, spontaneously reversible or irreversible) have to be distinguished from each other.[3]

V. Conflicts

Material gathered during treatment can be utilized to grade the severity of a disturbance according to the type of conflict which has given rise to it.

(a) External conflicts between the child and his immediate environment before identification and internalization have taken place.

(b) Internalized conflicts between ego, superego, and id after the ego agencies have taken over and represent to the id the demands of the external world.

(c) Internal conflicts between the drives such as love-hate, passivity-activity, femininity-masculinity.

While conflicts of the first kind are open to modification by alterations in the environment, the two other kinds of conflicts are accessible only to internal, analytic intervention.

[3] This outline was subsequently elaborated. See Anna Freud (1963b), ch. 24 in this volume, and Volume VI, pp. 93-107.

VI. Some General Characteristics Affecting the Chances
   of Spontaneous Recovery and Favorable Reaction to
   Treatment

Finally, the personality of the child should be scrutinized
for certain general tendencies, the absence or presence of
which will affect recovery, i.e., act as curative factors within
the structure or as their opposites. Such tendencies are, for
example, the following:

   (a) the level of frustration tolerance;

   (b) the level of anxiety tolerance and the means used to
master anxiety;

   (c) the relative preponderance of progressive versus regressive tendencies in situations of stress, unpleasure, or
anxiety.

SIGNIFICANCE OF THIS RESEARCH

The perfecting and testing of our diagnostic draft by application to all cases under psychoanalytic observation and
treatment in our Clinic may be important for a variety of
reasons:

   (a) In contrast to other diagnostic schemes or cate-
gorizations, the Developmental Profile seems to us to provide a comprehensive guide to the individual and to guard
the diagnostician against viewing the child from one aspect only, whether this aspect concerns his object relations
(for example, "autism"), his social adaptation (for example,
"delinquency"), or his intellectual achievements (for example, "mental deficiency").

   (b) In contrast to most other diagnostic schemes, our
Developmental Profile provides a guide to both the ill and

the healthy parts of the child's personality, making no difference between them so far as completeness and depth of scrutiny are concerned.

(c) With normal or near-normal children, our Developmental Profile can be applied to increase knowledge of the variations of normality.

(d) Owing to the Profile's emphasis on development in contrast to emphasis on symptomatology, deviations from the norm become visible in the scheme before they have reached the status of pathological formations, i.e., before they can be classified as symptoms. This enables the diagnostician to spot future pathology at an early date, to establish links and interrelations between the beginning, mild, and the full-grown, severe states of mental disorder, and to initiate treatment before pathology becomes ingrained.

(e) The Diagnostic Profile of a child carried out on the developmental lines indicated above allows for some prediction of future normality or abnormality, especially when not only the specific drive and ego elements but also the "general characteristics" of the personality are taken into account.

(f) The suggested repetition of Developmental Profiles at stated intervals before and after treatment enables us to assess treatment gains in developmental terms instead of in terms of behavior and symptomatology. (Those changes in the personality which have occurred due to maturation during and after treatment need to be deducted from the result, of course.)

Part II
(1964)

In 1962 we initiated a project called "Assessment of Pathology in Childhood." In this study the psychopathology of children was investigated from the point of view of *deviation* from normal personality development and of its *interference* with the normal progression of development. As our tool for such assessments a Developmental Profile of children based on psychoanalytic thinking was set up, tested by application to child cases of all types and ages, and evaluated critically as to its usefulness for highlighting both the ill and the healthy parts of the child's personality, making no difference between them so far as completeness and depth of scrutiny are concerned.

As the natural outcome of these studies in which developmental considerations took precedence throughout over considerations of symptomatology and manifest abnormal behavior, we developed a hierarchy of childhood disorders ranging from more or less complete intactness to more or less complete disruption of progressive development with drive and ego fixations, regressions, and distortions characterizing the intermediate points of the diagnostic scheme, approximately as follows:

I. Behavior disturbances in essentially healthy children whose personality falls within the wide range of "variations of normality";

II. Symptoms of a transitory nature which can be classed as by-products of developmental strain;

III. Permanent drive regression to previously established fixation points which leads to conflicts of a neurotic type and gives rise to infantile neuroses and character disorders;

IV. Drive regression as above plus simultaneous ego and superego regressions which lead to infantilisms, borderline, delinquent, or psychotic disturbances;

V. Primary deficiencies of an organic nature or early deprivations which distort development and structuralization and produce retarded, defective, and nontypical personalities;

VI. Destructive processes (of organic, toxic or psychic, known or unknown origin) which have effected or are on the point of effecting a disruption of mental growth.

The terms in which this diagnostic categorization was expressed were left intentionally wide and general to await further scrutiny and allow for clarification and rearrangement within the scheme.

PRESENT AIMS

We now propose to continue the previous investigation under the new title of "Assessment of Pathology in Childhood, Part II: Problems of Differential Diagnosis." This project is intended to take as its point of departure the diagnostic categories arrived at in the previous study, to undertake their further critical clarification, to improve their delimitation from each other, and to subdivide the individual groups by allocating specific clinical pictures to them. These tasks are meant to be carried out with the Developmental Profile and the Lines of Development being used as diagnostic tools and guidelines as before. When assessing cases, the pathology of the child should be seen on the one hand against the background of normal childhood development and on the other hand in the light of the better known psychopathology of adult life. For both purposes the diagnostician's attention has to go beyond the overt clinical picture of a case to the metapsychological (i.e., genetic, dynamic, economic, structural, adaptive) factors which lie behind it, and he has to use the latter, not the former, as standards for his differentiations, predictions, and comparisons.

THREE EXAMPLES OF STUDY PLANS

Investigations to be undertaken under the proposed project are exemplified in what follows by means of three different outlines for study for which the following topics have tentatively been selected:

1. Clarification and Subdivision of Diagnostic Category II (Symptoms of a Transitory Nature);
2. Disturbances of Narcissism as a suggested new Diagnostic Category (split off from III, the Infantile Neuroses);
3. Comparison of the Infantile with the Adult Neuroses (Diagnostic Category III).

Example 1
Clarification and Subdivision of Diagnostic
Category II (Symptoms of a Transitory Nature)

Symptom formation in childhood does not necessarily carry the same significance which it has in adult life, where "symptoms . . . give us our bearings when we make our diagnosis" (S. Freud, 1916-1917, p. 271). Although symptoms in children sometimes are lasting and have to be regarded as the first sign of permanent pathology, this is by no means always the case. In many instances, symptoms are no more than transient manifestations of strain which appear whenever a particular phase of development makes especially high demands on the child's personality. After adaptation to this particular phase has been achieved, or when its peak has passed, these overtly pathological manifestations (if they are not mishandled by the parents) disappear again without leaving much trace, or they make way for others. In either case, what they leave behind need be no more than an area of heightened vulnerability. Such "spontaneous cures," as they would be called in adult life, or "outgrowing of difficulties," as it is called in childhood, include a number of disturbances such as the following:

1. Certain *sleep* disorders of the second year of life, especially difficulties of falling asleep, so far as these are based on the child's increasing emotional attachments and on his ego growth.[4] Both these latter advances make the toddler cling more tenaciously to the object world and its interests and act against the withdrawal of libido to the self, which is a necessary prerequisite for falling asleep. Such difficulties disappear again spontaneously when the child's object relationships become less ambivalent and more secure and when his ego becomes sufficiently stabilized to permit regression to the undifferentiated state necessary for sleep.

Although the young child's sleeping difficulties resemble descriptively the sleeping disorders of the adult depressive or melancholic patient, the underlying metapsychological picture can be shown to be different, and the childhood disturbance should therefore in no way be considered as a forerunner of the adult one.

2. There is a long sequence of *eating* disturbances and food fads in childhood which belong legitimately to the consecutive stages of the Developmental Line toward independent eating and which are outgrown one after the other as the child moves forward. They are well known as the food refusals tied to the time of weaning from breast or bottle; the fluctuations of intake which the toddler uses as weapons in his battle with the mother; the food avoidances which are due to warded-off cannibalistic fantasies, to defenses against anal messing (disgust), or, in the oedipal period, against fantasies of impregnation.[5] All of these dis-

[4] See Volume IV, ch. 30.
[5] See Volume IV, ch. 2 and ch. 21.

turbances are tied to specific developmental levels and as such are transitory. The metapsychological formula underlying them is different from, for example, serious pathological syndromes such as anorexia nervosa, for which they are in no way a preparation.

3. The earliest *anxieties* of the child, often called the "archaic" fears which take darkness, loneliness, thunder, etc., as their object. They are often discussed as phobias, which is incorrect since, unlike the true phobias of the phallic phase, they are not based on displacement of fear from external objects or internal agencies. Instead, they are the product of ego weakness and immaturity and disappear with the developmental increases in the ego functions and especially the decrease of magical thinking.

4. The early *temper tantrums* which represent motor discharges of chaotic affective states and lose their usefulness as soon as new pathways for discharge have been opened up into speech and the secondary thought processes.

Diagnostically, it is important not to confuse these outbursts with the anxiety attacks, i.e., panic states, of older phobic children who are forced by external interference to meet the object or situation of fear which they are trying to avoid. Although metapsychologically different, the developmental symptom of the temper tantrum and the anxiety attack of the phobic child are descriptively almost identical.

5. The bedtime *ceremonials* and other rituals which correspond on the one hand to the defenses set up as a result of toilet training and on the other hand to a specific developmental phase of quasi-obsessional thought organization. They normally disappear when these phases have been lived through, except in those instances where too much

libidinal investment is made in them by the child with consequent later regression to them.

6. The increased *castration anxiety*, the death fears and wishes, together with the defenses used against both, which dominate the scene at the height of the oedipus complex. These normally fade out when the child enters the latency period.

7. The *loss of personality gains*, of social adaptations and of sublimations, which occurs regularly in preadolescence due to the drive and ego regressions which are bound up with this period.

8. The near-psychotic or near-dissocial *"borderline" symptomatology* which can frequently be seen as an accompaniment to the adolescent process and which normally disappears when adolescence has run its course.

The factors which these eight clinical pictures have in common are, first, their definite dependence on one particular developmental phase and, secondly, their transitory nature. For the rest there are also significant differences in their etiological formulas which further inquiry and closer study will have to elucidate. Present investigations undertaken at our Clinical Concept Research Group suggest that such precursors of the later infantile neurosis proper might be profitably named, distinguished from each other, and classified according to the type of stress to which the child is exposed and according to the extent to which the demands made on him are part either of the external or internal world.

The suggestion is to distinguish between:

(a) *developmental disturbances or interferences*, defined as instances when external demands are made on the child which are neither reasonable nor age-adequate and with which the child's ego cannot cope, or cannot cope without upset and distress;

(b) *developmental conflicts,* defined as being experienced by every child to a greater or lesser degree either when certain specific environmental demands are made at appropriate developmental phases or when developmental and maturational levels are reached which create specific conflicts;

(c) *neurotic conflicts,* defined as arising between drive activity and internalized demands, i.e., superego precursors.

Example 2
Disturbances of Narcissism as a Suggested New Diagnostic Category

Recently, the suggestion has been made by the Clinic's Index Research Group that it is worthwhile to investigate more closely a number of child cases which do not fit into the diagnostic categories I, II, IV, V, and VI, and which are therefore placed by exclusion in category III, although the disturbances presented by them cannot legitimately be described as classical infantile neuroses or as classical disorders of character.

In the infantile neurosis which truly belongs in category III, we assume pathology to be located in the child's libidinal and aggressive relationships with his parental objects. Drive regression occurs at the height of the oedipus complex and throws the child back to previously important pregenital positions. Since ego and superego remain intact at higher levels of development at this juncture, they raise objections to the crudely infantile forms of object love and hate which have emerged, and internal conflicts arise which lead to symptoms or the formation of fixed character traits. Only where such conflicts are eased or resolved through interpretation in treatment and where regressions are reversed is the child restored to the path of progressive development and to object relationships which are normal for his age.

In the group of children alluded to above, on the other hand, pathology seems to be located in the libidinal cathexis of their own selves (or their ideal image of themselves). This disturbance has a developmental history which can be traced and symptoms are formed, not as compromise formations between id and ego, but as a consequence of the failure to establish a satisfactory equilibrium in regard to what may be called their narcissistic supplies. In the course of events, the relations to the parental objects and the demands they make on them are affected secondarily by their precarious narcissistic equilibrium. Children of this kind are liable to special stresses and certain of their symptoms may be viewed as attempts to restore a narcissistic balance in the face of strain.

It is being suggested, accordingly, that these disturbances should not be forced into the framework of the infantile neuroses (category III) or into that of the ego regressions and disturbances (category IV) in spite of certain overt similarities to both groups. Either categorization would do violence to their specific character. Instead, separate provision might be made for them in our diagnostic scheme, perhaps under the title of "Disturbances of Narcissism," of which the depressive reactions of children are probably the most familiar clinical representatives.

Work to be done on cases of this new group includes an

investigation into the interactions between the individual's libidinal and aggressive relations to himself and to his objects, as well as the tracing back of the disorder to its roots, which may have to be looked for in the earliest mother-child relationship.

Example 3
Comparison of the Infantile with the Adult
Neuroses (Diagnostic Category III)

In contrast to the developmental conflicts and disturbances which are characteristic of childhood and exclusive to it, the infantile neuroses have been described since the beginnings of psychoanalysis as being on a par with their adult counterpart—and even more: their protoype and model. In the basic psychoanalytic literature we find pronouncements that the neurosis of childhood has the significance "of being a type and a model" of adult neurosis (S. Freud, 1909a, p. 147); that the analysis of children's neuroses "afford us . . . as much help towards a proper understanding of the neuroses of adults as do children's dreams in respect to the dreams of adults" (S. Freud, 1918, p. 9); that their study "protects us from more than one dangerous misunderstanding of the neuroses of adults" (S. Freud, 1916-1917, p. 363); that "analysis regularly reveals it [a neurosis of later years] as a direct continuation of the preceding infantile illness" (*ibid.*, p. 364).

Further, a close correspondence has repeatedly been shown to exist between the manifest symptomatology of the infantile and the adult neuroses. In *hysteria,* what is common to both are free-floating anxiety and anxiety attacks; conversion into physical symptoms; vomiting and

food refusals; animal phobias, agoraphobia; only claustro-
phobia is rare in children, in whom instead situational phobias such as school phobia, phobia of the dentist, etc., play
a large part. On the side of the *obsessional* neurosis, both
children and adults show the painfully heightened ambivalence of feelings, the bedtime ceremonials, washing compulsions, repetitive actions, questions, and other rituals;
magic formulas and gestures or magic avoidance of certain
words and movements; compulsions to count and list, to
touch or avoid touch, etc. With the *inhibitions*, inhibited
play and learning in childhood correspond to the later inhibitions of work; inhibitions of exhibitionism, of aggression, of competition, etc., produce the same crippling effect
on the individual's personality whether they occur within
the earliest or the later social settings. In the neurotic
characters, there is little difference between the budding
hysterical, obsessional, or impulsive character in childhood
and their later full-grown counterparts.

More important still than these manifest correspond-
ences is the identity which has been shown to exist between
the infantile and the adult neuroses with regard to their
dynamics. For both, the classical etiological formula runs
as follows: initial developmental progress to a comparatively high level of drive and ego development (i.e., for the
child, to the phallic oedipal; for the adult, to the genital
level); an intolerable increase of anxiety or frustration on
this position (for the child, of castration anxiety within the
framework of the oedipus complex); regression from the
age-adequate drive positions to pregenital fixation points;
emergence of infantile, pregenital sexual-aggressive impulses, wishes, fantasies; anxiety and guilt with regard to
them, mobilizing defense on the part of ego and superego;

defense activity leading to compromise formations; resulting character disorders or symptoms, determined in detail by the quality and levels of the fixation points to which regression has taken place, the content of the warded-off impulses, and the quality of the defenses which are being used.

Nevertheless, in spite of these impressive similarities and identities between the neuroses of children and adults, child psychiatrists and child analysts also have to be alert to the differences between the two manifestations and must take account of the latter, especially for their prognostic pronouncements. While in adults the individual neurotic symptom usually forms part of a genetically related personality structure, this is not the case in children, where symptoms occur more often in isolation or are coupled with other symptoms and character traits of a different nature and origin. Thus, even well-defined obsessional features such as bedtime ceremonials or counting compulsions can be found in children with otherwise uncontrolled, restless, impulsive, hysterical personalities; or, conversely, hysterical conversions, phobic trends, in character settings which are obsessional. Single delinquent acts happen in children who are otherwise socially adapted and conscientious. Children who are out of parental control for neurotic reasons can be surprisingly well adapted in school, or vice versa, etc.

There are reasons, furthermore, why a particular type of infantile neurotic disorder cannot automatically be assessed as the forerunner of the same type of mental illness in adult life. Comparisons of the clinical material offer much evidence for this assumption. For example, the impulsive behavior of a four-year-old may in its manifestations be identical with that of a juvenile or adult delinquent so far as aggression, appropriation of other people's belongings, disregard for their feelings are concerned. But for all these similarities there is no reason to expect that the early "delinquency" is prognostically a sign for later delinquent development. On the contrary: the young child, in the course of his development, may ward off his aggression, etc., and by virtue of his ego defenses become an obsessional neurotic patient, not a delinquent.

In contrast, there are young children with truly compulsive symptoms who resemble adult obsessionals in every way but who may be predestined not to become obsessional adults but to develop psychotic illnesses instead. With them, the early compulsive symptoms are the first ominous signs of an inner disharmony which is so severe that it will later lead to a total disintegration of the personality.

Children with early anxiety hysteria, on the other hand, may later turn into true obsessionals, provided that they cease to control their anxiety by means of bodily conversions and phobic mechanisms and instead use intellectual means such as counting, magic formulas, undoing and avoiding, within the thought processes, etc.

Under these conditions it is not at all easy for the diagnostician to assess the position or to make prognostic predictions. He can only conclude that the symptomatology of the infantile neurosis and its comparison with the adult neurosis is well worth more attention and needs more detailed investigation.

SIGNIFICANCE OF THIS RESEARCH

A detailed clinical and theoretical investigation into the psychopathology of children as set out above may be important and useful for a variety of reasons:

1. Improved differential diagnoses between the various groups of disorders will enable clinics to make better use of their therapeutic facilities by differentiating between children

    (a) who suffer from developmental disturbances only and should be left untreated and whose parents should be counseled as to their reasonable management;

    (b) who suffer from an infantile neurosis, for which child analysis is the treatment of choice;

    (c) who suffer from a disturbance of their narcissistic equilibrium or fall into diagnostic categories IV or V, for whom the psychoanalytic method of treatment has to be modified in various ways;

    (d) who belong in diagnostic category VI, for whom psychoanalytic or psychotherapeutic methods of approach will probably not be effective.

2. Detailed comparisons between infantile and adult disturbances of all diagnostic groups (as illustrated above for the neuroses) will lead to more assurance in the prognostic opinions which are demanded from child psychiatrists and child analysis at the diagnostic stage.

3. Earlier differentiations, especially between delinquent and neurotic development, will lead to the appropriate choice of therapy, which should be made at the earliest possible date in childhood and not in adolescence, when

the juvenile delinquent is often wholly beyond psycho-analytic or psychotherapeutic help and much valuable treatment time is spent on him without tangible results.

4. The detailed study of many clinical pictures will high-light the contributions made to them on the one hand by the course of normal maturation and development, on the other hand by environmental influences, and will offer suggestions as to modifying the latter. This attempt has already been carried out with regard to two disorders, namely, dissociality and homosexuality (see Volume VI).

5. The results of the proposed studies will be available not only to psychoanalysts and child psychiatrists in child guidance clinics but also to workers in the social services for children in general such as schools, residential institutions, social agencies, juvenile courts, etc., where they can help considerably in the understanding of disturbed behavior and can become the basis for deciding on placement and other dispositions for children who are out of parental control and in need of educational, therapeutic, or judicial intervention.

Part III
(1966 [1965])

In our ongoing project called "Assessment of Pathology in Childhood," the emphasis throughout was laid on seeing childhood pathology against the background of a hypothetical developmental norm and to assess its severity from the points of view of deviation from and interference with normal development. Insofar as we viewed childhood disturbances against the background of mental disorders in adult life, the primary focus of our inquiries was on the ways in which childhood disturbances differ from the pathology of adults.

PRESENT AIMS

We now propose to widen our survey and attempt to assess the impact of childhood disturbances on the mental disorders in adult life. There is the widespread belief in the analytic field that, at least as far as the neuroses are concerned, the infantile neurosis is the prototype and forerunner of the adult neurosis. Moreover, since the mental disturbances of adults are invariably built on the basis of mental upsets in early years, it is frequently taken for granted that this statement is reversible and that mental upsets in childhood are invariably followed by their counterparts in later life. In fact, both statements need closer scrutiny, since it happens just as often that they are not borne out by clinical experience.

During our own work, our attention has been alerted to the facts that mental upsets occur more frequently in children than they do in adults; that in early, more often than in later life, they may affect only isolated functions or areas, leaving the rest of the personality intact; that so far as causation and upkeep are concerned, disorders in childhood are more dependent on the environment than disorders of adults are later; that their symptomatic expression is more open to change; and that the symbolic meaning underlying the symptoms is not always the same in the two periods, even where the manifest pathology itself appears to be identical.

In accordance with these clinical findings, we now suggest carrying out comparisons between infantile and adult mental disorders from the following four aspects:

(1) range and spread of pathology;
(2) involvement of the environment;

(3) lability or stability of symptoms;

(4) significance of symptomatology.

Seeing the characteristic qualities of childhood disturbances against the background of adult pathology as was outlined in Part II (Example 3), implies the necessity to follow more systematically the gradual unfolding of certain psychopathological conditions through the main phases of their clinical history. So far as we consider early disturbances as forerunners of later ones, for purposes of study and clarification *three critical stages* in the development of any pathological entity can be distinguished from each other, viz., consecutively:

(a) as age-adequate transient by-products of normal mental growth;

(b) as pathological elements within a potentially transient infantile neurosis;

(c) as permanent parts of a neurotic character structure or of a neurotic, psychotic, perverse or delinquent syndrome.

To correlate these three stages with each other throws new light on the transformations and modifications of symptomatology as they occur during an individual's lifetime. In addition, it widens our experience of the various mental disorders as individual clinical structures with natural histories of their own. In the clinical research undertaken so far, we have concentrated mostly on one or another of these stages, or at best two. We propose now to study the correlation with each other of all three stages along the line from transient to permanent pathology.

EXAMPLES OF STUDY PLANS

Sleep Disorders

In my previous discussion (Part II) as well as that by Nagera (1966), the vulnerability of sleep in the earliest part of life (stage a) has been described as one of the normal by-products of the child's immaturity of apparatus (in the first months of life); of his dependency on his objects (first and second year); of his ego growth (toddler stage); of his age-adequate conflicts (anal and phallic phases, latency period). In the second stage (stage b), overstimulation by the environment and the conflicts of the infantile neuroses result in deviations from the sleep norm such as nightmares, sleep-walking, etc. The study needs to be taken further to explore the significance of these early manifestations for the later severe abnormalities of sleep (stage c) which reach their height in extreme sleeplessness (or its opposite) in some adult neuroses and psychoses (depression, melancholia).

Rages and Temper Tantrums

Our earlier studies (e.g., Koch and Sandler, 1966) attempted to arrive at the underlying causation and significance of this disturbing symptom. This study (representing stage b of the disorder) needs to be amplified in two directions. On the one hand, correlation is needed with the temper tantrums of the toddler age before the full establishment of speech, i.e., at a time when the outburst represents an age-adequate, motor-affective outlet for internal strain, frustration-distress, primitive conflict, etc. (stage a). In the other direction, the line needs to be followed further, from the mere "tempers" in which the direction of the aggression alternates between self and objects, to the uncontrollable outbursts of rage in adults (stage c) which are discharged exclusively against the external world and which, if put into action, culminate in the so-called "crimes of passion."

Transvestitism

In cooperation with some analytic colleagues in the adult field, and through the courtesy of a local Court and its probation officer, this manifestation is being approached by us on all three levels:

At stage a, as the familiar children's game of "dressing up," which is being observed in our nursery school. In this form it serves a variety of role-plays and fantasies in which the sex differences play no part or are transcended easily.

At stage b, as secret or overt transvestite activities in a number of boy patients in young latency age. In their case, the transvestite behavior was traced back in treatment to various causes, such as the mother's original wish for a girl child, the boy's envy of a preferred sister, the boy's attempt to recapture a lost female object by identification with her. Unexpectedly, the arousing of sexual excitement via the female garments did not play a conspicuous part at this stage.

At stage c, as the full-blown sexual perversion of adult life, examined in some cases in analytic treatment.

Fears and Phobias

Clinical observation shows how the developmentally earliest fears of darkness, solitude, thunder, etc. (stage a) fade out with the strengthening of certain ego functions. Manifestly similar anxieties, although different in underlying meaning, appear subsequently (stage b) within the infantile neuroses, where they are dealt with by means of phobic mechanisms. In the further course, three different developments may take place:

    (i) The infantile phobia may fade out in its turn, with no other pathology appearing in its stead;

    (ii) the phobia may retain its essential character and persist into adult life in the framework of an anxiety hysteria;

    (iii) the phobia may make place for an obsessional neurosis of adulthood for which it has merely figured as the forerunner (stage c).

The modifications and transformations which are relevant to this disturbance are studied currently in our Clinical Concept Group, with special regard to the change of phobic object from childhood to adulthood (e.g., animal phobias and school phobias in stage b, agoraphobia in stage c).

Other Examples

Similar correlations could be carried out with regard to disturbances of femininity, feeding disorders, obsessional manifestations, delinquent disturbances, etc.

SIGNIFICANCE OF THIS RESEARCH

A further clarification of the diagnostic field in childhood, a comparison of infantile with adult disorders, and a study of transformation of pathology in its course from the near-normal developmental forms to the severest adult abnormalities are essential prerequisites for a realistic orientation in the field of mental health.

The psychoanalytic treatment and investigation of adults have enabled us increasingly to reconstruct the external events and internal processes in early years which contribute to or cause pathology. Conversely, the analytic treatment and investigation of childhood disorders can open up a path to early detection and prediction of pathological potentialities in later life. In fact, it is this very combination of retrospective and prognostic thinking on which effective measures for the prevention of mental illness will have to rely increasingly in the future.

4

Metapsychological
Assessment of the
Adult Personality
The Adult Profile
(1965)

The need for a Profile of adult patients has made itself felt in our clinical work for some time, especially for those cases where a child and one or the other parent are in treatment simultaneously.

Our original Profile schema was devised for neurotic child

This paper was written in collaboration with Humberto Nagera and W. Ernest Freud. First published in *The Psychoanalytic Study of the Child*, 20:9-19, 1965. The original paper contained an example of the application of the Adult Profile to a specific case, prepared by Humberto Nagera (pages 19-41), which has not been included here.

patients in order to facilitate the organization of the material available about them under psychoanalytically meaningful headings (before, during, or after therapy). When the Profile was subsequently applied beyond the scope of the neurosis, a number of sections had to be amplified to embrace all the details relevant to the individual's specific pathology. In the case of the blind, this involved above all the headings concerned with phase development, fixation and regression (see Nagera and Colonna, 1965). In the case of the borderline children, the sections containing information about cathexis of self and cathexis of objects have already been provided with subdivisions to trace in more minute detail the location of pathology (see Ruth Thomas et al., 1966). When the Profile schema was applied to the characterization of the adolescent, it had to be widened to accommodate the variations of superego development, ideal formation, and the identity problems which form an essential part of the adolescent's upheaval (see Laufer, 1965).

While the Profile schema as such profited from these expansions and gained so far as its scope of application was concerned, the basic rationale underlying it remained untouched. For all the categories of disturbance enumerated above, assessment by Profile is made on the basis of developmental considerations, i.e., the individual is examined for his position on the progressive sequences relevant to drive development, ego and superego development, and the age-adequate developments of internal structuralization and adaptation to the environment. Pathology is evaluated in all instances according to its interference with orderly and steady progress in these respects.

This basic rationale changes with the application of the

Profile schema to the adult personality. In this instance, assessment is concerned not with an ongoing process but with a finished product in which, by implication, the ultimate developmental stages should have been reached. The developmental point of view may be upheld only insofar as success or failure to reach this level or to maintain it determines the so-called maturity or immaturity of the adult personality. For the rest, normality is judged by the quality of functioning (in sex, work, and sublimations), the pleasure in life derived from it, and by the quality of the individual's object and community relations. Pathology reveals itself through permanent symptomatology which interferes with any of the above aims, by suffering for internal causes, by the individual's incapacity to relate realistically to his environment, or by both.

Since childhood and adult Profiles are not identical in orientation, the comparison between such assessments of parent and child will have to be restricted to the sections which are most similar. Nevertheless, the schemas may prove invaluable for the correlation of items such as the importance within the individual structure of particular drives, the quality of the defense organization, the content of ideal self and superego, the developmental phase governing the quality of object relationships, etc.

As regards the application of what follows to individual case material, the analytic clinician has to be advised as well as warned. It would be a grave misunderstanding of what the authors have in mind if the Profile were treated as a questionnaire, if it were allowed to dominate the interviewer's attitude during diagnostic examination, if it were shared with the patient, or if its headings were merely filled in with information given by him. What the metapsychological Profile sets out to be is of a completely different order—namely, a framework for the analyst's thinking, and a method to organize findings after they have been elicited, assimilated, and digested by him. Where a Profile is set up after diagnostic investigation, it is only natural that there will be many blanks and unanswered questions in the analyst's mind; these will be filled gradually as an analysis proceeds, to be most completely answered when analytic treatment has been terminated. Profiles set up at these different junctures will reflect the analyst's growing familiarity with the material and, by their increase in completeness, give evidence of his advances in awareness of existing problems, complications, and solutions.

METAPSYCHOLOGICAL ASSESSMENT OF THE ADULT PERSONALITY ADULT PROFILE

(List the material on which the Profile is based.)

I. REASON FOR REFERRAL

Symptoms, anxieties, inhibitions, difficulties, abnormalities, breakdowns in functioning, acting out in the environment, inability to fulfill inherent potentialities, arrests in development leading to faulty ego and supergo structuralization, etc.

An attempt is to be made, where possible, to distinguish between the manifest and the latent reasons for which the patient seeks help.

II. DESCRIPTION OF THE PATIENT AS DIRECTLY OR INDIRECTLY CONVEYED IN THE INTERVIEW

Personal appearance, moods, manner, affects, attitudes, etc.

III. FAMILY BACKGROUND (PAST AND PRESENT) AND PERSONAL HISTORY

(As provided by patient or derived from other sources.)

IV. POSSIBLY SIGNIFICANT ENVIRONMENTAL CIRCUMSTANCES

(Interviewer's as well as patient's evaluation where available:)

(a) in relation to the timing of referral;
(b) in relation to the overall causation of the disturbances as evaluated by the patient himself as well as by the interviewer;
(c) in relation to the links between individual and family pathology and their interaction.

V. ASSESSMENT OF DRIVE AND EGO-SUPEREGO POSITIONS

A. *The Drives*

1. *Libido.*—Examine and state
 (a) *Libidinal Position*
  Describe the present libidinal position of the patient against the ideal normal position that he should have reached. Ideally, for women, a passive feminine position; for men, an active masculine one, with no more

than the normal admixture in terms of bi-sexuality. At the time of assessment it is important to determine if the highest level has ever been reached, if it is being maintained, or if it has been abandoned regressively for an earlier one. Where the adult position has not been reached, it is important to assess the quality and quantity of interference contributed by previous phases.

(b) *Libido Distribution*
   (i) *Cathexis of the Self*
      whether the self is cathected, and whether there is sufficient narcissism (primary and secondary), invested in the body, the ego, and the superego, to ensure regard for the self, self-esteem, a sense of well-being, without leading to overestimation of the self. If possible, consider the regulation of narcissism; note whether this is brought about through identification, object dependence, magical means, work, etc. In the adult, some information in relation to the cathexis of the self can be obtained in areas such as the patient's personal appearance, clothes, etc. (while the child's appearance in this respect reflects the adult's attitude toward him).
   (ii) *Cathexis of Objects* (past and present; animate and inanimate)
      The disturbances observed here should be described from the point of view of

their predominant origin in one of the following phases: narcissistic, need-fulfilling, object constancy, preoedipal, oedipal, postoedipal, adolescence. As in previous sections, evaluation should start at the highest level, i.e., at the level where the objects are considered and treated as partners in their own right. State:

—whether the individual in question has been able to choose his or her *sexual partner* and how far his object needs are met by the partner;

—whether the attitude necessary for *motherhood* and *fatherhood* has been achieved and on what level;

—whether and how far the infantile oedipal relationships have been outgrown or still dominate the picture;

—what part is played by *other human relationships* such as friendships, alliance to groups, or their avoidance, working relationships, etc.;

—above all, what part is played on the one hand by heterosexual object cathexes and on the other hand by homosexual object cathexes;

—whether too much libido is withdrawn from the real object world and sexual satisfaction sought in masturbation (accompanied by object-directed fantasies);

—whether and how deeply the individual is attached to objects which serve as substitutes for or extensions of ties with other human beings such as *animals, property, money,* etc.

2. *Aggression*

Note to what degree aggression is under control while being at the service of the personality in sexual life, work, and sublimatory activities.

Examine the defenses against aggression for relevant information. Aggression thus has to be assessed:

(a) according to quantity, i.e., presence or absence in the manifest picture;

(b) according to quality, i.e., correspondence with a given libidinal position;

(c) according to the direction or distribution, i.e., toward the object world (within or outside the family) or the self or both. In the latter case, state whether directed to the body or through the superego to the ego;

(d) according to the methods and defense activity used in dealing with it.

B. *Ego and Superego*

(a) Examine and state the intactness or defects of the ego apparatuses serving perception, memory, motility, etc.

(b) Examine and state in detail the intactness, or otherwise, of ego functions, as they are at present (memory, reality testing, synthesis, control of motility, speech, secondary thought processes, etc.). If possible compare the present state of ego functions with functioning before the onset of the disturbance.

(c) Examine and state whether danger is experienced by the ego as coming from the external world, the id, or the superego, and whether as a consequence anxiety is felt predominantly in terms of fear of annihilation, separation anxiety, fear of loss of love, castration fear, guilt, etc.

(d) Examine in detail the status of the defense organization and consider:

—whether defense is employed specifically against individual drives, affects, and anxieties (to be identified here) or more generally against drive activity and instinctual pleasure as such;

—whether the patient's defense organization is mature, i.e., dependent on his own superego structure;

—whether it has remained immature, or regressed to presuperego stages, i.e., whether id control is dependent on the object world;

—whether the defense mechanisms predominantly used are archaic or of a higher order (for example, denial, projection versus reaction formation, sublimation);

—whether defense is balanced, i.e., whether the ego has at its disposal the use of many of the important mechanisms or is restricted to the excessive use of specific and primitive ones;

—whether defense is effective, especially in its dealing with anxiety, whether it results in equilibrium or disequilibrium, lability, mobility, rigidity, or symptom formation within the structure.

(e) Note all secondary interferences of defense activity with ego functioning, i.e., the price paid by the individual for the upkeep of the defense organization.

(f) Examine the status of the superego with regard to:

—its degree of structuralization (arrested, faulty, mature, etc.);

—its sources (where obvious);

—its functions (critical, aim- and direction-giving, satisfying);

—its effectiveness (in relation to ego and id);

—its stability (under the impact of internal and external pressure);

—the degree of its secondary sexual or aggressive involvement (in masochism, in melancholia, etc.).

C (A + B). *Reaction of the Total Personality to Specific Life Situations, Demands, Tasks, Opportunities, etc.*

Drive and ego development that were viewed separately for purposes of investigation in the earlier sections of the Profile are here seen in interaction with each other, as well as in reaction to specific situations, such as: the totality of the patient's attitude to his sex life; his success or failure in work; attitude to social and community responsibilities; his disturbed or undisturbed capacity for enjoying companionship, social relationships, and the ordinary pleasures of life; his vulnerability and ability or failure to withstand disappointments, losses, misfortunes, fateful events, environmental changes of all kinds, etc.

VI. ASSESSMENT OF FIXATION POINTS AND REGRESSIONS

As character disturbances, neuroses, and some psychotic disturbances—in contrast to the atypical personalities—are assumed to be based on fixations at various early levels and on drive regressions to them, the location of these points is one of the vital concerns of the diagnostician. At the time of initial diagnosis such areas are betrayed:

(a) by the type of the individual's object relationships, the type of drive activity, and the influence of these on type of ego performance in cases where these are manifestly below adult level;

(b) by certain forms of manifest behavior which are characteristic of the given patient and allow conclusions to be drawn about the underlying id processes which have undergone repression and modification but have left an unmistakable imprint. The best example is the overt obsessional character where cleanliness, orderliness, punctuality, withholding and hoarding, doubt, indecision, slowing up, etc., betray the special difficulty experienced by the patient when coping with the impulses of the anal-sadistic phase, i.e., a fixation at that phase. Similarly, other character formations or attitudes betray fixation points at other levels or in other areas. Unrealistic concerns for health, safety of the marital partner, children, parents or siblings show a special difficulty of coping with death wishes; fear of medicines, food fads, etc., point to defense against oral fantasies; shyness to defense against exhibitionism, etc.;

(c) by the patient's fantasy activity. Some adult patients may occasionally be more willing than children to communicate some of their fantasy life at the diagnostic stage. Personality tests may reveal more of it (during analysis the patient's conscious and unconscious fantasy provides, of course, the fullest information about the pathogenically important parts of his developmental history);

(d) by those items in the symptomatology where the relations between surface and depth are firmly established, not open to variation, and well known to the diagnostician (such as the symptoms of the obsessional neurosis with their known fixation points); in contrast, symptoms with multiple causation such as anxiety attacks, insomnia, vomiting, some forms of headaches, etc., convey no clear genetic information at the diagnostic stage.

VII. ASSESSMENT OF CONFLICTS

By examining the conflicts which are predominant in an individual's personality, assessments can be made of
—the level of maturity, i.e., the relative independence of the patient's personality structure;
—the severity of disturbance, if any;
—the intensity of therapy needed for alleviation or removal of the disturbance.

According to quality, conflicts, which should be described in detail, may be graded as follows:

(a) *External Conflicts*
In the adult direct clashes between id and external demands occur only where ego and superego development are defective. Conflicts between the total personality and the environment (refusal to adapt to, creative attempts to modify the environment) can occur at any stage after adolescence and are not pathogenic.

(b) *Internalized Conflicts*
In the fully structured mature adult, disharmonies between instinctual wishes and external demands are mediated via ego and superego and appear as internalized conflicts. Occasionally such conflicts are externalized and appear in the guise of conflicts with the environment.

(c) *Internal Conflicts* between insufficiently fused or incompatible drive representatives (such as unsolved ambivalence, activity versus passivity, masculinity versus femininity, etc.).

VIII. ASSESSMENT OF SOME GENERAL CHARACTERISTICS WITH A BEARING ON THE NEED FOR ANALYTIC THERAPY AND THE ABILITY TO PROFIT FROM IT

An all-round metapsychological view of the patient will assist the analyst in assessing on the one hand the patient's need for internal change, and on the other hand his chances to effect this in psychoanalytic treatment.

As regards the need for internal change the following points may be considered relevant:

—whether the patient's id and ego agencies have been separated off from each other too completely by excessive use of repression, and whether better communication needs to be established between them;

—whether the ego's sphere of influence has been restricted unduly by the defenses and needs to be enlarged;

—whether ego mastery over the impulses is weakened for other than defensive reasons (ego defects, psychotic core, etc.) and whether improvement will depend in the first instance on the strengthening effect that therapy has on the ego resources;

—whether the superego structure is archaic and, through analysis of its sources, needs to be replaced by a more mature one;

—whether the libidinal and aggressive energies

or only libido or aggression are bound up in countercathexes, conflicts, and symptom formation, and need to be released for constructive use.

The following characteristics, attitudes, and circumstances seem of relevance to either a positive or negative reaction to analytic therapy:

On the positive side:

—whether there is insight into the detrimental nature of the pathology, including the desire to be cured;

—whether there is ability for self-observation, self-criticism, and capacity to think and verbalize;

—whether the patient has a sufficiently high level of object relationship and a sufficient quantity of free object libido to establish a meaningful transference relationship to the analyst, and whether this relationship will also serve as a treatment alliance and withstand all the ups and downs of the resistances;

—whether there is enough frustration tolerance to cope with the necessary restrictions on wish fulfillment in the transference setting;

—whether there is enough tension tolerance to cope with the additional anxiety likely to be released by exposing conflicts and weakening defenses during the analytic process;

—whether the patient has on previous occasions shown ability to persevere in the face of difficulties;

—whether there are (past or present) areas of established sublimations which attest to the patient's capacity to displace and neutralize and to accept substitute satisfactions;

—whether in the absence of established sublimations there is evidence of a sublimation potential which has been interfered with by pathology;

—whether there is flexibility of libido (as contrasted with adhesiveness);

—whether there is a positive, optimistic general outlook on life (as contrasted with a crippling pessimism).

On the negative side:

—whether there is dangerously low tolerance for frustration and anxiety, coupled with the unwillingness to renounce secondary gains of the pathology;

—whether the patient's pathology is part of a pathological family or professional setting and cannot be altered without causing major upheavals and breakups in the external life situation;

—whether there are extreme self-punishing, self-destructive, and masochistic attitudes that are satisfied through the pathology and oppose improvements, i.e., which cause negative therapeutic reactions.

5

Psychoanalysis and
Family Law
(1966 [1964])

The data systematically collected and studied in the psychoanalytic treatment of children are relevant to childhood development in its normal and abnormal aspects. Such data can be applied usefully to a better understanding of the individual's success or failure to relate to his family as well as to the wider community. In fact, they already are being used for this purpose in the educational, medical, and legal services for children in a number of countries.

With regard to legislation, the studies of the Hampstead

From an application to the Walter E. Meyer Research Institute of Law, New York, 1966 [1964].

Clinic throw light on a number of subjects which fall within the scope of Family Law:

(1) Distortions of personality development which follow on the young child's *separation* from either mother or father after disorganization of the family. Clinical data elicited in this respect can act as guides in the determination of *custody*.

(2) The relevance of *chronological age* to the determination of *custody*.

(3) The relevance of *divided loyalties* to distortions of personality development and the lesson to be learned from such data in the granting of *visiting rights*.

(4) The links between *mental illness* of a parent and the appearance of neurotic, psychotic, or delinquent pathology in the child; how far the latter outcomes warrant *state intervention* as a preventive measure.

(5) The link between *multiple placement* in early childhood and later *delinquent* development. How far a systematic presentation of the convincing clinical data in this respect could lead to new guides governing foster care placements in which *continuity of care* is the overriding principle.

(6) The *adopted* child's specific problems in relation to his natural parents, typical distresses, danger moments, and critical chronological ages; the elicited facts to be used in adoption proceedings and the counseling of adoptive parents.

(7) A study of discipline and its beneficial or harmful effect on the socialization of the child with special regard to the question of corporal punishment and the Law of Torts.

(8) A study of criminal events within the family (assault, murder) and their traumatic effect on the child.

(9) Attempt at a psychoanalytic definition of the "best interests" of the child, as represented by fulfillment of the needs for (a) affection, (b) stimulation, (c) unbroken continuity of care.

6

Services for
Underprivileged Children
(1966)

I recently had the opportunity to attend two conferences
in the United States, one at Hillcrest Hospital, Washington, D.C., the other at Yale University, sponsored jointly
by the Children's Bureau in Washington and the Yale
Child Study Center in New Haven, Connecticut. Both
conferences were concerned with the urgent need for help
to children and adolescents who have to be considered
casualties, either for social or for psychological reasons.
What was under debate was the form in which such help
could be given to the best advantage.

In the Hillcrest Symposium, the point was raised (by Dr.

From an application to The Taconic Foundation, New York,
July 25, 1966.

Anny Katan, Cleveland) that even the best efforts of Operation Head Start could not achieve the desired results in those cases where young children were underdeveloped and deprived to a degree which prevented them from profiting from nursery school education, and that in these instances therapeutic help is needed before nursery school education can take over. At the Yale conference the question was discussed whether children who are deprived of effective family support, for whatever reason, are served best by residential care, foster care, or day-care arrangements (i.e., nursery school).

I maintained that any child's normal development is based on the fulfillment not of a single need but of a whole series and hierarchy of needs, stemming from all sides of his personality. Children need the opportunity to develop their affections toward suitable objects in their environment; they need to feel that they themselves are important to these people; they need appropriate stimulation from birth onward to develop their inborn potentialities, and to become able to participate in and adapt to the culture in which they live; they need an environment in which the objects of their love and the sources of their stimulation are stable and permanent factors, at least so far as the early years of childhood are concerned.

A normal and happy family can, with luck, fulfill all these conditions, but most families fail to do so for one reason or another; however, no residential institution, very few foster families, and no nursery school, even the best, can hope to come up to the young child's requirements in this respect. On the other hand, in many instances, the right combination of family care, foster care, residential care, and day care could provide what is required if the best and most helpful elements were extracted from each and made use of for the child in the right measure and at the appropriate time. Even destitute families would function better if day care came to their permanent help, and if residential care could be asked for in short-term emergencies. Foster care would break down less frequently if it were supplemented regularly by nursery school attendance, which not only benefits the child but also relieves the foster mother from twenty-four-hour attendance to her ward. Stimulation, which is usually lacking in the underprivileged family, is most appropriately offered in day care in the nursery school.

I was glad to feel that my suggestion to provide for the needs of children by a combined service of this kind met with the approval of most of the Conference members.

NEED FOR ACCURATE ASSESSMENT OF THE CHILD'S STATUS

It cannot be emphasized too much that the success of any help given to children in this manner depends on the careful assessment of the relevant environmental and internal factors in the individual case. Much knowledge is needed about each child to prevent mistakes such as separating children from their families and placing them in residential care if this, instead of being helpful to them, endangers their last emotional links with the environment and promotes harmful withdrawal; or such as accepting children into the group conditions of a nursery school if what they need is therapeutic help in an individual setting; or such as placing in foster care young adolescents who will revolt against any kind of family setting and respond favorably only to a therapeutic community, etc. Much effort, time, and money can be spent with disappointing results if the specific qualities of a child's urgent need do not coincide with the particular measure which the authorities or agencies apply to it.

ASSESSMENT WORK CARRIED OUT IN THE HAMPSTEAD CLINIC

In connection with problems of this nature which are arising increasingly in the Children's Services, I would like to emphasize that in the Hampstead Clinic we have built up an elaborate scheme for the very purpose of assessing a child's developmental status from the emotional, intellectual, moral, and social points of view. We determine, within this scheme, which particular deficiency is characteristic of a particular child's background and what impact this has had on the inner life of the child. We try to pinpoint where in the child's personality his deviation from the norm is most conspicuous. On the basis of such assessment we try to conclude which of the available measures is most likely to arouse a favorable response in the child and to act as a therapeutic as well as a preventive agent.

CHANGE OF NURSERY SCHOOL POPULATION

As previously reported, we operate, in addition to our clinical facilities, a small nursery school for children who are assessed as ready and able to profit from group life and educational measures. In the past years this school served predominantly children from our own middle-class neighborhood whose background was financially stable and satisfactory, but, in most instances, emotionally unstable and unsatisfactory (broken marriages, neurotic or otherwise inefficient parents, overprotective or neglectful mothers, etc.). Teaching our students, we emphasized in each particular case the particular hazards and harmful effects exercised by the environment and the measures needed to ensure normal progressive development and appropriate social adaptation in the individual case.

From the autumn term 1966 onward we are exchanging this nursery school population for children from a neighboring district who are socially and financially deprived and understimulated, i.e., in most cases children of immigrants to England who are very insecurely settled owing to racial and cultural differences. This will give us an excellent opportunity to collect more material about the effect of the parents' cultural uprootedness and insecurity on the children's home, school, and social problems. With these children we are especially interested in studying in detail the interactions between emotional and intellectual development, i.e., how far the lack of a loving, secure family background influences the unfolding of the learning capacities; and conversely, how far the absence of appropriate intellectual stimulation has repercussions on the child's emotional development.

We hope that our own work with a small number of underprivileged children will bring results which can be applied to the large numbers dealt with in the official children's services here and in the U.S.

Appendix

The various research projects outlined in the preceding chapters have in the meantime resulted in several publications by the author herself as well as by various members of the research team. They are listed below under a series of headings that correspond to the principal areas of research. The list includes only those reports that, since 1957, have appeared in print. Many other reports are available in mimeographed form, but they are still undergoing revision as new findings obtained in these ongoing projects become available.

It should be emphasized, however, that the major publication resulting from the investigations carried out at the Hampstead Child-Therapy Clinic is the author's own book,

Normality and Pathology in Childhood:
Assessments of Development

[Volume VI in this series of Anna Freud's Writings],

which is singled out here rather than listed under each heading. It would have to appear in all of them.

Editor's note

ADOLESCENCE

Freud, A. (1958), Adolescence (see ch. 9 in this volume).

Sprince, M. P. (1962), The Development of a Preoedipal Partnership between an Adolescent Girl and Her Mother.

Frankl, L. & Hellman, I. (1963), A Specific Problem in Adolescent Boys.

Rosenblatt, B. (1963), A Severe Neurosis in an Adolescent Boy.

Hellman, I. (1964), Observations on Adolescents in Psycho-Analytic Treatment.

Laufer, M. (1964), Ego Ideal and Pseudo Ego Ideal in Adolescence.

Sprince, M. P. (1964), A Contribution to the Study of Homosexuality in Adolescence.

Laufer, M. (1965), Assessment of Adolescent Disturbances: The Application of Anna Freud's Diagnostic Profile.

Freud, A. (1966), Adolescence as a Developmental Disturbance (see Volume VII).

Laufer, M. (1966), Object Loss and Mourning during Adolescence.

Laufer, M. (1968), The Body Image, the Function of Masturbation, and Adolescence: Problems of the Ownership of the Body.

BORDERLINE CASES

Freud, A. (1956), The Assessment of Borderline Cases (see ch. 18 in this volume).

Singer, M. B. (1960), Fantasies of a Borderline Patient.

Kut Rosenfeld, S. & Sprince, M. P. (1963), An Attempt to Formulate the Meaning of the Concept "Borderline."

Kut Rosenfeld, S. & Sprince, M. P. (1965), Some Thoughts on the Technical Handling of Borderline Children.

Thomas, R et al. (1966), Comments on Some Aspects of Self and Object Representation in a Group of Psychotic Children: An Application of Anna Freud's Diagnostic Profile.

MOTHERLESS CHILDREN

Hellman, I. (1962), Hampstead Nurseries Follow-up Studies: I. Sudden Separation and Its Effect Followed over Twenty Years.

Gyomroi, E. L. (1963), The Analysis of a Young Concentration Camp Victim.

BLIND CHILDREN

Burlingham, D. (1961), Some Notes on the Development of the Blind.

Sandler, A.-M. (1963), Aspects of Passivity and Ego Development in the Blind Infant.

Burlingham, D. (1964), Hearing and Its Role in the Development of the Blind.

Burlingham, D. (1965), Some Problems of Ego Development in Blind Children.

Nagera, H. & Colonna, A. B. (1965), Aspects of the Contribution of Sight to Ego and Drive Development: A Comparison of the Development of Some Blind and Sighted Children.

Sandler, A.-M. & Wills, D. M. (1965), Preliminary Notes on Play and Mastery in the Blind Child.

Wills, D. M. (1965), Observations on Blind Nursery School Children's Understanding of Their World.

Burlingham, D. (1967), Developmental Considerations in Occupations of the Blind.

Burlingham, D. & Goldberger, A. (1968), The Re-education of a Retarded Blind Child.

Colonna, A. B. (1968), A Blind Child Goes to the Hospital.

OTHER PHYSICAL HANDICAPS

Lussier, A. (1960), The Analysis of a Boy with a Congenital Deformity.

Thomas, R., Folkart, L., & Model, E. (1963), The Search for a Sexual Identity in a Case of Constitutional Sexual Precocity.

SIMULTANEOUS ANALYSIS OF
MOTHER AND CHILD

Hellman, I., Friedmann, O., & Shepheard, E. (1960), Simultaneous Analysis of Mother and Child.

Freud, A. (1960), Introduction to K. Levy's paper (see ch. 30 in this volume).

Levy, K. (1960), Simultaneous Analysis of a Mother and Her Adolescent Daughter: The Mother's Contribution to the Loosening of the Infantile Object Tie.

Sprince, M. P. (1962), The Development of a Preoedipal Partnership between an Adolescent Girl and Her Mother.

OBSERVATIONAL COMPARED
TO ANALYTIC DATA

Freud, A. (1957), The Contribution of Direct Child Observation to Psychoanalysis (see ch. 7 in this volume).

Freud, A. (1958), Child Observation and Prediction of Development: A Memorial Lecture in Honor of Ernst Kris (see ch. 8 in this volume).

Burlingham, D. & Barron, A. T. (1963), A Study of Identical Twins: Their Analytic Material Compared with Existing Observation Data of Their Early Childhood.

Freud, A. (1967), A Discussion with René Spitz (see Volume VII).

THE HAMPSTEAD INDEX

Sandler, J. (1960), On the Concept of Superego.

Sandler, J. (1962), The Hampstead Index as an Instrument of Psycho-Analytical Research.

Sandler, J. et al. (1962), The Classification of Superego Material in the Hampstead Index.

Sandler, J. & Rosenblatt, B. (1962), The Concept of the Representational World.

Sandler, J., Holder, A., & Meers, D. (1963), The Ego Ideal and the Ideal Self.

Sandler, J. & Nagera, H. (1963), Aspects of the Metapsychology of Fantasy.

Freud, A. (1965), Preface to Bolland & Sandler's monograph (see ch. 31 in this volume).

Bolland, J. & Sandler, J. et al. (1965), *The Hampstead Psychoanalytic Index: A Study of the Psychoanalytic Case Material of a Two-Year-Old Child.*

Joffe, W. G. (1965), Notes on Pain, Depression, and Individuation.

Sandler, J. & Joffe, W. G. (1965), Notes on Childhood Depression.

PREVENTION

Robertson, Joyce (1962), Mothering as an Influence on Early Development: A Study of Well-Baby Clinic Records.

Freud, A. (1964), Psychoanalytic Knowledge and Its Application in Children's Services (see ch. 27 in this volume).

Freud, A. (1965), [Chapter entitled] Conclusion. In *Children in the Hospital*, by T. Bergmann and A. Freud (see ch. 25 in this volume).

ASSESSMENT OF PATHOLOGY IN CHILDHOOD

The Diagnostic Profile

Freud, A. (1962), Assessment of Childhood Disturbances.*

Freud, A. (1963), The Concept of Developmental Lines.*

Freud, A. (1963), Regression as a Principle in Mental Development.*

Nagera, H. (1963), The Developmental Profile: Notes on Some Practical Considerations Regarding Its Use.

Freud, A., Nagera, H., & Freud, W. E. (1965), Metapsychological Assessment of the Adult Personality: The Adult Profile (see ch. 4 in this volume).

Laufer, M. (1965), Assessment of Adolescent Disturbances: The Application of Anna Freud's Diagnostic Profile.

Nagera, H. & Colonna, A. B. (1965), Aspects of the Contribution of Sight to Ego and Drive Development: A Comparison of the Development of Some Blind and Sighted Children.

Thomas, R. et al. (1966), Comments on Some Aspects of Self and Object Representation in a Group of Psychotic Children: An Application of Anna Freud's Diagnostic Profile.

Freud, W. E. (1967), Assessment of Early Infancy: Problems and Considerations.

* Although these papers were written during the time period covered by this volume, they have not been included in Volume V because they also form integral parts of Volume VI, *Normality and Pathology of Childhood*.

Freud, W. E. (1968), Some General Reflections on the Metapsychological Profile.

Clinical Studies in Psychopathology

Casuso, G. (1957), Anxiety Related to the "Discovery" of the Penis: An Observation.

Freud, A. (1957), Introduction to Casuso's paper (see ch. 28 in this volume).

Freud, A. (1957), Introduction to A.-M. Sandler et al.'s paper (see ch. 29 in this volume).

Sandler, A.-M., Daunton, E., & Schnurmann, A. (1957), Inconsistency in the Mother as a Factor in Character Development: A Comparative Study of Three Cases.

Bergen, M. E. (1958), The Effect of Severe Trauma on a Four-Year-Old Child.

Frankl, L. (1961), Some Observations on the Development and Disturbances of Integration in Childhood.

Frankl, L. (1961), A Child and His Symptoms.

Frankl, L. (1963), Self-Preservation and the Development of Accident Proneness in Children and Adolescents.

Frankl, L. & Hellman, I. (1964), The Ego's Participation in the Therapeutic Alliance.

Nagera, H. (1964), On Arrest in Development, Fixation, and Regression.

Nagera, H. (1964), Autoerotism, Autoerotic Activities, and Ego Development.

Robertson, Joyce (1965), Mother-Infant Interaction from Birth to Twelve Months: Two Case Studies.

Robertson, Joyce (1965), Three Devoted Mothers.

Sandler, J. & Joffe, W. G. (1965), Notes on Obsessional Manifestations in Children.

Freud, A. (1966), Preface to Nagera's monograph (see ch. 32 in this volume).

Nagera, H. (1966), *Early Childhood Disturbances, the Infantile Neurosis, and the Adult Disturbances.*

Nagera, H. (1966), Sleep and Its Disturbances Approached Developmentally.

Holder, A. (1968), Theoretical and Clinical Notes on the Interaction of Some Relevant Variables in the Production of Neurotic Disturbances.

Part II

This section corresponds to Part I in Volume IV. It consists of papers addressed primarily to psychoanalysts.

Several papers written and published during the period covered by the current volume (1956-1965) belong in this section:

Assessment of Childhood Disturbances (1962)
Regression as a Principle in Mental Development (1963)
The Concept of Developmental Lines (1963)
Diagnostic Skills and Their Growth in Psychoanalysis (1965)

These papers have been omitted here to avoid duplication: they form an integral part of *Normality and Pathology in Childhood* (Volume VI), which represents the author's major psychoanalytic contribution deriving from work done during this time period.

Editor's note

7

The Contribution of
Direct Child Observation
to Psychoanalysis
(1957)

The value of direct child observation for psychoanalysis has
not been under review since 1950, when it was discussed
in a meeting of analysts and child analysts in Stockbridge, Mass., under the title of "Problems of Child Development" (see Symposium, 1951). Members of the present panel may wish to take as one of their starting points
the "Opening Remarks on Psychoanalytic Child Psychology" made by Ernst Kris on that occasion and published in
Volume VI of *The Psychoanalytic Study of the Child*
(1951). There, Ernst Kris makes two distinctions which

Read at the 20th Congress of the International Psycho-Analytical Association, Paris. It is here published for the first time.

may be helpful in limiting the scope of our present symposium: one, the distinction between the analytically trained observer, on the one hand (i.e., the analyst in the temporary role of direct observer), and the nonanalytic, academic observer, on the other; and, secondly, the distinction between the research or observation setting, in which the observer himself plays a vital part (such as the analytic session itself, or any life situation which the observing analyst shares with the child), and the artificially constructed test or research setting, in which the observing psychologist remains an objective and noninterfering outsider.

I take it for granted that the members of this panel will be concerned almost exclusively with the analytic observer and with observation settings of the first kind.

THE CASE FOR AND AGAINST DIRECT OBSERVATION

I propose to limit myself to a discussion of the justification of direct child observation, rather than to a discussion and enumeration of its results. On the basis of my personal experience I assume that the stand which analysts take on this theoretical question depends largely on the opportunities for practical work which have come their way. When I took part in the Stockbridge Symposium, I came fresh from several years of work in a children's institution which offered opportunities for long-term observations of children on an almost twenty-four hour basis. Naturally, I was impressed by the additions to our insight, especially with regard to the processes of maturation, which such an opportunity provides, and I made use of the occasion to report in detail on those confirmations and modifications of and contradictions to our analytic knowledge by which I had been struck.

To the present discussion, on the other hand, I come from several years' work in a children's clinic which gives me the possibility to follow the analytic treatment of large numbers of children's cases of all ages and descriptions. I am, therefore, under the fresh impression of the overwhelming advantage of the analytic method itself over all other methods of observation and, as analysts tend to be, inclined to look down on all other ways and means of gaining access to the child's mind. Luckily, though, work in a children's clinic provides varied opportunities. For example, a study of exceptional behavior in children undertaken from both the observational and the analytic angles indicates the advantages and limitation of the two methods, used parallel, or set against each other.

THE DEFINITION OF "ANALYTIC" MATERIAL

For my part, I find it impossible to enter into a discussion of the value of direct observation without reference to analysis itself and the classification of material as it emerges in the analytic hour. There is no doubt that in this setting, too, direct, or common, observation has its place. Recent developments in psychoanalytic technique have gone in the direction of even grading what the patient has to offer according to its analytic validity; to assign a comparatively low value to the observation of conscious memories, attitudes, behavior, and the associations belonging to them; and to focus their analytic attention on only those manifestations which are direct or indirect expressions of transference. I leave appreciation of this selectiveness aside, to be discussed elsewhere.[1]

For the present, I propose to concentrate on the historical fact that, long ago, when the analytic technique came into being, the decision had to be made whether analysts should restrict their field of observation to the material offered by the patients themselves, about themselves, or to supplement it with information offered by the relatives and even the analyst's own direct observations of the family environment. That the former course was decided on, despite obvious disadvantages, happened on the basis of deeply rooted theoretical convictions.

Analytic work has always proceeded, and still proceeds, in analogy to dream interpretation. We expect patients to offer us manifest content, i.e., material which has undergone a secondary, distorting, elaboration in their conscious minds. It then becomes the task of the analyst, together with the patient, to undo the distortions which the latent content has undergone and to arrive gradually at the underlying id strivings with which we are concerned. It is obvious from this definition of the analytic technique that the smoothness of the procedure depends on the presence of a functioning ego which, in the first instance, distorts id material and, in the second instance, cooperates in undoing secondary processes.

Thus, analysts meet technical difficulties in all those cases where the ego is deteriorated or out of action, as it is in the psychoses; where it is immature, as in all children;

---

[1] [This point was taken further in a paper entitled "Diagnostic Skills and Their Growth in Psycho-Analysis" (1965), which was not included in this volume; see also Volume VI, ch. 1.]

or where it is in the preverbal stage of development, as it is in infants. In the classical situation, we expect the material to pass through the sieve of the patient's self-observation, no matter how much it changes or how much of it is held back during this process.

Where this cannot happen, the analyst feels the need for additional forms of observation to supplement the analytic insight and technique. This may explain why in most forms of child analysis, analysts find it difficult to work without adding to the child's own material the daily observations of behavior which the mother makes between analytic sessions. It may also explain our attitude to much of our ignorance concerning the first year of life. With regard to this period of life, when the subject's self-observation is wholly nonexistent, the temptation is great to fill the gaps by means of direct observation.

PITFALLS AND SAFEGUARDS IN DIRECT OBSERVATION

It is unlucky for the direct observer that some secondary processes which distort and disguise id content (such as the primitive defenses) develop earlier than other ego functions (such as self-observation) which channelize and summarize material. The direct observer of young children is therefore faced with an overwhelming mass of pictures of manifest behavior which must not be taken at their face value, but for the unraveling of which there seems to be no key.

To this quandary, analysts are seen to react in one of two ways. Some interpret what they see in analogy to material seen in the analytic situation. This, to me, seems wrong since it equals "wild" analysis, or the interpretation of manifest dreams without the personal associations of the dreamer. Others declare themselves defeated, and acknowledge that there is a gap between internal material and surface behavior which cannot be bridged except by means of transference manifestations in the analytic session. This, to me, seems too pessimistic. I submit the idea that, if care is exercised, certain correct guesses are possible which lead directly from specific forms of surface behavior to specific underlying unconscious elements. This, if proved, would constitute "direct observation" in the psychoanalytic sense.

To use once more the analogy with dream interpretation: besides the elements in the manifest dream which have to be unraveled with the help of associations, there are others which can be translated directly, i.e., the symbols which represent fixed relations between the surface and the depth. There are, further, typical manifest elements such as dreams of flying, nakedness, etc., which betray their latent content. What we learn from dreams holds good, further, for specific symptoms and specific elements of character. It is true that manifest behaviors such as stealing, lying, oversensitiveness, bed wetting, etc., may have any of a large number of unconscious meanings and are not open to translation without analytic work. But the same is not true of attitudes such as orderliness, punctiliousness, obstinancy, which invariably and unmistakably point to the conflicts of the anal sphere which lie behind them. I now contend, for the purpose of this discussion, that we know more invariable connections of this kind than are represented by the elements of the oral, anal, or urethral character, and that use can be made of such pictures when they are observed.

Actually, this is precisely what happens whenever the diagnosis of a child's case had to be made, since in this procedure the average child is usually wholly uncooperative. For purposes of diagnosis we "observe" the child and often, without realizing it, we are led in our guesses by a mass of behavioristic data, some of which are open to translation. Working on the subject of diagnosis of childhood disturbances, I have on several occasions attempted to enumerate such data, selected carefully from children's behavior with regard to feeding, sleep, bodily illness, play, etc. These data, observed mostly in older children can, I believe, be extended to provide clues to the happenings during the first years of life, and checked against our analytic assumptions gained from reconstruction.

CONCLUSION

So much for my personal contribution to the panel. Other contributors will probably approach this topic by completely different routes. It is to be hoped, above all, that some members will concentrate not on the justification of the procedure, but on its results.

8

Child Observation and Prediction of Development

A Memorial Lecture in Honor of Ernst Kris (1958 [1957])

I am grateful to my American friends and colleagues for inviting me to join this Memorial Meeting held in honor

Read at the Ernst Kris Memorial Meeting held by the New York Psychoanalytic Society and Institute and the Western New England Psychoanalytic Society and Institute at the New York Academy of Medicine on September 2, 1957. First published in *The Psychoanalytic Study of the Child*, 13:92-116, 1958. In part also in: *The Family and the Law*, by Joseph Goldstein and Jay Katz. New York: Free Press, 1965, pp. 953-959, 1002, 1017, and in: *Psychoanalysis, Psychiatry and Law* by Jay Katz, Joseph Goldstein, and Alan M. Dershowitz. New York: Free Press, 1967, pp. 399-402.

of Ernst Kris and for letting me share the feelings of appreciation, of indebtedness, and of loss which move us all, thinking of his death.

I welcome the decision that this commemoration should take the form of a symposium, dealing with all the ramifications and implications of Ernst Kris's work. This offers the opportunity to each contributor in turn to select what seems to him personally the most important and intriguing aspect of his activities and to argue the principal points, as it were, still in discussion with him.

ERNST KRIS'S "NOTES ON THE DEVELOPMENT AND SOME CURRENT PROBLEMS OF PSYCHOANALYTIC CHILD PSYCHOLOGY"

In this spirit I select as my starting point a paper written by Ernst Kris as his contribution to a panel discussion on "Psychoanalysis and Developmental Psychology" and published under the indifferent title of "Notes on the Development and Some Current Problems of Psychoanalytic Child Psychology" (1950a). This was the period when Ernst Kris began to be involved in the methods of direct child observation carried out by analysts and to plead for the legitimacy of such procedures within the framework of psychoanalytic investigations. It was this concern which prompted him a year later to arrange for and introduce the so-called Stockbridge discussion attended by many child analysts and analysts which dealt with the same subject (see Symposium, 1951).

The Two Phases of Psychoanalytic Child Psychology:
The Double Approach to Investigation

In the paper selected here for discussion, Ernst Kris began by distinguishing between two phases in the development of psychoanalytic child psychology. He placed the dividing line between them somewhere in "the early twenties" and listed as the salient new points in the second phase the new theory of anxiety, the introduction of the structural point of view, the recognition of aggression as an independent drive, and the legitimacy of a psychoanalytic ego psychology. He emphasized the special relevance which this division into two phases has for the relationship between the two sets of data on which our present psychoanalytic child psychology is based: those gained by reconstruction during analytic treatment, and those gained by direct observation. He showed that, in the first phase, the data furnished by direct observation remained of only marginal interest, more important for the applications of psychoanalysis (such as education, re-education, etc.) than for analysts themselves, whereas in the second phase, they attained the dignity of an analytic study proper and became increasingly capable of integration with material derived from reconstruction in the analyses of adults and of children.

In this connection Ernst Kris contradicted, quite rightly, a pessimistic statement of mine concerning the function of direct child observation. I had taken the attitude that such work is useful since it serves to prove or disprove the correctness of our reconstructions but "that it will not break new ground." Ernst Kris took the opposite attitude in an emphatic manner. He stated: "It would be erroneous to generalize . . . that all that the observational study of infant and child will ever be able to provide is a test of psychoanalytic hypotheses, their confirmation, or their falsification . . . this is not the sole and dominant function of child observation" (p. 41). If it is used rightly, and if its relation to psychoanalysis is fully utilized, "observational and reconstructive data [would] be comparable"; and while the former would certainly not replace the latter, they would implement, supplement, control, and enlarge the picture in various ways. He went on to state what he considered the optimal conditions for child observation: not short-time intensive observation periods, i.e., spot observations; not observation limited to cross-sections; but organized, systematic longitudinal studies of the life histories of a selected number of individual children, supplemented and checked at various points by analytic investigation. What he had in mind was a double approach, on the one hand by analytic reconstruction, on the other hand by direct observation, the resulting data to be compared and correlated; in short, the research technique for which the Child Study Center at Yale has since become renowned (see Marianne Kris, 1957).[1]

Ernst Kris as Historian, Research Worker, and Clinician

So far Ernst Kris has shown us in this paper two aspects of his work with which we are familiar. One is in his capacity of chronicler and historian of psychoanalysis as a scientific movement and as a theory, a role in which he had already excelled in his widely known Introduction to the Fliess letters (1950b). The other is his leaning toward aca-

[1] See also Ritvo and Solnit (1958, 1960) and Ritvo et al. (1963).

demic thoroughness and exactitude, in his capacity of psychologist who is intent on collecting facts, and on checking, rechecking, and verifying them increasingly. The greater the reliability of his basic data, the stronger was his hope that he might win standing and recognition for them even with those scientific workers outside the analytic field who dismiss reconstructive data as scientifically unproved and irrelevant.

We all know from personal experience Ernst Kris's remarkable capacities for the study of detail. He demonstrated this on many occasions in the more remote past in his work as an art historian, where he dealt with minute differences and similarities in identifying objects, and, more recently, in his analytic work, when he patiently followed mental processes from their instinctual roots to the highest sublimations, disentangling their vicissitudes on the long and intricate paths through the structure of the personality. But, unlike most other analytic workers who possess this ability, he never lost himself in detail. He never permitted his preoccupation with a particular subject to subtract from his interest in what he felt to be the whole—that is, in this instance, the important role which, in his opinion, psychoanalytic child psychology was destined to play in psychoanalytic theory and therapy.

Instructive as these two points are for the student of the subject, neither the historical distinctions nor the plea for direct observation in the form in which it should be employed are exclusive to this paper. On the contrary, the former subject was taken up by him and dealt with on a wider scale for purposes of the Stockbridge discussion one year later, the latter brought into representative form in the paper read after his death at the Paris Congress 1957, in which his research program for the Child Study Center at Yale was described and justified (M. Kris, 1957).

So far we remain on familiar ground. But there is an additional aspect which, for me, lends a specific and exciting character to these "Notes on the Development. . . ." Ernst Kris proceeded to take up in them what prompted his research and, surprisingly enough, the motives given are neither those of academic nor of metapsychological inquiry. He appears suddenly in his third role: that of clinician and therapist. And, without stating it explicitly, but still clearly enough, he reveals that what he actually meant to do —and did at Yale—was to put his observational-reconstructive research to clinical use for the purpose of investigating the variations of mental health on the one hand and the earlier recognition of pathology on the other.

Prediction and the Diagnostic Dilemma

I owe Ernst Kris an apology for the fact that it took me a long time to come to terms with the word "prediction," which he used to designate the aims of his research. To me, and to many other colleagues, this term was misleading since it conveyed only a vague meaning and brought with it the suspicion of theoretical speculation regarding the future. Such a concern is basically alien to the analytically trained mind since our interest in past events looms larger than all other preoccupations. What we were slow to recognize, in spite of all the evidence contained in these "Notes," was that prediction meant to Ernst Kris clinical foresight of development and that what motivated him in his theoretical observational studies was nothing more or less than a passionate concern with one of our most pressing practical problems: the question of the assessment and diagnosis of the disturbances of childhood.

Ernst Kris was well aware of the difficulties of diagnosis which beset the child analyst and of the manner in which we all flounder, more or less helplessly, in the mass of childhood disturbances which come to our notice via parents, pediatricians, school, child guidance clinics, and analytic practice. He regretted, as we all do, that our assessments are inexact, that our diagnoses usually come too late, when the disturbance has become massive and ingrained, and that the dividing line between normality and pathology is too easy to miss. He knew that our diagnostic categories had become all the more inadequate since the concept of an "infantile neurosis" had gradually ceased to serve us as a focal point.

The new ego psychology had made us acquainted with a further number of variations and deviations of structure, had added the atypical and autistic developments to our list, and played havoc with earlier seemingly secure distinctions such as those between emotional and intellectual disorders, the latter now merely appearing as an adjunct or a function of the former. Investigations into the first year of life and the consequences of the earliest mother-child relationship had revealed that much may be acquired by the infant that had previously been considered as innate, thus putting out of action some more of our basic diagnostic categories. No wonder that the result was a chaotic one and that child psychiatrists and analysts have difficulty in finding their way in a field which is crowded by manifestations such as disturbances of vital functions (sleeping, eating, learning); retardation of ego activities (motility, speech); failures of management (toilet training); fixations and regressions (especially affecting smooth transition in phase development)—all this in addition to the more familiar anxieties, inhibitions, defenses, neurotic, psychotic, and borderline manifestations.

It was this situation which, I believe, Ernst Kris was trying to remedy by placing the fact finding in observational research at the service of diagnosis. He was trying, to use his own words, "to predict from observational data that pathology exists in a given child" (p. 37). He wondered, "how soon can we spot it from the child's behavior, from that of the family unit, or from the history of mother and child?" It became his ambition "to recognize . . . symptomatology before it becomes manifest, . . . to spot danger before it appears" (p. 34).[2]

The Difficulties of Prediction

Naturally, I do not mean to imply that Ernst Kris deceived himself about the difficulties of clinical foresight, or that he took prediction lightly. His own pronouncements are sufficient evidence to the contrary, backed up further by the convincing illustrations of his work, presented by Marianne Kris (1957). It was Ernst Kris himself who drew our attention to the hopelessness of such clinical foresight in what he had described as the first phase of psychoanalytic child psychology. While we knew no more of the predestined sequences of development than the libidinal phases

[2] It is interesting to note in this respect that more than twenty years earlier Aichhorn (1932) distinguished in a similar manner between "latent" and "manifest" dissociality. The former would correspond to the symptomatology "before it becomes manifest" and represent the "danger before it appears." See also Aichhorn (1948).

and some "crucial conflicts and typical danger situations related to the maturational sequence" (p. 27), prediction was not possible. There were too many unknown factors which determined the outcome of the child's reactions to his experiences and their genetic, economic, and dynamic interrelations.

It is true that all this seemed to change in the second phase. It became possible, as Ernst Kris remarks, "to view the interaction of libidinal and aggressive drives in each of the typical danger situations of childhood; . . . to take the stages of ego and superego development into account . . . to correlate [in a number of instances, at least] the use of certain mechanisms of defense to certain situations and developmental phases" (p. 27). Further, we came to understand the extent to which conflict, danger, and defense are "essential and necessary concomitants of growing up," as well as "the adaptive function of defense" (p. 28). If we add to this the increasing insight into "the uniqueness of the mother in human life," i.e., into the preoedipal experiences of the infant, we have a large number of added factors which can be taken into account in our assessment of a child's immediate condition or his prospects for the future.

In spite of these advances (and I feel sure that Ernst Kris would agree with this qualifying statement), there remain a number of factors which make clinical foresight, i.e., prediction, difficult and hazardous. I name three of them here. (1) There is no guarantee that the rate of maturational progress on the side of ego development and drive development will be an even one; and whenever one side of the structure outdistances the other in growth, a variety of unexpected and unpredictable deviations from the norm will follow. (2) There is still no way to approach the quantitative factor in drive development, or to foresee it; but most of the conflict solutions within the personality will, in the last resort, be determined by quantitative rather than by qualitative factors. (3) The environmental happenings in a child's life will always remain unpredictable since they are not governed by any known laws. Marianne Kris (1957) has given us an interesting example how this unmovable obstacle to prediction can be taken into account in the longitudinal study and even used formally to test the skill of the "predicting" observer.

Ernst Kris himself testified to the presence of the unknown or unknowable forces at work in development in the following sentences: "The self-healing qualities of further development are little known." And we do not know how much "latency, prepuberty, or adolescence do to mitigate earlier deviation or to make the predisposition to . . . disturbances manifest" (p. 38).

PRACTICAL APPLICATIONS OF THE DOUBLE APPROACH TO INVESTIGATION

It is time, I believe, to put argumentation aside and to scrutinize the double approach to investigation (observational as well as reconstructive) for its impact on our clinical work with children, as we already experience it, or expect to experience it in the future. The items of material which I use for the purpose will seem a miscellaneous collection, selected at random, as they are, from the daily range of problems in a children's clinic, concerning treatment, diagnosis, prognosis, understanding and assessment of developmental and environmental factors, their relative value and their interactions.

The Value of Early Diagnosis for Treatment Purposes

To take treatment first. Ernst Kris envisaged that the integration of observational with reconstructive data will teach us more about typical sequences in child development and that, in turn, such additional knowledge will enable us to foresee and anticipate pathology, at least in typical cases.

If this comes true, it will, indeed, revolutionize the conditions for child analysis and any known form of analytic child therapy. Even where we stand now, we have ample evidence that the date at which we take therapeutic action is of extreme importance. With children, usually, the interval between the outbreak of trouble and the onset of treatment is comparatively long. In the past this was due to the parents' distrust and fear of analysis which caused them to experiment with every conceivable educational or medical device before turning, at last, and often too late, to analytic help. At present the causes are of the opposite kind, so many parents seeking help for their children that the waiting lists for treatment are unduly long. However that may be, experience has taught us that the beginning of therapy, immediately after the appearance of trouble, will shorten the duration of treatment by many months. This has been proved repeatedly in connection with disturbances such as sleeping and eating disorders, phobias, inhibitions, and sudden regressive moves in development, such as loss of active aggression, of phallic qualities, or—earlier—of speech. It is easier, therapeutically, to intervene in a process of symptom formation in the fluid state than to deal with hardened symptoms. There is no child analyst, I believe, who would not welcome the next step forward to a state of affairs which places therapeutic intervention even earlier,

namely, at a time before symptom formation has been resorted to at all.

To mention some examples of my own experience:

(i) I had the opportunity, several years ago, to meet a
small boy with a facial tic one or two days after its appearance, to guess its meaning, and to dissolve it almost immediately by means of analytic interpretation. In this intervention I was guided not only by the clinical data provided by
the child, but by the lucky chance of an additional "longitudinal" observation of his life history. He was one of the
former war children whose family fortunes and misfortunes
I had followed from a near distance. I knew about his
intimacy with his mother in infancy when he was alone
with her; his unrelenting hostility to his father when the
latter returned, injured, from the war; his immense jealousy when a sibling was born; and his complete lack of
manifest anxiety when his mother fell ill and died in connection with her next pregnancy. A year after the mother's
death, the child, aged six years, developed the tic following
a slight nosebleed. The tic was two-timed and consisted of
a quick sniffing up and blowing down through the nostrils,
repeated at short intervals.

It seemed legitimate to me to combine past and present
information for the purpose of analytic action. There
seemed no doubt that the tic represented the culmination
and attempted solution of many conflicts of his past history: fear of injury to his body, heightened by the death
wishes against father and sibling, now turned against himself; his unconscious strivings for femininity and the fear of
them; his resentment about being neglected and "rejected"
by his mother; his taking upon himself the mother's role

in stopping the bleeding (by sniffing up) and testing the result again and again for reassurance (by blowing down). It was this latter meaning, I believe, which determined the selection of the symptom. The child had withdrawn libido from the object world, following his threefold disappointment in the mother (return of father, arrival of sibling, her death), and had cathected his own body instead, thereby giving inflated, hypochondriacal importance to his body ailments. His tic represented a pathological way of playing mother-and-child with his own body; he took over the role of the mother in a comforting and reassuring capacity, while his body represented himself in the role of the frightened and suffering child.

It is instructive to subject this very abbreviated case history to Ernst Kris's lines of reasoning. I think he would have argued quite rightly as follows:

Was it really necessary to let this child wait for help until there was a manifest outbreak of pathology in the form of symptom formation? Is this not one of those typical sequences which, according to our knowledge of life histories, was bound to lead to pathology? Could we not have spotted pathology in this case "before it appeared," merely (as quoted above) "from the child's behavior, from that of the family unit, from the history of mother and child"? There is only disadvantage, he would have maintained, in waiting with therapy until the whole host of conflicting ideas and impulses in the child are compressed into a symptom, and one, moreover, which is notoriously difficult to remove by analysis once it has established itself and been allowed to persist for any length of time.

(ii) The second example which I have to offer is not

dissimilar. In this case, the longitudinal observation was provided for me by the analysis of a relative in whose life the child was important, and who, in the analytic material, conveyed a multitude of major and minor facts concerning her development. This little girl was, in the eyes of her parents, an ideal child, healthy, happy, affectionate, and intelligent, apparently wholly unneurotic. They were all the more perturbed when, suddenly, at the age of six, in the second year of an otherwise undisturbed school attendance, she developed a school phobia with violent outbreaks of anxiety. After a short period of battle, during which they tried in vain to take her to school in spite of protest, they had to declare themselves defeated and acquiesce in her remaining home.

I was less surprised by the appearance of pathology. Even though to unskilled eyes all had proceeded smoothly in the child's development, I, in my role as "shadowy observer" of the family, to quote an apt phrase of Ernst Kris's, had thought otherwise. I had thought the child too consistently affectionate, with a conspicuous absence of aggression and hostility. Her relationship to her mother had followed too persistently the preoedipal pattern, and the step to the oedipal change (positive cathexis of the father and aggressive rivalry with the mother) was too slow in coming. There had been at least one unwarranted upset in her preschool years about a "naughty" boy on the playground whom she wanted to avoid. Further, approximately six months before the outbreak of the phobia, very slight changes of character had taken place: the child's happiness had become less radiant, her clinging to the mother had become slightly more insistent, some anxiousness concerning the topics of death and illness had become apparent.

The mother, although not analyzed herself, began to consult with me concerning the child's state. Her reports on the little girl's talk, play, and imaginary games were faithful and correct. This, together with the slight danger signals listed above, helped me to understand the unconscious content of the phobia. Here was an example of a typical infantile neurosis organized around the oedipal experience. On the one side was the child's sadistic conception of intercourse and impregnation as assault and victimization; from this originated her fear of the feminine role and her rejection of it. On the other side was her drive toward femininity which lead inexorably toward rivalry with her beloved mother and death wishes against her. Both threats together inhibited libidinal progress and fixated the child to the less conflicting and less anxiety-arousing preoedipal relationships. However, since the maturational forces in this potentially normal child would not permit a mere arrest in development, the danger situation and conflict were removed from home, where they belonged, and transferred to the school, where the anxiety had to be rationalized and became attached successively to playmates, teachers, achievement tests, etc.

After so much had become evident, I was able to guide the mother to interpret to the child carefully and very gradually; aggression, death wishes, sexual curiosity, fantasies about parental intercourse became manifest in the child's consciousness during the next weeks. With their appearance, the phobia disappeared, and the child returned to school. More important still, she abandoned the preoedipal position and moved forward to the normal triangular oedipal relationship.

If we compare this case with the foregoing one, we find

that foresight of pathology was a more subtle matter; the danger signs were slighter, although, for the initiated, no less typical. Following Ernst Kris, we as analysts and analytic observers may be convinced that this child too needed earlier help and that, this given, the disrupting and disturbing phobia need never have appeared. But this raises a further problem, to be added to our former argumentation concerning prediction. What are the chances for the observer to convey such convictions of future pathology to a child's environment? With the present spread of knowledge about child development, many parents have become enlightened as to the inevitableness of mood swings, conflicts, anxieties in the normal course of events. How much further will such enlightenment have to proceed to help them to distinguish these normal forms of upset from the more ominous ones?

(iii) It is interesting to note that there also exist cases in which the described positions of parents and professional diagnostician are reversed, so that the latter sees no cause for alarm while the former are on the alert for danger. This usually happens when one of the parents or both have undergone a therapeutic analysis, or when the knowledge of some hereditary illness in the family causes watchfulness.

I mention two unconnected instances of this kind seen recently, both boys in early latency. Several years previously, their fathers had undergone successful analyses and after a hard struggle freed themselves from disturbing neuroses affecting their efficiency in sex life and in work. In each case the child, after a promising and active start in life, was showing the first slight signs of slackening: a decrease of success in school; a slight slowing up of actions;

a new complaining tone in the voice; some lack of courage when facing pain; complaints of being teased by playmates. In each case the mother stoutly denied that there were any changes or grounds for worry. The fathers, on the other hand, had no difficulty in recognizing the first typical indications of retreat from phallic masculinity and regression to the passive-feminine strivings of the anal phase. They saw ominous signs of their own psychosexual difficulties repeating themselves in their sons, and they advocated treatment.

I had no doubt that their observations were correct and their demands justified; but I was interested to see that even in an analytically enlightened children's clinic they had a difficult task to convince a reluctant staff that they were not merely chasing phantoms.

The truth is that, as knowledge stands at present, it is difficult to draw the line between prediction of pathology based on authentic danger signals and a diffuse and indiscriminate overanxiousness, all too easily aroused by every slight deviation from the optimal and from the norm.

What we need to decide the issue is the further systematic inquiry into the possibilities and the limitations of clinical foresight. We look for the answers to the research on prediction carried on in the Child Study Center at Yale, now under Marianne Kris (1957).

Some Features of the Early Mother-Child Relationship

In the paper with which we are concerned, Ernst Kris designates as "the area in which observational techniques have contributed most during recent decades—the early features of the mother-child relationship." We may add that this is also the place where the results of the double approach to investigation are most obvious to analysts and least controversial for them.

I take as a case in point the concept of the "good" and "bad" mother. These terms came into use as a result of Melanie Klein's analysis of the infant's experiences in connection with the mother's breast: the satisfying "good" breast preparing the way for the image of the "good" mother, the empty or frustrating breast creating in the same manner the image of the "bad" mother. Melanie Klein demonstrated how far these actual experiences of the suckling infant become increasingly complicated and overlaid by the processes of introjection and projection which occur simultaneously; they intensify the bad images by adding to the experienced frustration the projections of the child's own aggressive and destructive impulses.

In our usual analytic perspective, with which I, personally, feel more familiar, the same process is represented, not by the concept of a double *internal image*, but by that of a double trend of impulses, such as love and hate, linked together and directed toward one and the same object—in short, by the well-known concept of *human ambivalence*.

Dealing with the same clinical data, Ernst Kris has shown that these two aspects still leave room for a third, which can be added to the former presentations as the result of longitudinal observations. In a paper from the Yale Child Study Center at Yale, he and his co-authors (see Coleman, Kris, Provence, 1953) discussed the "adaptive element in parent-child relationship" and postulated that these variations in parental attitudes, which can be noted even during early infancy, play a part in the development of the

child's personality. I think we may assume that besides
having other consequences, they also add a considerable
amount of external reality to the internal forces which are
responsible for the contrasting images of the mother or
the contrasting feelings toward her. To follow Ernst Kris's
meaning as closely as possible: much appears in later analysis as a unified picture which has been organized as such
due to the particular manner in which human memory functions. What in the analytic recall appear as simultaneous
past happenings may in actual experience have been successive events. Thus, the actual variations in the attitude
of a mother (loving, indulgent, possessive, critical, demanding, frustrating) and the infant's reactions to them may become telescoped, superimposed on each other, and help
toward the creation of the composite and conflicting mother
images as we meet them in analysis.

There is another aspect of the early mother-child relationship which has profited greatly from the observational
study of recent years, namely, the infant's reaction to the
depression or emotional withdrawal of the mother. Ernst
Kris has stated that this hypothesis could not be gained
by observation; it was only confirmed by it. At the same
time he stressed the advantages of the double approach in
this respect, i.e., that the observational studies of Margaret
Ribble (1943), Margaret Fries (1946), and Spitz (1945,
1946)[3] have helped us "fully to realize that in extreme cases
the lack of adequate object relationship in infancy may
threaten the infant's life, may cause serious and even irreversible changes in areas of maturation and create psychosomatic disturbances, the extent and impact of which is

[3] We should add to this list of authors the name of John Bowlby, London.

not as yet fully known" (1950a, p. 31). Actually, the addition of the observational to the reconstructive method has raised this discovery, in the course of less than twenty years, from the status of a hypothesis to that of a near-certainty.

On the other hand, our beliefs in this respect do not yet imply that we are able, or even willing, to take action. There are few situations in a child's development where it is more difficult to interfere. An emotionally withdrawn mother who is partially or wholly unable to satisfy her infant's emotional needs is not able to profit from guidance or advice, owing to the very depth of her disturbance. She may profit from treatment, but by the time beneficial results make themselves felt, her child's infancy may be past history. In some cases it may be possible to arrange for the addition of a substitute mother within the family (whether grandmother, aunt, or paid help); in other instances this will prove impossible for practical reasons.

Add to this that we live in a period when it has become an invidious task to separate the mother-child couple. Even for severely disturbed mothers, a modern mental hospital may nowadays make arrangements to admit them together with their infants or young children.[4] This is a step based on insight into the precarious libido situation in the mother, for whom the child and his care may represent the last precious thread which ties her to reality and to the object world. But what proves beneficial for the mother's treatment and recovery need not necessarily be of advantage to the child. Closeness to a mother in a depressive phase or during a schizophrenic episode may give rise in the infant, not necessarily to immediately visible pathology, but to the

[4] Such a scheme had recently been initiated by Dr. Tom Main in the Cassel Hospital, Richmond, Surrey.

kind of aftereffect which shows up years later and reveals itself in adult analysis as the starting point for mental trouble.

To return once more to the observational setting:

In the medicopsychological baby service attached to our Hampstead Child-Therapy Clinic, our pediatrician, Dr. Josefine Stross, periodically sees an infant (from the age of two months onward) whose mother shows indications of an unsatisfactory attitude toward the child. There is an apparent lack of genuine warmth, no visible pride in the baby's appearance or clothing, a reluctance to fondle or to play with the child's body, and a marked clumsiness in distinguishing between the child's needs (whether for nourishment, body comfort, company or entertainment). At the same time the baby is adequately and conscientiously cared for in bodily matters, and there is no question of neglect in its official sense. The mother's attitude to life is revealed, on inquiry, as a depressed and withdrawn one, although not to the degree on which psychiatric diagnoses are based. The baby's responses are predominantly normal, so far, although his social reactions (smiling responses, etc.) were at times somewhat below the expected age level.

This is where our quandary begins. Our feeling, based on knowledge of typical development, indicates that subtle harm is being inflicted on this child and that the consequences of it will become manifest at some future date. But is this foresight backed by sufficient evidence to justify intervention? Further: what are the criteria for choosing between different ways of intervening, such as treatment of the mother (which may be unwelcome to her), introduction of a second mother figure (which may prove impracticable), or, if it comes to an extreme, separation of mother and child (which may harm the mother)? Or is the answer that in such cases we may have to wait with interference until the relations between cause and effect in mental matters have become as firmly established and removed from doubt as they are today on the physical side, for example, when one is dealing with tubercular infection through the mother?

The Assessment of Sublimations

It is hardly possible to discuss Ernst Kris's work without referring at least to some aspects of sublimation. He was deeply and repeatedly involved in the problem of sublimation, which he recognized as one of the important pathways toward the understanding of artistic creativity.

Together with Heinz Hartmann, he increased our insight into the metapsychology of the process of sublimation. Starting out from the concept of sublimation as a displacement of drive energy, the two authors added to this the notion of a qualitative change in the energy itself, a change which places the activity maintained by it under the domination of the ego (desexualization, neutralization). They distinguished, further, between a permanent investment of the ego with such neutralized energy (described by Hartmann [1955] as the "reservoir"), and the temporary or transitory additions to it, provided by displaced instinctual strivings (described by Kris as the "flux"). The first of these, I believe, comes nearest to what we used to describe as the individual's "capacity for sublimation." To avoid confusion between displacement of goal on the one hand and energy transformation on the other, Kris suggested in 1952 to reserve the term sublimation once more for the former and to use the new term "neutralization" exclusively for the latter.

When, finally, in 1955 Ernst Kris added some observational studies of sublimation in young children to his reconstructive work in analysis, he did so in the hope of throwing further light on a number of problems concerning both displacement and transformation of energy. He attempted to trace how far successful fusion between libido and aggression in the earliest object relationships influences neutralization; he examined the influence of early identifications on the neutralizing process; he followed sublimations in the making; and he watched their increase and decrease in the unformed and immature personality.

It is these latter attempts which lead back once more to our problems of early diagnosis and to the assessment of normality and pathology at a given moment of development. The presence or absence of sublimations and, more than that, the degree to which the capacities for sublimation and neutralization have been developed in a child are highly significant for this individual's chances to remain "normal." Not only that the sublimated activities themselves have significance for social adaptation and for determining the width and scope of the personality as a whole; much more important still is the fact that the capacity for sublimation implies the ego's readiness to accept substitute satisfactions of symbolic value[5] when the way to the originally desired sexual and aggressive aims is blocked. This diminishes pressure from the drives and acts as some protection against the building up pathogenic frustrations with the resultant anx-

[5] This point invites comparison with the writings of Susan Isaacs (1935), Melanie Klein (1932), Marion Milner (1952), C. F. Rycroft (1956), and others in London.

ieties, defenses, regressive moves, which lead to symptom formation.

With so much metapsychological insight at our disposal, we should find it easy in diagnoses to assess the incidence and probable stability of sublimations present in a child. Actually, this is not the case. In diagnostic work we find that attempts at sublimation, i.e., displacements of drive energy, in young children are notoriously labile and transitory; so are neutralizations of drive energy which may revert to their crude instinctual nature whenever the child is overstimulated, exasperated or fatigued. Further, what is true for the very young, is equally true for older children with borderline disturbances. In both instances, the lines of demarcation between id and ego are insufficiently defined and the ego is badly protected against intrusions from the id. Consequently, it remains difficult in the clinical picture to distinguish between the beginnings of true sublimations which will prove of lasting value, sexualizations of ego functions and activities, or even compulsive interests which initiate pathology.

The following are some examples to illustrate the difficulties of clinical discrimination in this respect.

Example 1 is taken from the case of a boy who at the age of thirteen underwent a change of personality marked by withdrawal from the environment, overwhelming fantasy activity, inability to learn, some confusion about his orientation in reality.[6] He was taken into treatment as a

---

[6] These items are taken with the permission of Sara Kut Rosenfeld from her reports given in the case conferences of the Hampstead Child-Therapy Clinic (see Kut Rosenfeld and Sprince, 1963).

typical borderline case with uncertain prognosis. He was found to be entirely preoccupied with an elaborate insect world which he controlled by means of his intellect. In the center of this was his interest in bees and wasps whose habits he studied in great detail, his main researches being directed toward the composition and action of their stings. It testified to the defect in his reality testing that he maintained that his only close friend "actually claimed to own such a sting himself."

In this case, the sexual nature of the fantasy, its use for defensive purposes, and its central position in a complicated pathological state are obvious, of course. In the long analysis which followed, it became possible to trace the history of the "collapsible sting-tooth-penis" fantasy from its early oral and preoedipal aspects in the relationship to the mother to its phallic, oedipal meaning. It also became possible to disentangle the boy's confusion between internal and external reality and to show the manner in which denial, projection, identification, intellectualization, and ego restriction had been employed jointly to produce the wasp fantasy as their final result.

On the other hand, this obviously pathological structure also contained various aspects of a true sublimation. Apart from the initial *displacement* of sexual curiosity to the study of the insect world, the boy had achieved a remarkable degree of *neutralization* of energy in pursuing the displaced interest, which enabled him to read, abstract, summarize, and classify. Although during the treatment he remained emotionally on the borderline between neurosis and a prepsychotic state, this neutralization of energy became increasingly independent of internal pressures, so far as his chosen subjects, biology and botany, were concerned. Thus, what impressed us in the diagnostic interviews as a central symptom may finally prove to be the only reliable link between his ego and the external world.

Example 2 is not dissimilar, a boy of ten and three quarter years, again taken into treatment as a borderline case in the Hampstead Child-Therapy Clinic.[7] He had lived for several years in identification with an underground train and spent his days withdrawn from reality, either imitating the action of such trains or actually walking on underground lines, thereby endangering his life. His intellectual activity (which was somewhat below average[8]) spent itself on reading maps and memorizing the names of stations, streets, etc.

I quote this case for the reason that even this threatening spread of pathology in a child contained some elements of sublimation and neutralization which proved important for prognosis. It is true that the displacement of interest from the cavities of the human body to the system of underground tunnels hardly deserved to be called a sublimation at the time of diagnosis; it is equally true that his preoccupation with maps and names at that period was wholly in the service of his obsession. Nevertheless, the latter achieved some degree of neutralization; in an ego which otherwise functioned poorly, memorizing became a strong point, extending from street names to the names of people, etc. I found it interesting to read five years later, after his treatment, a report given on him by a vocational guidance de-

[7] The items of this case are taken with the author's permission from her reports in case conferences of the Hampstead Child-Therapy Clinic (see Singer, 1960).

[8] According to intelligence tests he had an IQ of 78 before treatment and an IQ of 101 after treatment.

partment. By this time many other manifestations of his deep-seated pathology had disappeared from the surface; but the industrial psychologist in his write-up remarked, among other things, that this boy had "a soft spot for maps" and he recommended (among other possibilities) "work in delivery or collection," thus treating the former obsession (of which he was ignorant, of course) as the basis of a neutralized, ego-directed activity.

Perhaps, in time, we shall learn to spot such potentially helpful props for the ego and links with reality even where they appear in the midst and at the service of severe pathology.

Example 3 is of a different nature. I quote it from the longitudinal observation of a small boy, undertaken by his father, himself a well-known educator (Hill, 1926, p. 47). According to the father's notes, this boy first showed interest in *water* at the age of twelve months, when he began to do without diapers during daytime; he was occasionally found patting a pool of water he had made on the floor. "Little pools of rain-water also interested him, and he thoroughly enjoyed smacking the water in the bath or wash-hand basin. At fourteen months he was very interested in turning water-taps on and off. When taken to the water-closet he watched the rush of water with great interest. At two years of age he spent hours controlling water supplies, filling and emptying buckets, tins, jars, tea-pots, hot-water bottles. He wanted to know where the water came from to the water-closet bowl. When he was taken to a gentleman's lavatory outside, he always insisted on seeing the hole down which the water went, and the cistern which supplied the water. At two and a half years he was tracing every pipe he could see; water-supply pipes, drain pipes, rain-pipes, gas pipes. Hours were spent lighting and turning out gas jets." Before he was three, the father had to take the cover off the water-closet cistern to satisfy his curiosity. "He spent about half an hour every day for a fortnight, standing on a ledge up at the cistern. . . . He filled the cistern to the overflow, and wanted to know the function of every detail of the mechanism." The father goes on to show how the child's interest spread from here to fireplugs, fire engines, water pumps, the gas works, and the sewage works. In nursery school, at the age of four and a half years, when told the story of Moses in the Bulrushes and asked to draw a picture of Moses in his cradle, he supplied the cradle with a long line, representing "a drain pipe" leading away from it.

For the direct observer of children, a behavioral picture of this kind gives rise to a number of important questions. He will have no difficulty in diagnosing the underlying presence of powerful pregenital interests with special preponderance of curiosity directed toward the urinary function and (as in Example 2) the inside of the human body. He will feel less certain about the degree of desexualization of curiosity (i.e., neutralization) achieved by the child. Accordingly, he will be unsure whether what he sees should be assessed as the beginning of a true sublimation which will enrich the ego, or as the beginning of a fixation to a primitive pregenital level which will restrict it and sooner or later lead to pathology. Is it the correct procedure to assist the boy in his researches (as his father has done) or should he be helped to detach himself from his overriding interest in the subject and develop toward further levels, as treatment would do in all probability?

In the case in question the answer has been supplied by the further life history of the boy. In the thirty years since the observation was made, he has developed into a physicist of unusual ability and standing, the recorded incidents evidently representing the first steps in the direction of this lasting sublimation. This, to my mind, does not signify that other, almost identical pictures, seen for diagnosis, could not lead to opposite results. In spite of all theoretical advances concerning the subject of sublimation, we are still— with Ernst Kris—impressed by the fluidity and uncertainty of these developmental processes. Perhaps we shall learn that it is not the sublimatory process itself from which we can take our cue, identical states or forms of sublimation possibly leading to different results; rather, we have to look for our evidence to accompanying circumstances and conditions in that total picture of the personality. For example, persistent water play of the kind described above may acquire a different and less favorable aspect when it is accompanied by bed wetting.

However that may be, correct assessment of sublimation in the very young remains a difficult matter; so does the prognosis for the future and the appropriate handling of the child based on our judgments. As matters stand now, we are still apt to do too little for those children in whom fixations and pathological development are in the making. On the other hand, there is also the danger that we may interfere too much or too soon and thereby (as somebody expressed it jokingly in discussion) "nip future physicists in the bud."

The Assessment of Traumatic Events

There is still a further (and for this paper last) area where prediction in Ernst Kris's use of the term might prove invaluable for our clinical concerns. I refer to the traumatic experiences of early childhood and the assessment of their impact on development.

Ernst Kris alluded to this subject in his "Notes on the Development . . . ," by discussing the differences between the data on life history gained by direct observation and those supplied by psychoanalytic reconstruction. He stressed the objective unselected character of the former and stated that, in contrast, "Data obtained by psychoanalysis are naturally selective . . . contain more precise information on areas of conflict involvement than on areas free of . . . conflict, [and] indicate what had been important in an etiological sense and when it had become important" (p. 41).

He considerably enlarged on these statements in 1956 in a paper in which he dealt with the dynamics of memory. Here, he traced events from their actual occurrence in a child's life, through the changes to which they are subjected in the mind, to their reappearance on the surface in analysis. As a result of such comparisons he went so far as to state that the traumatic significance of an event is not laid down at the time of its occurrence but that "the further course of life seems to determine which experience may gain significance as a traumatic one" (p. 73).

It is useful to keep these statements in mind when we inquire into the etiology of a child's disturbance. The life history of a child patient, as supplied by the parents, is the result of external observation. At best, it contains objective facts; more often, of course, it is given subjectively, with omissions, distortions, and selections of facts which are determined by the parents' own emotional needs and limitations. Therefore, the biographical material cannot (or should not) be used for guidance as to the pathogenic importance of past events. The material is "weighted" (to use a term of Ernst Kris's) according to the parents' and not according to the child's internal stresses.[9]

There is no difficulty in confirming this with clinical material. One mother, for example, dated her boy's disturbance to a car accident of the father which had been traumatic for both parents; the child's analysis, on the other hand, showed that in his mind this event was completely overshadowed by the departure of a beloved maid, which had occurred at the same time and had proved traumatic for him; in turn, this latter event had been dismissed from the mother's memory as unimportant.

Many mothers cite the loss of a grandparent as a decisive event in the child's life; here, subsequent analysis usually shows that the child has ignored the death as such, but has reacted violently to the mother's mourning, depression, and emotional withdrawal which followed the event.

Where bodily illnesses are concerned, the mothers will report those as significant which were objectively dangerous or aroused their own anxiety; the child, on his part, may react pathologically to any minor disturbance of health on the basis of pain, discomfort, anxiety, dietary and motor restrictions which are felt to be intolerable, enforced passivity. A similar variance in evaluation exists concerning time: separations may seem short and therefore negligible by

[9] The life history of an adult patient, as supplied by himself, is the product of his own memory and therefore illuminating.

adult standards and still be interminable, and therefore traumatic for the child (see T. Bergmann and A. Freud, 1966; and ch. 25 in this volume).

On the whole, such comparisons between biographical and analytic material constitute an instructive object lesson with regard to the gap existing between external and internal (psychic) reality.

I agree with Ernst Kris that we cannot predict from outside observations, and at the time of occurrence, which events will prove important for future pathology. I should like to add that we do not know either which aspect or element of a given experience will be selected for cathexis and emotional involvement (see ch. 14 in this volume).

The latter statement is borne out by our analyses of children who were subjected to war and concentration camp experiences. Where we expected to unearth buried memories of death, destruction, violence, hatred, etc., we usually found the traces of separations, motor restrictions, deprivations (of toys, pleasures), together with all the usual emotional upsets which are inseparable from any child's life. I was impressed in this respect by the story of a boy who, at four and a half years, had escaped with his family from enemy-occupied territory. A subsequent analysis showed which element of the experience had been singled out for traumatic value: he had suffered a severe shock from the fact that the invaders had deprived his father of his car. This, to him, meant that the father had been robbed of his potency. Beside this all-important oedipal experience, everything else (loss of home, security, friends) paled into insignificance.

One last example which may serve for many. This comes from the case of a little girl who, at the age of four years, had witnessed her father murdering her mother in a delusional attack of jealous rage. The child's analysis, undertaken six months later, was recorded by her therapist, Mary E. Bergen, under the title of "The Effect of Severe Trauma on a Four-Year-Old Child" (1958). In this paper the author traced in detail the child's attempt to assimilate "an act of violence which in a few minutes had swept away her parents and home and irrevocably changed the course of her life" (p. 407). It is the merit of this record that it illuminates, under the microscope of analysis, how one element of the horrifying event after the other became involved with the child's own fantasy world, thereby receiving weight through emotional cathexis. Thus, the girl's preoedipal sense of frustration, jealousy, and rage, and her search for an ideal, "good" mother, found guilty fulfillment in her move to a new foster home. Her death wishes against three younger siblings served her identification with the violent, but loved, father. On the oedipal level, the murder of the mother gave reality to the guilt-laden wish to remove the rival parent. Actually, all the elements of the oedipal position appeared in full force: love for the father, rivalry with the mother, guilt for wishing to separate the parents and set them quarreling, the effects of prolonged witnessing of the primal scene. The latter determined the child's deep involvement with that particular moment of the tragedy when the threatened and frantic woman tried to remove the child from the scene of murder by screaming at her: "Get out of here!" In the analysis, this detail was shown to symbolize the crowning insult, the mother being experienced as trying to exclude the child angrily from the parents' intimacy.

I cannot help wondering whether—without analysis—it would have been the fate of this particular detail to be singled out for permanent traumatic significance.

CONCLUSION: THE RELATION BETWEEN PREDICTION AND PREVENTION

In the foregoing paper I undertook to follow some of Ernst Kris's lines of reasoning where his observational studies are concerned. I shall consider the attempt successful if it should serve to reduce the reluctance of many analysts to accept child observation and prediction of development as relevant concerns and convince them of the bearing of such studies on clinical and diagnostic work.

It is implicit in such an acceptance of Ernst Kris's work to adopt a changed attitude to the concept of prevention as well.

The wish to use analytic insight not only for therapeutic but for preventive purposes has played its part since the beginnings of analysis. We used to think that prevention was served best by applying analytic knowledge to the principles of upbringing. But we have learned since that even the wisest handling of a child cannot prevent stress, conflicts, and occasional pathology, all of which are inseparable from the hazards of development; thus, we need the readiness for therapeutic action.

It is on this point that Ernst Kris's statements about "prediction of pathology" and early "spotting of danger" fall into place. Prediction will serve prevention if it teaches us (to use his own words) "which therapeutic steps are appropriate to each age level and its disturbance, or to each typical group of disturbances."

9

Adolescence
(1958 [1957])

ADOLESCENCE IN THE PSYCHOANALYTIC THEORY

I return to the subject of adolescence after an interval of twenty years. During this time much has happened in analytic work to throw added light on the problems concerned and to influence the conditions of life for young people, whether normal or abnormal. Nevertheless, in spite of partial advances, the position with regard to the analytic study of adolescence is not a happy one, and especially un-

Read on the occasion of the Thirty-fifth Anniversary of the Worcester Youth Guidance Center on September 18, 1957. First published in *The Psychoanalytic Study of the Child*, 13:255-278, 1958. Also in: *Recent Developments in Psychoanalytic Child Therapy*, ed. Joseph Weinreb. New York: International Universities Press, 1960, pp. 1-24. Partially in: *The Family and the Law*, by Joseph Goldstein and Jay Katz. New York: Free Press, 1965, pp. 907-908. German translation: Probleme der Pubertät. *Psyche*, 14:1-24, 1960.

satisfactory when compared with that of early childhood. With the latter period, we feel sure of our ground, and in possession of a wealth of material and information which enables us to assume authority and apply analytic findings to the practical problems of upbringing. When it comes to adolescence, we feel hesitant and, accordingly, cannot satisfy the parents or educational workers who apply for help to us and to our knowledge. One can frequently hear it said that adolescence is a neglected period, a stepchild, where analytic thinking is concerned.

These complaints, which come from two sides, from the parents as well as from the analytic workers themselves, seem to me to warrant closer study and investigation than they have received so far.

Adolescence in the Psychoanalytic Literature

The psychoanalytic study of adolescence began, as is well known, in 1905 with the relevant chapter of the *Three Essays on the Theory of Sexuality*. Here, puberty was described as the time when the changes set in which give infantile sexual life its final shape. Subordination of the erotogenic zones to the primacy of the genital zone; the setting up of new sexual aims, different for males and females; and the finding of new sexual objects outside the family were listed as the main events. While this exposition explained many features of the adolescent process and behavior which had been unexplained before, the newly developed notion of the existence of an infantile sex life could not but lower the significance of adolescence in the eyes of the investigators. Before the publication of the *Three Essays*, adolescence had derived major significance from its role as the beginning of sex life in the individual; after the discovery of infantile sexuality, the status of adolescence was reduced to that of a period of final transformations, a transition and bridge between the diffuse infantile and the genitally centered adult sexuality.

Seventeen years later, in 1922, Ernest Jones published a paper on "Some Problems of Adolescence" which dwelt on a "correlation between adolescence and infancy" as its most distinctive point. Following the pronouncement in the *Three Essays* that the phase of development corresponding to the period between the ages of two and five must be regarded as an important precursor of the subsequent final organization, Jones showed in detail how "the individual *recapitulates and expands* in the second decennium of life the development he passed through during the first five years . . ." (p. 398). He ascribed the difference in "the circumstances in which the development takes place" but went as far as propounding "the general law . . . that adolescence recapitulates infancy, and that the precise way in which a given person will pass through the necessary stages of development in adolescence is to a very great extent determined by the form of his infantile development" (p. 399). In short: "these stages are passed through on different planes at the two periods of infancy and adolescence, but in very similar ways in the same individual" (p. 399).

Jones's important but isolated contribution to the problem coincided with a peak in the publications of Siegfried Bernfeld in Vienna, a true explorer of youth, who combined work as a clinical analyst and teacher of analysis with the unceasing study of adolescence in all its aspects of individual and group behavior, reaction to social influences, sublimations, etc. His most significant addition to the analytic theory was the description of a specific kind of male adolescent development (1923), the so-called "protracted" type which extends far beyond the time limit normal for adolescent characteristics, and is conspicuous by "tendencies toward productivity whether artistic, literary or scientific, and by a strong bent toward idealistic aims and spiritual values. . . ." As the solid background for his assumptions, Bernfeld published, in cooperation with W. Hoffer, a wealth of material consisting of self-observations of adolescents, their diaries, poetic productions, etc.

While Bernfeld accounted in this manner for the elaborations of the normal adolescent processes by the impact of internal frustrations and external, environmental pressures, August Aichhorn, also in Vienna, approached the problem from the angle of dissocial and criminal development. His work lay with those young people who respond to the same pressures with failure to adapt, faulty superego development, and revolt against the community. His book *Wayward Youth* (1925) acquired world renown as the outstanding pioneering attempt to carry psychoanalytic knowledge into the difficult realm of the problems of the young offender.

Familiar with Bernfeld's views, and having been intimately connected with Aichhorn's studies, I contributed in 1936 two papers under the titles "The Ego and the Id at Puberty" and "Instinctual Anxiety during Puberty."[1] In my case, interest in the adolescent problems was derived from my concern with the struggles of the ego to master the tensions and pressures arising from the drive derivatives, struggles which lead in the normal case to character forma-

---

[1] See Chapters 11 and 12 in *The Ego and the Mechanisms of Defense* [Volume II].

tion, in their pathological outcome to the formation of neurotic symptoms. I described this battle between ego and id as terminated first by a truce at the beginning of the latency period and later breaking out once more with the first approach of puberty, when the distribution of forces inside the individual is upset by quantitative and qualitative changes in the drives. Threatened with anxiety by the drive development, the ego, as it has been formed in childhood, enters into a struggle for survival in which all the available methods of defense are brought into play and strained to the utmost. The results, that is, the personality changes which are achieved, vary. Normally, the organization of ego and superego alter sufficiently to accommodate the new, mature forms of sexuality. In less favorable instances, a rigid, immature ego succeeds in inhibiting or distorting sexual maturity; in some cases, the id impulses succeed in creating utter confusion and chaos in what has been an orderly, socially directed ego during the latency period. I made the point that, more than any other time of life, adolescence with its typical conflicts provides the analyst with instructive pictures of the interplay and sequence of internal danger, anxiety, defense activity, transitory or permanent symptom formation, and mental breakdown.

Interest increased in the postwar years and brought a multitude of contributions, especially from the United States. Fortunately for the student of the subject, Leo A. Spiegel published in 1951 a lengthy "Review of Contributions to a Psychoanalytic Theory of Adolescence." Although his attempt to construct an integrated theory out of often widely divergent parts could hardly be successful, the paper serves a most useful purpose by abstracting, reviewing, and classifying the material. He grouped the publications under headings such as:

"Classification of Phenomenology" (Bernfeld, Hartmann, Kris, and Loewenstein, Wittels)

"Object Relations" (Bernfeld, Buxbaum, H. Deutsch, Erikson, Fenichel, A. Freud, W. Hoffer, Jones, A. Katan, Landauer)

"Defense Mechanisms" (Bernfeld, H. Deutsch, Fenichel, A. Freud, Greenacre, E. Kris)

"Creativity" (Bernfeld, A. Freud)

"Sexual Activity" (Balint, Bernfeld, Buxbaum, H. Deutsch, Federn, Ferenczi, S. Freud, Lampl-de Groot)

"Aspects of Ego Functioning" (Fenichel, A. Freud, Harnik, Hoffer, Landauer)

"Treatment" (Aichhorn, K. R. Eissler, A. Freud, Gitelson, A. Katan, M. Klein, Landauer, A. Reich).

A detailed bibliography attached to the review contained altogether forty-one papers by thirty-four authors, covering apparently every theoretical, clinical, and technical aspect of the subject.

But in spite of this impressive list of contributors and contributions the dissatisfaction with our knowledge of the field remained unaltered, nor did our own, or the parents', confidence in our analytic skill with adolescent patients increase. There was now much published evidence to the contrary; nevertheless, adolescence remained, as it had been before, a stepchild in psychoanalytic theory.

Some Difficulties of Fact Finding Concerning Adolescence

There are, I believe, two different causes which may, possibly, account for our bewilderment when faced with all the intricacies of the adolescent process.

When, in our capacity as analysts, we investigate mental states, we rely, basically, on two methods: either on the analysis of individuals in whom that particular state of mind is in action at the moment, or on the reconstruction of that state in analytic treatment undertaken at a later date. The results of these two procedures, used either singly or in combination with each other, have taught us all that we, as analysts, know about the developmental stages of the human mind.[2]

It happens that these two procedures, which have served us well for all other periods of life, prove less satisfactory and less productive of results when applied to adolescents.

RECONSTRUCTION OF ADOLESCENCE IN ADULT ANALYSIS

As regards reconstruction, I am impressed how seldom in the treatment of my adult cases I succeed in reviving their adolescent experiences in full force. By that I do not mean to imply that adult patients have an amnesia for their adolescence which resembles in extent or in depth the amnesia for their early childhood. On the contrary, the memories of the events of the adolescent period are, normally, retained in consciousness and told to the analyst without

[2] It may be worthwhile to remind the reader in this connection that our knowledge of the mental processes of infancy has been derived from reconstructions in the analyses of adults and was merely confirmed and enlarged on later by analyses or observations carried out in childhood.

apparent difficulty. Masturbation in preadolescence and adolescence, the first moves toward intercourse, etc., may even play a dominant part in the patients' conscious memories and, as we know well, are made use of to overlay and hide the repressed masturbation conflicts and the buried sexual activities of early childhood. Further, in the analyses of sexually inhibited men who deplore the loss of erective potency, it is fairly easy to recover the memories of the bodily practices carried out in adolescence—frequently very crude and cruel ones—which served at that time to prevent erections or to suppress them as soon as they occurred.

On the other hand, these memories contain no more than the bare facts, happenings, and actions, divorced from the affects which accompanied them at the time. What we fail to recover, as a rule, is the atmosphere in which the adolescent lives, his anxieties, the height of elation or depth of despair, the quickly rising enthusiasms, the utter hopelessness, the burning—or at other times sterile—intellectual and philosophical preoccupations, the yearning for freedom, the sense of loneliness, the feeling of oppression by the parents, the impotent rages or active hates directed against the adult world, the erotic crushes—whether homosexually or heterosexually directed—the suicidal fantasies, etc. These are elusive mood swings, difficult to revive, which, unlike the affective states of infancy and early childhood, seem disinclined to re-emerge and be relived in connection with the person of the analyst.

If this impression, which I gathered from my own cases, should be confirmed by other analysts of adults, such a failure—or partial failure—to reconstruct adolescence might account for some of the gaps in our appraisal of the mental processes during this period.

ANALYSIS DURING ADOLESCENCE

Discussing the contributions dealing with the analytic therapy of adolescents, Spiegel (1951) deplored what seemed to him an undue pessimism on the part of some authors. He pointed to the need of adapting the analytic technique to the adolescent patients' particular situation and expressed surprise at the absence of explicit discussions of an introductory phase "analogous to the one used with children and delinquents."

Actually, since 1951, some further papers on the subject of technique appeared in print. Two of them dealt with the opening phase (Fraiberg, 1955; Noshpitz, 1957), a third with the terminal one (Adatto, 1958). (See also Eissler, 1958; Geleerd, 1958.)

While these authors brought material to highlight the special technical difficulties encountered in the beginning and ending of therapy, work on adolescents done in our Hampstead Child-Therapy Clinic emphasized special technical difficulties met with in the very center of it, i.e., at the critical moment when preadolescence gives way to adolescence proper, when the revolt against the parents is anticipated in the transference and tends to lead to a break with the analyst, i.e., to abrupt and undesirable termination of treatment from the patient's side.

Thus, according to experience, special difficulties are encountered in the beginning, in the middle, and in connection with the end of treatment. Put in other words, this can only mean that the analytic treatment of adolescents is a hazardous venture from beginning to end, a venture in which the analyst has to meet resistances of unusual strength and variety. This is borne out by the comparison of adolescent with adult cases. In adult analysis, we are used to handle the difficult technical situations with certain hysterical patients who cannot bear frustration in the transference and try to force the analyst to enact with them their revived love and hate feelings in an actual personal relationship. We are used to guard against the obsessional patients' technique of isolating words from affect and of tempting us to interpret unconscious content while it is divorced from its emotional cathexis. We attempt to deal with the narcissistic withdrawal of the borderline schizophrenics, the projections of the paranoid patients who turn their analyst into the persecuting enemy, the destructive hopelessness of the depressed who claim disbelief in any positive outcome of the analytic effort; the acting-out tendencies and the lack of insight of the delinquent or psychopathic characters. But in the disturbances named above, we meet either the one or the other of these technical difficulties, and we can adapt the analytic technique to the resistance which is specific to the type of mental disorder. Not so in adolescence where the patient may change rapidly from one of these emotional positions to the next, exhibit them all simultaneously, or in quick succession, leaving the analyst little time and scope to marshal his forces and change his handling of the case according to the changing need.

OBSTACLES IN THE LIBIDO ECONOMY: COMPARISON WITH
THE STATES OF MOURNING AND UNHAPPY LOVE

Experience has taught us to take a serious view of such major and repeated inadequacies of the analytic technique. They cannot be explained away by individual characteristics of the patients under treatment or by any accidental or environmental factors which run counter to it. Nor can they be overcome simply by increased effort, skill, and tact on the part of the analyst. They have to be taken as indications that something in the inner structure of the disturbances themselves differs markedly from the pattern of those illnesses for which the analytic technique was originally devised and to which it is most frequently applied (Eissler, 1950). We have to gain insight into these divergences of pathology before we are in a position to revise our technique. Where the analyses of children, of delinquents, and of certain borderline states are concerned, this has already happened. What the analytic technique had to provide for in these cases were the immaturity and weakness of the patients' ego; their lower threshold for the toleration of frustration; and the lesser importance of verbalization with increased importance of action (acting out) for their mental economy. It remains to be pointed out what corresponding factors are characteristic of the adolescent disorders, i.e., to what specific inner situation of the patients our technique has to be adjusted to make adolescents more amenable to analytic treatment.

So far as I am concerned, I am impressed by a similarity between the responses of these young patients and those of two other well-known types of mental upset, namely, the reactions to treatment during unhappy love affairs and during periods of mourning. In both these states, there is much mental suffering and, as a rule, the urgent wish to be helped; in spite of this, neither state responds well to analytic therapy. Our theoretical explanation of this comparative intractability is the following: being in love as well as mourning are emotional states in which the individual's libido is fully engaged in relation to a real love object of the present, or of the most recent past, the mental pain being caused by the difficult task to withdraw cathexis and give up a position which holds out no further hope for return of love, that is, for satisfaction. While the individual is engaged in this struggle, insufficient libido is available to cathect the person of the analyst, or to flow back regressively and reinvest former objects and positions. Consequently, neither the transference events nor the past become meaningful enough to yield material for interpretation. The immediate object (of love, or of mourning) has to be given up before analytic therapy can become effective.

To my mind, the libidinal position of the adolescent has much in common with the two states described above. The adolescent too is engaged in an emotional struggle—moreover, in one of extreme urgency and immediacy. His libido is on the point of detaching itself from the parents and of cathecting new objects. Some mourning for the objects of the past is inevitable; so are the "crushes," i.e., the happy or unhappy love affairs with adults outside the family, or with other adolescents, whether of the opposite or of the same sex; so is, further, a certain amount of narcissistic withdrawal which bridges the gap during periods when no external object is cathected. Whatever the libidinal solution at a given moment may be, it will always be a preoccupation with the present time and, as described above, with little or no libido left available for investment either in the past or in the analyst.

If this supposition as to the libido distribution in the adolescent personality can be accepted as a correct statement, it can serve to explain some of our young patients' behavior in treatment, such as: their reluctance to cooperate; their lack of involvement in the therapy or in the relationship to the analyst; their battles for the reduction of weekly sessions; their unpunctuality; their missing of treatment sessions for the sake of outside activities; their sudden breaking off treatment altogether. We learn here by contrast how much the continuity of the average adult analysis owes to the mere fact of the analyst being a highly cathected object, quite apart from the essential role played by the transference in the production of material.

There are, of course, those cases where the analyst himself becomes the new love object of the adolescent, i.e., the object of the "crush," a constellation which will heighten the young patient's keenness to be "treated." But apart from improved attendance and punctuality, this may mean merely that the analyst is brought up against another of the specific difficulties of the analyses of adolescents, namely, the urgency of their needs, their intolerance for frustration, and their tendency to treat whatever relationship evolves as a vehicle for wish fulfillment and not as a source of insight and enlightenment.

Under these conditions it is not surprising that besides analytic therapy many alternative forms of treatment for adolescents have been evolved and practiced, such as manipulation of the environment, residential treatment, the setting up of therapeutic communities, etc. Valuable as these experimental approaches are from the practical point of view, they cannot, of course, be expected to contribute directly to our theoretical insight into the unconscious contents of the adolescent's mind, the structure of his typical disturbances, or into the details of the mental mechanisms by which these latter are maintained.

CLINICAL APPLICATIONS

What follows is an attempt to apply at least some of our hard-won insights to three of the most pressing problems concerning adolescence.

Is the Adolescent Upset Inevitable?

There is, first, the ever-recurrent question whether the adolescent upheaval is welcome and beneficial as such, whether it is necessary, and, more than that, inevitable. On this point, psychoanalytic opinion is decisive and unanimous. The persons in the child's family and school who assess his state on the basis of behavior may deplore the adolescent upset which, to them, spells the loss of valuable qualities, of character stability, and of social adaptation. As analysts, who assess personalities from the structural point of view, we think otherwise. We know that the character structure of a child at the end of the latency period represents the outcome of long-drawn-out conflicts between id and ego forces. The inner balance achieved, although characteristic of each individual and precious to him, is preliminary only and precarious. It does not allow for the quantitative increase in drive activity, or for the changes of drive quality which are both inseparable from puberty. Consequently, it has to be abandoned to allow adult sexuality to be integrated into the individual's personality. The so-called adolescent upheavals are no more than the external indications that such internal adjustments are in progress.

On the other hand, we all know individual children who as late as the ages of fourteen, fifteen, or sixteen show no such outer evidence of inner unrest. They remain, as they have been during the latency period, "good" children, wrapped up in their family relationships, considerate sons of their mothers, submissive to their fathers, in accord with the atmosphere, ideas, and ideals of their childhood background. Convenient as this may be, it signifies a delay of normal development and as such is a sign to be taken seriously. The first impression conveyed by these cases may be that of a quantitative deficiency of drive endowment, a suspicion which will usually prove unfounded. Analytic exploration reveals that this reluctance to "grow up" is derived not from the id but from the ego and superego aspects of the personality. These are children who have built up excessive defenses against their drive activities and are now crippled by the results, which act as barriers against the normal maturational processes of phase development. They are, perhaps more than any others, in need of therapeutic help to remove the inner restrictions and clear the path for normal development, however "upsetting" the latter may prove to be.

Is the Adolescent Upset Predictable?

A second question which we are frequently asked to answer concerns the problem whether the manner in which a given child will react in adolescence can be predicted from the characteristics of his early infantile or latency behavior. Apart from the more general affirmative answer given by Ernest Jones (1922), only one among the authors named above has made clear and positive assertions in this respect. Siegfried Bernfeld (1923), discussing the protracted type of male adolescence and its characteristics, established the links between this form of puberty and a specific type of infantile development based on the following three conditions: (a) that the frustration of infantile sexual wishes has been shattering for the child's narcissim; (b) that the incestuous fixations to the parents have been of exceptional strength and have been maintained throughout the latency period; (c) that the superego has been established early, has been delineated sharply from the ego, and that the ideals contained in it are invested with narcissistic as well as with object libido.

Other and less precise answers to the same question are scattered through the literature. We find the opinion that, in the majority of cases, the manifestations of the adolescent process are not predictable since they depend almost wholly on quantitative relations, i.e., on the strength and suddenness of drive increase, the corresponding increase in anxiety causing all the rest of the upheaval.

I suggested in 1936 that adolescence occasionally brings about something in the nature of a spontaneous cure. This happens in children whose pregenital activities and characteristics remained dominant throughout latency until the increase in genital libido produces a welcome decrease in pregenitality. This latter occurrence, on the other hand, can be matched by a corresponding one which produces the opposite effect: when phallic characteristics have remained dominant during latency, the increase in genital libido produces the effect of an exaggerated and threatening aggressive masculinity.

It seems to be generally accepted that a strong fixation to the mother, dating not only from the oedipal but from the preoedipal attachment to her, renders adolescence especially difficult. This latter assertion, on the other hand, has to be correlated with two recent findings of a different nature which we owe to work done in our Hampstead Child-Therapy Clinic. One of these findings is derived from the study of orphaned children who were deprived of the relationship to a stable mother figure in their first years. This lack of a mother fixation, far from making adolescence easier, constitutes a real danger to the whole inner coherence of the personality during that period. In these cases adolescence is frequently preceded by a frantic search for a mother image; the internal possession and cathexis of such an image seem to be essential for the ensuing normal process of detaching libido from it for transfer to new objects, i.e., to sexual partners.

The second finding mentioned above is derived from the analyses of adolescent twins, in one case children whose twin relationship in infancy had been observed and recorded in minute detail (Burlingham, 1951). In their treatments it transpired that the "adolescent revolt" against the love objects of infancy demands the breaking of the tie to the twin in no lesser degree than the breaking of the tie to the mother. Since this libidinal (narcissistic as well as object-directed) cathexis of the twin is rooted in the same deep layer of the personality as the early attachment to the mother, its withdrawal is accompanied by an equal amount of structural upheaval, emotional upset, and resulting symptom formation. Where, on the other hand, the twin relationship survives the adolescent phase, we may expect to see a delay in the onset of maturity or a restrictive hardening of the character of the latency period similar to the instances mentioned above in which the childhood love for the parents withstands the onslaught of the adolescent phase.

To return to the initial question: it seems that we are able to foretell the adolescent reactions in certain specific and typical constellations but certainly not for all the individual variations of infantile personality structure. Our insight into typical developments will increase with the number of adolescents who undergo analysis.

Pathology in Adolescence

This leaves us with a third problem which, to my mind, outweighs the preceding ones so far as clinical and theoretical significance is concerned. I refer to the difficulty in adolescent cases to draw the line between normality and pathology. As described above, adolescence constitutes by definition an interruption of peaceful growth which resembles in appearance a variety of other emotional upsets and structural upheavals.[3] The adolescent manifestations come close to symptom formation of the neurotic, psychotic, or dissocial order and merge almost imperceptibly into borderline states, initial, frustrated, or fullfledged forms of almost all the mental illnesses. Consequently, the differential diagnosis between the adolescent upsets and true pathology becomes a difficult task.

For the discussion of this diagnostic problem I leave most other authors in the field to speak for themselves and summarize my own impressions based on past and present clinical experience.

[3] Adolescence is, of course, not the only time in life when alterations of a physiological nature cause disturbances of mental equilibrium. The same happens in later years in the climacterium; and recently Grete L. Bibring (1959) has given a convincing description of similar damage to the equilibrium of mental forces during pregnancy.

In 1936, when I approached the same subject from the aspect of the defenses, I was concerned with the similarity between the adolescent and other emotional disturbances rather than with the differences between them. I described that adolescent upsets take on the appearance of a neurosis if the initial, pathogenic danger situation is located in the superego with the resulting anxiety being felt as guilt: that they resemble psychotic disturbances if the danger lies in the increased power of the id itself, which threatens the ego in its existence or integrity. Whether such an adolescent individual impresses us, then, as obsessional, phobic, hysterical, ascetic, schizoid, paranoid, suicidal, etc., will depend on the one hand on the quality and quantity of id contents which beset the ego, on the other hand on the selection of defense mechanisms which the latter employs. Since, in adolescence, impulses from all pregenital phases rise to the surface and defense mechanisms from all levels of crudity or complexity come into use, the pathological results—although identical in structure—are more varied and less stabilized than at other times of life.

Today it seems to me that this structural description needs to be amplified, not in the direction of the similarity of the adolescent to other disorders but in that of their specific nature. There is in their etiology at least one additional element which may be regarded as exclusive to this period and characteristic of it: namely, that the danger is felt to be located not only in the id impulses and fantasies but in the very existence of the love objects of the individual's oedipal and preoedipal past. The libidinal cathexis of them has been carried forward from the infantile phases and was merely toned down or inhibited in aim during latency. Therefore, the reawakened pregenital urges, or—worse still

—the newly acquired genital ones, are in danger of making contact with them, lending a new and threatening reality to fantasies which seemed extinct but are, in fact, merely under repression.[4] The anxieties which arise on these grounds are directed toward eliminating the infantile objects, i.e., toward breaking the tie with them. Anny Katan (1937) has discussed this type of defense, which aims above all at changing the persons and the scene of conflict, under the term of "removal." Such an attempt may succeed or fail, partially or totally. In any case, I agree with Anny Katan that its outcome will be decisive for the success or failure of the other, more familiar line of defensive measures which are directed against the impulses themselves.

A number of illustrations will serve to clarify the meaning of this assumption.

DEFENSE AGAINST THE INFANTILE OBJECT TIES

   Defense by Displacement of Libido: There are many adolescents who deal with the anxiety aroused by the attachment to their infantile objects by the simple means of flight. Instead of permitting a process of gradual detachment from the parents to take place, they withdraw their libido from them suddenly and altogether. This leaves them with a passionate longing for partnership which they succeed in transferring to the environment outside the family. Here they adopt varying solutions. Libido may be trans-

---

[4] An important clinical instance of this can be found in adolescent girls with anorexia nervosa. Here the infantile fantasies of oral impregnation receive added impetus from the new real possibilities of motherhood opened up by genital development. Consequently, the phobic measures adopted against the intake of food on the one hand and identification with the mother on the other hand are overemphasized to a degree which may lead to starvation.

ferred, more or less unchanged in form, to parent substitutes, provided that these new figures are diametrically opposed in every aspect (personal, social, cultural), to the original ones. Or the attachment may be made to so-called "leaders," usually persons in age between the adolescent's and the parents' generation, who represent ideals. Equally frequent are the passionate new ties to contemporaries, either of the same or of the opposite sex (i.e., homosexual or heterosexual friendships) and the attachments to adolescent groups (or "gangs"). Whichever of these typical solutions is chosen, the result makes the adolescent feel "free" and revel in a new precious sense of independence from the parents who are then treated with indifference bordering on callousness.

Although the direction taken by the libido in these instances is, in itself, on lines of normality, the suddenness of the change, the carefully observed contrast in object selection, and the overemphasis on the new allegiances mark it as defensive. This course represents an all-too-hasty anticipation of normal growth rather than a normal developmental process.

It makes little further difference to the emotional situation whether the libidinal flight is followed by actual flight, i.e., whether the adolescent also "removes" himself bodily from his family. If not, he remains in the home in the attitude of a boarder, usually a very inconsiderate one so far as the older and younger family members are concerned.

On the other hand, the withdrawal of cathexis from the parents has most decisive consequences for the rest of the defensive processes. Once the infantile objects are stripped of their importance, the pregenital and genital impulses cease to be threatening to the same degree. Consequently, guilt and anxiety decrease and the ego becomes more tolerant. Formerly repressed sexual and aggressive wishes rise to the surface and are acted on, the actions being taken outside the family in the wider environment. Whether this acting out will be on harmless, or idealistic, or dissocial, or even criminal lines will depend essentially on the new objects to whom the adolescent has attached himself. Usually, the ideals of the leader of the adolescent group or gang are taken over wholeheartedly and without criticism.

Adolescents of this type may be sent for treatment after their actions have brought them into conflict with their schools, their employers, or the law. As far as psychoanalytic therapy is concerned, they seem to offer little chance for the therapeutic alliance between analyst and patient without which the analytic technique cannot proceed. Any relationship to the analyst and, above all, the transference to him would revive the infantile attachments which have been discarded; therefore, the adolescent remains unresponsive. Moreover, the escape from these attachments has suspended the feeling of internal conflict, at least temporarily; consequently, the adolescent does not feel in need of psychological help. Aichhorn had these points in mind when he maintained that adolescents of the dissocial and criminal type needed a long period of preparation and inner rearrangement before they could become amenable to analytic treatment. He maintained that the latter would be successful only if, during this preparation in a residential setting, the adolescent made a new transference of object love, reawakened his infantile attachments, internalized his conflicts once more—in short, became neurotic.

To try and analyze an adolescent in this phase of successful detachment from the past seems to be a venture doomed to failure.

Defense by Reversal of Affect: A second typical reaction to the same danger situation is, although less conspicuous outwardly, more ominous in nature inwardly. Instead of displacing libido from the parents—or, more likely, after failing to do so—the adolescent ego may defend itself by turning the emotions felt toward them into their opposites. This changes love into hate, dependence into revolt, respect and admiration into contempt and derision. On the basis of such reversal of affect the adolescent imagines himself to be "free," but, unluckily for his peace of mind and sense of conflict, this conviction does not reach further than the conscious surface layer of his mind. For all deeper intents and purposes he remains as securely tied to the parental figures as he has been before; acting out remains within the family; and any alterations achieved by the defense turn out to his disadvantage. There are no positive pleasures to be derived from the reversed relationships, only suffering, felt as well as inflicted. There is no room for independence of action, or of growth; compulsive opposition to the parents proves as crippling in this respect as compulsive obedience to them can prove to be.[5] Since anxiety and guilt remain undiminished, constant reinforcement of defense is necessary. This is provided in the first place by two methods: denial (of positive feeling) and reaction formations (churlish, unsympathetic, contemptuous attitudes). The behavioral picture that emerges at this stage is that of an uncooperative and hostile adolescent.

[5] Ferenczi pointed to this effect of "compulsive disobedience" many years ago.

Further pathological developments of this state of affairs are worth watching. The hostility and aggressiveness, which in the beginning serve as a defense against object love, soon become intolerable to the ego, are felt as threats, and are warded off in their own right. This may happen by means of projection; in that case the aggression is ascribed to the parents, who as a consequence become the adolescent's main oppressors and persecutors. In the clinical picture, this appears first as the adolescent's suspiciousness and, when the projections increase, as paranoid behavior.

Conversely, the full hostility and aggression may be turned away from the objects and employed inwardly against the self. In these cases, the adolescents display intense depression, tendencies toward self-abasement and self-injury, and develop, or even carry out, suicidal wishes.

During all stages of this process, personal suffering is great and the desire to be helped intense. This in itself is no guarantee that the adolescent in question will submit to analytic therapy. He will certainly not do so if treatment is urged and initiated by the parents. Whenever this happens, he will consider analysis as their tool, extend his hostility or his suspicions to include the person of the analyst, and refuse cooperation. The chances are better if the adolescent himself decides to seek help and turns to analysis, as it were, in opposition to the parents' wishes. Even so, the alliance with the analyst may not be of long duration. As soon as a true transference develops and the positive infantile fantasies come into consciousness, the same reversal of affect tends to be repeated in the analytic setting. Rather than relive the whole turmoil of feelings with the analyst, many adolescent patients run away. They escape from their positive feelings, although it appears to the analyst that they break off treatment in an overwhelmingly strong negative transference.

Defense by Withdrawal of Libido to the Self: To proceed in the direction of increasing pathology: Withdrawal of libido from the parents, as it has been described above, does not itself determine its further use or fate. If anxieties and inhibitions block the way toward new objects outside the family, the libido remains within the self and may be employed to cathect the ego and superego, thereby inflating them. Clinically this means that ideas of grandeur will appear, fantasies of unlimited power over other human beings or of major achievement and championship in one or more fields. Or the suffering and persecuted ego of the adolescent may assume Christlike proportions with corresponding fantasies of saving the world.

On the other hand, the cathexis may become attached only to the adolescent's body and give rise to the hypochondriacal sensations and feelings of body changes that are well known clinically from the initial stages of psychotic illness.

In either case, analytic therapy is indicated as well as urgent. Treatment will dispel the appearance of severe abnormality if it reopens a path for the libido, either to flow backward and recathect the original infantile objects, or to flow forward, in the direction described above, to cathect less frightening substitutes in the environment.

What taxes the analyst's technical skill in these cases is the withdrawn state of the patient, i.e., the problem of establishing an initial relationship and transference. Once this is accomplished, the return from narcissistic withdrawal

to object cathexis will relieve the patient, at least temporarily.

I believe that there are many cases where the analyst
would be wise to be content with this partial success without urging further treatment. A further and deeper involvement in the transference may well arouse all the anxieties
described above and again lead to abrupt termination of
the analysis due to the adolescent's flight reaction.

Defense by Regression: The greater the anxiety aroused by the object ties, the more elementary and
primitive is the defense activity employed by the adolescent ego to escape them. Thus, at the extreme height of
anxiety, the relations with the object world may be reduced
to the emotional state known as "primary identification"
with the objects. This solution, with which we are familiar
from psychotic illnesses, implies regressive changes in all
parts of the personality, i.e., in the ego as well as in the
libido organization. The ego boundaries[6] are widened to
embrace parts of the object together with the self. This
creates in the adolescent surprising changes of qualities,
attitudes, and even outward appearance. His allegiance to
persons outside himself betrays itself in these alterations of
his own personality (i.e., his identifications) rather than in
an outflow of libido. Projections, together with these identifications, dominate the scene and create a give-and-take
between the self and the object which has repercussions on
important ego functions. For example, the distinction between the external and internal world (i.e., reality testing)
becomes temporarily negligible, a lapse in ego functioning

[6] See Federn (1952) and, following him, Freeman et al. (1958).

which manifests itself in the clinical picture as a state of confusion.

Regression of this kind may bring transitory relief to the ego by emptying the oedipal (and many of the preoedipal) fantasies of their libidinal cathexis,[7] but this lessening of anxiety will not be long-lived. Another and deeper anxiety will soon take its place, which I have characterized on an earlier occasion (Volume IV, ch. 10) as the fear of emotional surrender, with the accompanying fear of loss of identity.

DEFENSE AGAINST IMPULSES

Where the defenses against the oedipal and preoedipal object ties fail to achieve their aim, clinical pictures emerge which come nearest to the borderline of psychotic illness.

The "Ascetic" Adolescent: One of these, the "ascetic" adolescent, I have previously described as fighting all his impulses, preoedipal and oedipal, sexual and aggressive, extending the defense even to the fulfillment of the physiological needs for food, sleep, and body comfort. This, to me, seems the characteristic reaction of an ego driven by the blind fear of overwhelming id quantities, an anxiety which leaves no room for the finer distinctions between vital or merely pleasant satisfactions, the healthy or the morbid, the morally permitted or forbidden pleasures. Total war is waged against the pursuit of pleasure as such. Accordingly, most of the normal processes of instinct and need satisfaction are interfered with and become paralyzed. According to clinical observation, adolescent asceticism is,

[7] See in this connection M. Katan (1950).

with luck, a transitory phenomenon. For the analytic observer it provides precious proof of the power of defense, i.e., of the extent to which the normal, healthy drive derivatives are open to crippling interference by the ego.

On the whole, analytic treatment of the ascetic type does not present as many technical difficulties as one would expect. Perhaps, in these individuals, defense against the impulses is so massive that they can permit themselves some object relationship to the analyst and thus enter into transference.

The "Uncompromising" Adolescent: Another, equally abnormal adolescent is described best as the "uncompromising" type. The term, in this instance, does refer to more than the well-known conscious, unrelenting position adopted by many young people who stand up for their ideas, refuse to make concessions to the more practical and reality-adapted attitudes of their elders, and take pride in their moral or aesthetic principles. "Compromise," with these adolescents, includes processes which are as essential for life as, for example, the cooperation between impulses, the blending of opposite strivings, the mitigation of id strivings by interference from the side of the ego. One adolescent whom I observed in analysis did his utmost, in pursuit of this impossible aim, to prevent any interference of his mind with his body, of his activity with his passivity, his loves with his hates, his realities with his fantasies, the external demands with his internal ones, in short, of his ego with his id.

In treatment, this defense was represented as a strong resistance against any "cure," the idea of which he despised in spite of intense suffering. He understood correctly that mental health is based in the last resort on harmony, i.e., on the very compromise formations which he was trying to avoid.

THE CONCEPT OF NORMALITY IN ADOLESCENCE

Where adolescence is concerned, it seems easier to describe its pathological manifestations than the normal processes. Nevertheless, there are in the above exposition at least two pronouncements which may prove useful for the concept: (1) that adolescence is by its nature an interruption of peaceful growth; and (2) that the upholding of a steady equilibrium during the adolescent process is in itself abnormal. Once we accept for adolescence disharmony within the psychic structure as our basic fact, understanding becomes easier. We begin to see the upsetting battles which are raging between id and ego as beneficient attempts to restore peace and harmony. The defensive methods which are employed either against the impulses or against the object cathexis begin to appear legitimate and normal. If they produce pathological results, this happens not because of any malignancy in their nature, but because they are overused, overstressed, or used in isolation. Actually, each of the abnormal types of adolescent development, as it is described above, also represents a potentially useful way of regaining mental stability, normal if combined with other defenses, and if used in moderation.

To explain this statement in greater detail: I take it that it is normal for an adolescent to behave for a considerable length of time in an inconsistent and unpredictable manner; to fight his impulses and to accept them; to ward them off successfully and to be overrun by them; to love his parents and to hate them; to revolt against them and to be dependent on them; to be deeply ashamed to acknowledge his mother before others and, unexpectedly, to desire heart-to-heart talks with her; to thrive on imitation of and identification with others while searching unceasingly for his own identity; to be more idealistic, artistic, generous, and unselfish than he will ever be again, but also the opposite: self-centered, egoistic, calculating. Such fluctuations between extreme opposites would be deemed highly abnormal at any other time of life. At this time they may signify no more than that an adult structure of personality takes a long time to emerge, that the ego of the individual in question does not cease to experiment and is in no hurry to close down on possibilities. If the temporary solutions seem abnormal to the onlooker, they are less so, nevertheless, than the hasty decisions made in other cases for one-sided suppression, or revolt, or flight, or withdrawal, or regression, or asceticism, which are responsible for the truly pathological developments described above.

While an adolescent remains inconsistent and unpredictable in his behavior, he may suffer, but he does not seem to me to be in need of treatment. I think that he should be given time and scope to work out his own solution. Rather, it may be his parents who need help and guidance so as to be able to bear with him. There are few situations in life which are more difficult to cope with than an adolescent son or daughter during the attempt to liberate themselves.

SUMMARY

In the foregoing paper I have reviewed and summarized some of the basic literature on adolescence[8] as well as my own views on the subject. My former description of the defensive processes in adolescence has been amplified to include specific defense activities directed against the oedipal and preoedipal object ties.

[8] [Since this paper was written, several psychoanalytic studies of adolescence have been published. See Eissler (1958), Geleerd (1958), Hellman (1958), Erikson (1959), Solnit (1959), Lampl-de Groot (1960), Jacobson (1961, 1964), Blos (1962), Lorand and Schneer (1962), Sprince (1962), Frankl (1963), Rosenblatt (1963), Laufer (1964, 1965, 1966, 1968), Rexford (1966), H. Deutsch (1967), Kestenberg (1967-1968).]

10

Discussion of John Bowlby's Work on Separation, Grief, and Mourning

(1958, 1960)

PART I. "SEPARATION ANXIETY" (1958)

I should not have asked for speaking time tonight if John Bowlby in his paper had not referred repeatedly to the

The remarks contained in Part I are here published for the first time. They were presented before the British Psycho-Analytical Society, on November 5, 1958, when John Bowlby read his paper on "Separation Anxiety." Subsequently, Bowlby published a revised and longer version of this paper (1960a). The page references mentioned are to Bowlby's manuscript and not to the published version.

Part II is a discussion of Bowlby's paper on "Grief and Mourning in Infancy and Early Childhood" (1960b). It was first published in *The Psychoanalytic Study of the Child*, 15:53-62, 1960. The other discussants were Spitz (1960) and Schur (1960). For the response to these discussions, see Bowlby (1961b).

work on separation carried out in the Hampstead Nurseries during the war, work for which Dorothy Burlingham and I were responsible. On the one hand, Bowlby gave credit to our findings; on the other hand, he discounted or discredited our interpretations of the facts. I feel that these two attitudes, taken together, create a misleading impression of our work which I am anxious to correct.

Description of Material

Before entering into argument I want to meet a request (made by Dr. Bion at the last meeting) for more detailed characterization of the material on which the separation theories are based. So far as the Hampstead Nurseries were concerned, the material was gained from the close acquaintance with approximately eighty separated infants and young children (aged from ten days to five years) over a period of four years on a twenty-four-hour basis. Attention was paid to the communications of the children, whether preverbal or verbal, the expressions of their affects and moods, the manifestations of their libidinal and aggressive impulses and fantasies in behavior and in play, the progressive and regressive moves in their development, and, of course, to the whole range of their physical manifestations including the disturbances of health. This material was evaluated on the basis of analytic knowledge, namely, by comparison with the mental states seen or reconstructed in analysis.

THE QUESTION OF UNPREPAREDNESS FOR THE EVENTS

I turn from this digression to my first objection to Bowlby's statements. On page 13 of his paper he suggests that I and my co-workers found ourselves unprepared for the responses shown by the children after separation. I take this to imply that nothing in our theoretical equipment had led us to expect that infants might react badly when taken from their mothers. I have no hesitation in maintaining that the opposite was the case. We would never have opened the Hampstead Nurseries, a policy which ran counter to the government program of that period, nor would we have proclaimed free visiting years before this became an issue in hospitals, if it had not been for our conviction that evacuation without the mother and institutional care away from the mother were threats to the infant's mental health and would lead to serious repercussions. If anything came unexpected, it was perhaps the regularity and severity of the reactions which occurred. But even here our astonishment was rather of the type well known to every analyst who is "surprised" whenever a patient reacts "according to the book." (Whether in our case the "book" in question was really *Inhibitions, Symptoms and Anxiety* is an open question. Personally, I am inclined to think that the child's tie to the mother has always been an integral part of psychoanalysis and that we were familiar with it as such.)

AGREEMENT ABOUT OBSERVED FACTS

However that may be, there is no doubt that the clinical pictures we described tally with those given later by Bowlby and his co-workers. We saw the same sequence: a first stage of the child's loud protest, painful longing, and hope; a second stage of increasing anger and despair; and a third stage, which we called withdrawal and which we described as characterized by severe regressions, i.e., loss or disturbance of bodily and mental functions.

Bowlby raised the question why we failed to use the term

separation anxiety to denote the whole sequence. My answer is as follows: in the picture of separation distress which we described, anxiety as such played the least manifest part. According to our experience, anxiety came into play later, when the lost mother had returned or when a mother substitute had been accepted, i.e., anxiety came with the fear that the object loss might be repeated.

DISAGREEMENT ABOUT INTERPRETATION

Our agreement with Bowlby as to the facts is matched by a disagreement with regard to their significance. Bowlby dismissed our explanations as being based on a "secondary drive" theory. I am not quite certain about his usage of this term. If by any chance he meant to imply that we interpreted the distress shown by the children as derived from the actual or anticipated lack of fulfillment of body needs, I have to protest. This would constitute not only a misunderstanding of our theoretical position but, equally, a misunderstanding of the analytic concept of anaclitic object choice. The latter term does not imply that the child loves a person only while she feeds him, but that the direction in which libidinal cathexis is sent out to the environment is initially determined by the first experiences of satisfaction.

There is no time for it tonight, but on another occasion it might be worthwhile to compare the ethological theory advanced by Bowlby with the concept of anaclitic object choice. The former, which assumes a primary tie to the mother, elicited by acts of mothering, is a biological theory. The latter, the concept of anaclitic object choice, is a psychological assertion. As such it deals with the impact on the mind made by the acts of mothering, namely, with the pleasure-pain experiences which accompany primary instinctual reactions and form their mental content.

To describe our theoretical position in the Hampstead Nurseries correctly, Bowlby would have had to state that we interpreted the details of the separation distress on the basis of the libido theory, namely, as an unfortunate happening within the child's first experience of object love. Once an object is found and cathected by the infant, its disappearance is intensely painful. As described, for example, in *Inhibitions, Symptoms and Anxiety*, positive cathexis builds up and gives rise to states of intolerable longing. When the absence of the satisfying mother becomes prolonged, the positive inner image of her gradually changes to the negative, the aggressive elements of the normal ambivalence gaining the upper hand. Next, according to our assumption, object cathexis is withdrawn—not, as Bowlby assumes, denied. The infant becomes isolated and inaccessible within the environment. When the mother returns or a substitute takes her place, a new effort has to be made to recathect the object world. This happens again, now regressively, in the anaclitic manner, or, to use another term, in response to mothering.

It goes without saying that this simple scheme, which may fit the infant between the ages of six to sixteen months, becomes increasingly complicated as the object relationship as such becomes complicated by factors such as death wishes, ideas of punishment, guilt, the oedipal problems. In the analysis of older children, the further development of separation distress is studied best in the complex symptom commonly called homesickness.

While the comparative absence of the "primary instinctual responses" to separation in the first few months of life is difficult to explain on the basis of the ethological theory, it seems to fall into place more readily with the analytic assumptions. Object cathexis of the mother has to be rather firmly established and must be at least partially independent of need fulfillment before the full separation distress develops. Before this time (at least according to our observation) the infant reacts to separation from the mother less with affects and more by means of disturbance of bodily functions such as sleep, food intake, digestion.

FORM OF SEPARATION VERSUS FACT OF SEPARATION

To make one further point: on page 13 of his paper Bowlby quoted a remark of ours that the child reacts less to the fact of separation than to the form in which separation has taken place. He concluded from this that we consider the tie to the mother as a negligible factor. Again, I wish to protest and to maintain that this passage has to be understood within the framework of the theory from which it stems. That the loss of a highly cathected object is all the more traumatic and pathogenic the less we are prepared for it is a familiar concept for the analyst. With infants, a further factor has to be taken into account. While the first two stages of the separation distress (longing and despair) are the most overtly painful ones for the child, it is, to our knowledge, the third stage, that of withdrawal of cathexis, which is most productive of pathology. Our suggestion was that this stage might be avoided by careful preparation. If the separation of an infant from his mother has to occur at all, care should be taken to ensure a gradual transfer of cathexis from the original object to the substituting one. Whoever has handled young children knows that this can be effected.

Altogether, I cannot resist the temptation to remind people that the analytic theories of libido, aggression, and their blending in the object relationship carry us much further in the understanding of infantile manifestations than Bowlby believes or would lead his audience to expect.

PART II. "GRIEF AND MOURNING IN INFANCY AND EARLY CHILDHOOD" (1960)

Bowlby's paper on "Grief and Mourning in Infancy" offers to analysts a number of controversial points for discussion, amplification, or refutation. The following comments apply partly to the wider issues raised by his article, partly to those specific points in it where he makes direct reference to Dorothy Burlingham's and my account (1943) of the observations collected in the Hampstead War Nurseries.

Identity of Observations

There is little difference in the observed material collected during the war by the Hampstead Nursery team with regard to separated children and the observations made later by a Tavistock Clinic team with regard to hospitalized children. Actually, James Robertson, on whose observational studies Bowlby relies predominantly, was, and is, a valued and important member of both teams. With this identity of material, and partly of observers, in mind, an explanation is needed not only why the theoretical interpretations of the data on our two sides are divergent but also why misunderstandings in the discussion of the divergencies are persistent.

Difference in Theoretical Orientation

Referring back to Bowlby's earlier papers on "Separation Anxiety" (1960a) and "The Nature of the Child's Tie to His Mother" (1958), it becomes possible to point to a basic difference in orientation between his and our theoretical approach. Bowlby is concerned on the one hand with a biological theory which assumes the existence of an inborn urge tying an infant to the mother, on the other hand with the behavior resulting from this tie ("attachment behavior") or from the untimely disruption of the tie (separation anxiety, grief, mourning). For him, the gap between biological urge and manifest affect and behavior is bridged by certain actions and events occurring in the external world which activate inherited responses.

If this description of Bowlby's position can be accepted as correct, it may serve to explain some of our dissatisfaction in following his line of argumentation. Not that, as analysts, we do not share Bowlby's regard for biological and behavioral considerations; but taken by themselves, not in conjunction with metapsychological thinking, these two types of data do not fulfill the analyst's requirements. As analysts we deal not with drive activity as such but with the mental representations of the drives. In the case of the biological tie of infant to mother, this representation has to be recognized, I believe, in the infant's inborn readiness to cathect objects with libido. Equally, we deal not with the happenings in the external world as such but with their repercussions in the mind, i.e., with the form in which they are registered by the child. In the case of the activating events, it seems to me that they are experienced as events in the pleasure-pain series. It is true that this translation into psychological terms interferes with the simplicity and straightforwardness of Bowlby's scheme and introduces numberless complications. But these complications seem to me no more than a true reflection of the complexity of mental life, built, as we know it to be, on the drive derivatives and the dynamic interplay between them; on the sensations and perceptions arriving from the internal and external world; on the pleasure-pain experiences; on mental imagery and fantasies. Since Bowlby in his present paper extends his material on separated children far beyond the first year of life, we have to add as complicating factors to the enumerated primary manifestations all the later elaborations which are known as secondary mental processes, such as verbal and logical thinking, and the structural conflicts with their specific anxieties, guilt reactions, and defensive activities.

Theoretical Misconceptions

There are two points in Bowlby's paper which I find more suited than any others to highlight the misconceptions which arise due to the described difference in viewpoints.

MOTHER ATTACHMENT VERSUS PLEASURE PRINCIPLE

Discussing the problem of need satisfaction in the first year of life, Bowlby queries the role which we ascribe to this factor. He sets up a controversy between the tie to the mother and the action of the pleasure principle in terms of "primary and secondary drive" and criticizes us for reversing their order of importance, i.e., for regarding the tie to the mother as a secondary, the search for pleasure as a primary, instinctual urge. To my mind, this objection of his is based on a theoretical misunderstanding. We agree with Bowlby that the infant's attachment to the mother is the result of primary biological urges and ensures survival. But although the search for gratification is a tendency inherent in all drive activity, in our view the pleasure principle as such is not a drive representation at all, neither a primary nor a secondary one. In its metapsychological sense it is conceived as a principle which governs all mental activity in the immature and insufficiently structured personality. Since it embraces all mental processes, the tie to the mother is governed by it as well. But to assume a struggle for priority or first place between mother attachment and pleasure principle as if they were mental phenomena of the same order does not seem to me to apply.

Once this particular misunderstanding is removed, Bowlby's and our treatment of this subject are nearer to each other than appears at first glance. As suggested above, his conception of a biological tie resulting in certain patterns of behavior when activated by nursing care is paralleled in our way of thinking by the conception of an inborn readiness to cathect with libido a person who provides pleasurable experiences. It becomes evident that this latter theory is no more or less than the classical psychoanalytic assumption of a first "anaclitic" relationship to the mother, i.e., a phase in which the pleasurable sensations derived from the gratification of major needs are instrumental in determining which person in the external world is selected for libidinal cathexis.

Moreover, in both theories, in Bowlby's as well as in the classical one, the mother is not chosen for attachment by virtue of her having given birth to the infant but by virtue of her ministering to the infant's needs.

INFANTILE NARCISSISM

A second area where controvery seems to be based on mis-conceptions is the problem of infantile narcissism. Bowlby denies that narcissism can exist or does exist in infancy, i.e., at the period when he sees the child as wholly attached to the mother. Argumentation concerning this point is made difficult by the fact that Bowlby's use of the term differs from ours in important respects. He understands narcissism in the descriptive sense, as a state in which the infant is supposed to be withdrawn, self-sufficient, and independent of the object world, and he maintains that no normal infant displays behavior of this kind. While agreeing with this last assertion, we disagree on our side with his definition of the term. Metapsychologically speaking, the concept of infantile narcissism refers not to behavior but to an early phase of libido distribution and organization. There exists in this phase, according to this assumption, a state of libidinal equilibrium, similar to the equilibrium obtaining during intrauterine existence. The infant himself is unable to maintain this state and is dependent for its upkeep on the presence and nursing care of the mother who becomes the first object in the external world. It is characteristic of this phase that there is no libidinal exchange with the object as there will be in the later stages of true object love (loving and being loved). Instead, one-sided use is made of the mother for purposes of satisfaction. The object is drawn wholly into the internal narcissistic milieu—to use an expression introduced by W. Hoffer (1952)—and treated as part of it to the extent that self and object merge into one.

There is no other point where the clash between metapsychological and descriptive thinking becomes as obvious as it is here. It leads to the apparently paradoxical result that what in terms of the libido theory is the apex of infantile narcissism appears in Bowlby's descriptive terms as the height of "attachment behavior." But we agree with him, of course, that never again in his life will the child be found to be more clinging to the mother or more dependent on her presence.

Disagreement on Clinical Points

With the above-named major differences in theoretical outlook in mind, it becomes easier to discuss minor disagreements in clinical observations, their description, and their interpretation.

THE THREE PHASES OF BEHAVIOR AFTER
SEPARATION FROM THE MOTHER

In his exposition of the child's reaction after separation, Bowlby isolates three main phases which can be easily distinguished from each other by observation: a first phase of loud, angry, tearful behavior, which he calls *protest*; a second one of acute pain, misery, and diminishing hope, which he calls *despair*; and a third one in which the child behaves as if he had ceased to care, which he calls *denial*.[1] As regards the description of this sequence, there is no disagreement between observers such as the Tavistock or Hampstead teams or René Spitz. As regards the interpretation of the observed data, argumentation centers around the third and last phase. The question arises in which sense

[1] The discussion was prepared before Bowlby, in the final version of the published paper, adopted the term "detachment" in favor of "denial."

Bowlby uses the term "denial." If it is purely descriptive, it might imply no more than absence of manifest bereavement behavior; if used in the analytic dynamic sense, it would imply a defensive process directed either against the recognition of external reality (i.e., the absence of the mother), or against the affect of itself (i.e., an intolerably painful sense of bereavement). In neither case does it include the purely libidinal aspect which seems of the greatest importance to us. If we see the trauma of separation from the mother in terms of what happens to the libidinal cathexis of her image, we take the phases of protest and despair as manifestations of the child's attempt to maintain the libidinal tie with the absent object, the third phase as a sign that cathexis is not denied but actually withdrawn from the object.

I suggest, therefore, the use of the term *withdrawal* for Bowlby's third phase of bereavement behavior. It has the advantage of covering the manifest withdrawn behavior of the child as well as the internal process of libido withdrawal by which we believe this behavior to be caused.

DURATION OF BEREAVEMENT REACTIONS

In this paper Bowlby emphasizes the identity of the young child's grief and mourning with the reactions shown by the normal adult after object loss. While taking a similar view so far as the overt manifestations are concerned, we have been reluctant to assume a corresponding identity of the underlying processes in infants and adults. The process of mourning (*Trauerarbeit*) taken in its analytic sense means to us the individual's effort to accept a fact in the external world (the loss of the cathected object) and to effect corresponding changes in the inner world (withdrawal of libido from the lost object, identification with the lost object). At least the former half of this task presupposes certain capacities of the mental apparatus such as reality testing, the acceptance of the reality principle, partial control of id tendencies by the ego, etc., i.e., capacities which are still undeveloped in the infant according to all other evidence. We have hesitated, therefore, to apply the term "mourning" in its technical sense to the bereavement reactions of the infant. Before the mental apparatus has matured and before, on the libidinal side, the stage of object constancy has been reached, the child's reactions to loss seem to us to be governed by the more primitive and direct dictates of the pleasure-pain principle.

Considerations such as these were significant for our attempts to understand the most outstanding difference between the bereavement reactions of young children and adults. While the term of mourning traditionally assumed for normal adults is one year, such loyalty to the lost object would be considered abnormal in a young child. We stated, on the basis of what we saw in the Hampstead War Nurseries, that we expected bereavement behavior to last any length of time "from a few hours to several weeks or even a few months." On the basis of more systematic observations undertaken by James Robertson and Christoph Heinicke,[2] Bowlby queries the possibility of the "few hours" or similarly short periods and endorses the validity of the longer periods. But he agrees with us, seemingly, that the child's grief reactions do not normally approximate the duration usual for the adult.

In our minds, we linked the time needed to adjust to a

[2] See Heinicke and Westheimer (1965).

substitute object less with the chronological age of the child, and more with the level of object relationship and ego maturity reached by him before separation: the nearer to object constancy, the longer the duration of grief reactions with corresponding approximation to the adult internal processes of mourning.[3]

There is a further point which seems to me worth noting. Neither the Hampstead War Nurseries nor hospitals and other residential homes have offered ideal conditions for studying the length of time needed by young children to displace attachment from one person to another. We, as well as Bowlby, used data collected in circumstances where the children had to adapt not only to the loss of the mother but also to the change from family to group life, a transition very difficult to achieve for any young child. Whereas the mother herself had been the undisputed possession of the child in many cases, the nurse as substitute mother inevitably had to be shared with a number of contemporaries; also, inevitably, it is never one single nurse who substitutes for the all-day and all-night care of the mother.

If we wish to determine how long an infant needs to transfer cathexis from one mother figure to a substitute mother in the full sense of the word, we need to supplement our observations, excluding group or ward conditions. For all we know, the duration of grief might then be found to be either shorter or longer. Moreover, in the circum-

---

[3] Homesickness of older children is not included in this category. We reserve this term for a neurotic symptom to be found in latency children who cannot bear separation from their oedipal objects owing to a highly ambivalent attitude toward them. In these children, the repressed negative side of the ambivalent relationship is responsible for guilt reactions, fear of death of the parents, intolerable longing, etc.

stances which we studied, the infants were separated not only from their mothers but from their home background, which included separation from the father, siblings, all the inanimate familiar objects, sights, sounds, etc. From direct observation we know little or nothing about the duration of grief in those instances where the mother has to leave temporarily or permanently while the child remains at home.[4]

PATHOLOGICAL AFTEREFFECTS OF SEPARATION

As regards the pathology following early separations, Bowlby remarks quite rightly that we made no attempts to link these with the later states of depressive or melancholic illness. Actually, at the time of writing our study (1942, 1943), we had no access to material of this kind.[5] Since then, observational and analytic contact with a group of young concentration camp victims has provided additional data of some relevance. These children, who had undergone repeated traumatic separations from birth or infancy onward, achieved comparatively stable relationships during their latency period; but from preadolescence onward they

---

[4] [Since this paper was written, a number of studies that have a direct bearing on this issue have been published. See, e.g., Neubauer (1960), Bonnard (1961), Lewin (1961), Mahler (1961), Rochlin (1961, 1965), Shambaugh (1961), Scharl (1961), R. Furman (1964a, 1964b), Barnes (1964), McDonald (1964), Jacobson (1965), Sandler and Joffe (1965a), Gauthier (1965), Winnicott (1965), Zetzel (1965), Wolfenstein (1966), Nagera (1969), and the study on object loss currently being conducted at the Chicago Institute for Psychoanalysis under the leadership of Fleming.]

[5] In the meantime, I. Hellman (1962) has published a follow-up study of one of the children in the Hampstead War Nurseries. Her paper is focused specifically on the effect of sudden separation followed over twenty years.

displayed almost without exception withdrawn, depressive, self-accusatory or hostile mood swings. We expect that those among them who are now undergoing therapeutic analyses will in time supply us with more detailed information concerning the links between their early losses and their later pathology.[6] Meanwhile, to avoid the impression that we underestimated the pathogenic potentialities inherent in the separation trauma, I summarize in what follows some of our earlier findings.

Our wartime efforts concerning this subject did not go beyond a rough division between immediate and delayed, transitory and permanent consequences. Among the permanent damage done to the child, we emphasized, above all, the impairment in the capacity for and quality of object relationships which can be observed in cases where repeated changes of mother figure have taken place. Under such circumstances the child either becomes withdrawn (disinclined to cathect objects) or shallow and superficial in his object relations (i.e., never reaches or recaptures object constancy). On this point agreement between Bowlby and us is complete.

As regards some of the immediate pathological effects of separation, we were inclined to group them under headings such as the following:

Psychosomatic Conditions: These were frequent, especially in the youngest children, in the form of sleeping disturbances, feeding troubles, digestive upsets, especially constipation, an increased readiness to develop sore throats or succumb to respiratory infections.

[6] For the analytic study of one of these children, see Gyomroi (1963).

Regression in Instinct Development: On the libidinal side this consisted of a return to earlier levels, the more primitive manifestations being displayed toward the new objects (clinging, domineering, querulous anal or greedy, insatiable, dependent oral behavior), and in auto-erotic activities (sucking, rocking). On the aggressive side it resulted in the earlier, cruder forms of aggression coming to the fore (biting, spitting, hitting) or, worse still, in a defusion of libidinal and aggressive elements which allowed the latter to dominate the picture.

Regression in Ego Development: One of the most impressive and unexpected consequences of separation was undoubtedly the loss of ego functions such as speech, bowel and bladder control, and the beginning of social adaptation. According to our observations, the functions most endangered in this respect were those that had been most recently acquired.

Upsets in Libido Distribution: We have always considered the interval between loss of contact with the mother ("withdrawal," see above) and attachment to a substitute mother as the period most productive of pathology, especially if this interval is prolonged either for external reasons (lack of suitable substitute mother) or for internal reasons (inability to transfer cathexis). For the form of the pathological outcome it is decisive what happens during this interval to the libido withdrawn from the mother. It may be used to cathect (or recathect) the child's own body, resulting in disturbances of a psychosomatic or hypochondriacal nature; or it may be used for cathexis of the self-image where it may cause a variety of disturbances such as increased self-love, omnipotence, idea of grandeur, all due to narcissistic imbalance; or it may be employed to overcathect a crude inner fantasy world with the result that the child may become autistic, cut off from the environment, and wholly immersed in himself. The longer the interval lasts, the more difficult will it be to reverse these pathological developments.

Any assessment of the eventual pathological consequences of a separation trauma is inseparable, in our belief, from the assessment of the level of libido development at the time of its occurrence. Results vary according to the fact whether at the moment of separation the tie to the mother was still of a narcissistic nature, dominated by the search for instinctual satisfactions; or whether in the relationship to the mother the personal and affectionate elements had begun to predominate, transforming the attachment into object love; or whether the child had attained the level of so-called object constancy. In this last instance, the image of a cathected person can be maintained internally for longer periods of time, irrespective of the real object's presence or absence in the external world, and much internal effort will be needed before the libido is withdrawn. Such withdrawal happens gradually by means of the painful disengagement process known to us as mourning.

Conclusion

One more concluding remark: in the section entitled "The Occurrence of Mourning Behavior in Animals" of his paper, "Processes of Mourning" (1961a), Bowlby suggests tentatively that there are three main features which are specific to human as distinct from animal behavior: the long-drawn-out persistence of reactions oriented toward the lost object; the presence of hostility toward the self (which, I suppose, includes the guilt reactions); and the tendency to identify with the lost object. I should like to offer the suggestion that this useful distinction also lends itself to a sharper differentiation between the bereavement reactions of the youngest infants, on the one hand, and, on the other hand, the reactions to the separation trauma of young children with more highly developed and, accordingly, more complex mental processes and personality structures.

11

The Theory of the Parent-Infant Relationship

Contribution to the Discussion

(1962 [1961])

I think I would not use the time given to me here to the best advantage if I tried to amplify the papers given by Phyllis Greenacre (1960) and D. W. Winnicott (1960). I feel very happy with the manner in which Greenacre has centered her communications on a maturational point of

Discussion of the papers prepared by Phyllis Greenacre and D. W. Winnicott for the 22nd International Congress of Psycho-Analysis. Both papers were prepublished in 1960. The discussion remarks were presented at the Congress in Edinburgh on August 3, 1961, and first published in the *International Journal of Psycho-Analysis*, 43:240-242, 1962.

view, and also with the way in which Winnicott has centered his on parental care. They have done their own summing up, and no more is necessary. Perhaps it is left for me, then, and for those who follow me in discussion, to branch out from these two papers as a given starting point for more thought as it occurs to a psychoanalyst who deals with either adults or children, and works on similar lines.

The first point that occurs to me then is the following: for several years, since the preoccupation with the preverbal phase of development began in psychoanalytic circles, I have asked myself privately: "Are we here on new ground for a psychoanalyst? Or has this specific line of exploration been foreshadowed in psychoanalysis from its beginnings?" Both Greenacre and Winnicott have cited a number of quotations from Freudian writings to show the early beginnings of such interest. I shall add a few more, though I cannot be certain that I have found them all.

The phase of early dependence in child development then, if we approach it more closely, reveals itself as an old friend, and one commented on repeatedly. In Freud's writings it appears as "the biological factor": the young of the human race go through a long period of dependence and helplessness, and this period is held responsible for a number of important developments in later life, i.e., for the development of the oedipus complex, which, it is said there, could not come into being without the complete dependence and helplessness of the infant. You find this in a preface to Reik's book, *Ritual* (1919); and later in 1924 in "A Short Account of Psycho-Analysis." Dependence and helplessness of the human infant are likewise held responsible for the arousal of all neurotic development as such. This is especially to be found in *Inhibitions, Symptoms*

and Anxiety (1926a). The same factors, again, as the biological ones, are held responsible for the religious needs of
the human individual, and for the cultural struggle against
aggression, in *Civilization and Its Discontents* (1930).

But if our present direction of interest is no more than
a turning of our glance from the effects of dependence
onto the contents and processes in the period of dependence, it is still a turning point of decisive importance. By
taking this line we change the direction of our interest from
the illnesses themselves—neurotic or psychotic—to their
preconditions, to the matrix from which they arise, i.e., to
the era when such important matters as the selection of
neurosis and the selection of the types of defense are decided.

So much for the thoughts of an analytic investigator. Let
us turn from them to more practical considerations which
concern analytic technique and analytic therapy. I ask myself: What part does this period of dependence play in
analytic technique? How does it reach the analyst? How
much of it, and in which form? My first answer to this
question will probably not satisfy many people. I believe
that there is a certain part of this preverbal period which
does not concern the analyst as therapist, or rather, which
from the point of view of therapy is irreversible. To give an
example of this: Joyce Robertson (1962) will shortly pub-
lish a paper based on observations made in the Well-Baby
Clinic of our Hampstead Child-Therapy Clinic. She ex-
plores the effect of maternal care and of the various qualities of mothering on certain lines of development in the first
months of life; she shows how, so far as motility and aggression go, the infant responds with spurts of development or
arrests of development to the handling by the mother. I

very much hope that the contents of this paper as illustrations will satisfy Winnicott as well as Greenacre, and I shall be very glad, when it appears, to have comments from them on the content of the paper.

Concerning this same subject, I have expressed on other occasions the idea that at this early time of life the actions of the mother and her libidinal cathexis and involvement with the child exert a selective influence on the given potentialities in the child. They promote the growth of some, and hold back, or fail to stimulate and libidinize, the growth of other potentialities. This determines certain basic trends in the child concerning his motility, the earliness or lateness of his verbalization, etc. I was much impressed by an idea brought forward by Martin James (1962) that what we find here as the consequence of maternal care and earliest development has in the past been attributed to the constitution. I also agree fully with Michael Balint (1962), who calls the damage sustained at this time the "basic faults"; and with the words of Winnicott, who talks about the "inherited potential becoming an infant." I believe that it is only the infant that concerns the analyst in later therapy, not the inherited potential. So much for the earliest part of the period of dependence.

I fully agree that all the rest of it—and there is a great deal—reaches the analyst in a most meaningful way. But the answer that at present you find most often is that in therapy this period of dependence reaches us only in one form, namely, through the deep regression of the patient to his primitive, preverbal attitudes. I believe that this is not true. I think that although analysis, when it can be pursued deeply enough, reaches down to certain of these levels, there are at the same time various other ways in which we as therapists come in contact with the residues of the dependent phase.

I see especially three ways in which the various stages of dependence express themselves in the structure of the personality.

1. They express themselves in the forms and the remnants of all stages of object relationship, in life as well as in the transference.

2. They express themselves further by what is known in the child as "educational compliance," namely, the complete dependence on the object that makes the child amenable to the efforts of education. An independent being would never give up so much of life's satisfactions as the infant and child do owing to their dependence. This educational compliance changes in later life to social compliance.

3. They express themselves through the internalizations of all the dependencies, anxieties, and early satisfactions and dissatisfactions which the infant lives through in regard to his objects and which reach us through the internal conflicts and struggles of the individual, where they become "material" for the analysis.

I would like to add a few words to each of these three points. First, the object relationship: In his paper on "The Curative Factors in Psycho-Analysis" (1962) presented at this Congress, Gitelson showed us how the remnants of narcissistic object relationship that appear in the transference are on the one hand material, but on the other hand resistance, so far as the treatment alliance with the patient is concerned; that they have to be understood, but through understanding have to be changed into an object relationship which makes communication with the analyst a possibility. What Gitelson has done there for the narcissistic remnants of these early phases can be taken further to cover other residual elements. I feel that the symbiotic attitudes of the child which are left over for later life appear in the transference as the patient's wish for hypnosis, for complete merging with the analyst, and that they have to be analyzed as such.

I think that the elements of the need-fulfillment—i.e., the anaclitic—phase appear in analysis as the patient's wish for help, but a wish for help which allows of no co-operation from the side of the patient. As happened during the state of need fulfillment in infancy, the patient who reverts to this phase of childhood wants to be given—he does not want to give. We know that this anaclitic relationship of the patient to the analyst can act as a resistance which may lead to the breaking off of analysis since the analyst has to refuse to be the need-fulfilling object and make demands on the patient. Patients who in their object relationship have never progressed beyond the stage of need fulfillment are usually not ready to accept such refusals.

I think you will not misunderstand me if I say that the therapeutic alliance between analyst and patient is *not* carried by any of these earlier stages of object relationship, although all these earlier stages are "material." The therapeutic alliance is based, I believe, on ego attitudes that go with later stages, namely, on self-observation, insight, give-and-take in object relationship, the willingness to make sacrifices. It is the oedipal relationship which offers those advantages; thus, it serves as material for interpretation, as well as for cementing the alliance between analyst and patient.

As regards the second point, namely, the educational compliance, we may ask how this reaches us in the transference. I think it reaches us in the form of the dreaded compliance of the patient who is ready to undergo a transference cure but who cannot keep up any gain of the analysis in the absence of the relationship to the analyst. Transference cure and the readiness to accept suggestion seem to me elements which are the direct outcome of the phase of early infantile compliance.

I do not need to say much about the third point—the internalized processes—since they were treated at length in the various discussion groups and the various papers devoted to the internal conflicts between id, ego, and superego (see Symposium, 1962b). I only want to remind you once more that it is also the residues of the dependent phase which through internalization reach us in this form, externalized once more, in the transference. They do not only appear as internal conflicts, but come into being as demands, wishes, tendencies, conflicts, acted out toward the analyst.

Now for the conclusion. I have indicated before that where an individual has not developed toward the oedipus complex but has been arrested in his development in the preverbal phase or soon thereafter, within the processes that we have heard described here, we lack in analysis the background against which these early phases can be analyzed. I would end with an even more sweeping statement. I believe that where the phase of dependence has never been overcome and independence has not first been reached and then lost again, it is impossible to cure in analysis the state of dependency.

12

An Appreciation of
Herman Nunberg
(1964)

It seems to me entirely appropriate that Karl Menninger
and I share the assignment to honor Herman Nunberg on
his birthday. While I as a former co-member of his in the
Vienna Psychoanalytic Society represent his Austrian past,
Menninger as his co-member in the American Psychoanalytic Association stands for his American present. Nevertheless, in Nunberg's case, not too much needs to be made of
the change in geographical scene. In contrast to many
others among us who, like him, were uprooted in the middle of their professional careers, neither his working habits,

This paper was read, as an introduction to the first annual Herman Nunberg Lecture, at the New York Academy of Medicine,
on April 13, 1964. It is published here for the first time. [The lecture, entitled "The Greater Evil," was read by Karl A. Menninger.]

nor his pace, nor his attitude to life altered with the altered circumstances. He remained the same quiet, immersed, determined, highly critical, and inexorably careful
worker on either side of the Atlantic, and as such com-
manded the respect of the analytic world and the gratitude
of his patients.

If, in the foregoing, I have referred to myself as Nunberg's former co-member, not his colleague, this was not
done without intention. Although the importance of age
difference (slight as it is between us) dwindles with ad-
vancing years, something of the initial difference in professional status remains, and for me nothing does away with
the fact that Nunberg and I are not of the same analytic
generation. When we first met in the Vienna group, it is
true, this happened before official training institutes and,
with them, the gulf between training analysts and candidates came into being. But, if anything, this increased and
did not lessen the distance between the old-timers and the
newcomers, the experienced and the inexperienced. To
Nunberg's age group belonged (in alphabetical order)
Helene Deutsch, Paul Federn, Eduard Hitschmann, Lud-
wik Jekels; to mine, the Bibrings, Hartmann, Kris, Wilhelm Reich, Waelder. While Nunberg presented and discussed problems, I, as a silent listener, used to ask myself
enviously whether I would ever be as familiar with the
subject as he proved himself to be, able to teach and train
instead of learning, to write papers as he did, to treat patients as difficult as his, to play a part in the psychoanalytic
movement as he did, and show myself capable of influencing its course.

The part played by Nunberg in the *psychoanalytic movement* was, in fact, an important one, though, owing to his

unobtrusiveness, it is not known to many people. He had joined the Vienna Psychoanalytic Society in 1915, at a time when members were not "admitted," as they are today, but themselves decided to join on the basis of their previous publications and scientific convictions. From then onward his clinical and theoretical contributions formed an integral part of the Vienna's analytic life. Only three years later, in the Business Meeting of the International Psycho-Analytical Congress in Budapest, 1918, he took an unprecedented step, recorded in the *Minutes* modestly as "concerning the modalities for the acceptance of new members." This would have remained unrecognized in its importance if, at the Marienbad Congress in 1936, Max Eitingon had not revealed in a speech that Nunberg's proposal had consisted of the suggestion that "from now on nobody should become a member unless he has undergone a personal (training) analysis." As Eitingon stated: "As soon as that had been said by Nunberg, we all realized that something of extreme importance had been suggested, and it became a reality not very long afterwards." Thus, Nunberg had become, and has remained, the spiritual father of Training Analysis, an innovation which has become indispensable since then and has been instrumental in decisively altering the whole shape and direction of psychoanalytic training.

Nunberg was also involved in another significant moment in the history of psychoanalysis, although in this instance nothing came of it finally. In 1920, thanks to the active generosity of Max Eitingon, the Berlin Psychoanalytic Society founded its Polyclinic, which was to undertake training as well as therapeutic functions. I was present at the time when Eitingon came to Vienna to persuade Nunberg to join the new Institute. That Nunberg declined to leave Vienna was Berlin's loss but remained, of course, Vienna's gain.

For the rest, there are many analysts, now themselves elders in the movement, who owe the mainstay of their analytic education and of their scientific orientation to a training analysis carried out by Nunberg. In the further course of events, it was they, rather than their teacher, who became moving spirits in their various analytic societies. With the exception of his active participation over many years in the Education Committee of the New York Psychoanalytic Institute, of a period as president of the New York Psychoanalytic Society, and a similar one as President of the Psychoanalytic Research and Development Fund, Nunberg held himself aloof from committee work and active politics.

Nunberg's name *as author* appears for the first time in an article "On the Physical Accompaniments of Association Processes" (1910), published in C. G. Jung's *Studies on Word Association* (Chapter XIII), written in his preanalytic period, when he participated in the "Experiments in the Diagnosis of Psychopathological Conditions" carried out at the Psychiatric Clinic of Zurich University. So far as analytic publications are concerned, his entrance was made in 1912 with an introductory lecture on "The Unfulfilled Wishes According to Freud's Teachings," presented at the Second Congress of Polish Psychiatrists, Neurologists, and Psychologists in Cracow and published, subsequently, in *Neurologia Polska* (1913). This was followed in 1917 by a clinical presentation on "A Case of Hypochondriasis," reported in the *Internationale Zeitschrift für Psychoanalyse*.

From then onward his publications became numerous. What strikes me as their outstanding characteristic is the fact that, unlike others, Nunberg does not restrict himself to any one particular aspect of the personality or its pathology, but allows his interest to range freely over the whole structure, id, ego, and superego, singling out basic problems as they are highlighted for him by his clinical material.

As regards the exploration of *the id*, three of his papers remain essential for entering into an understanding of the psychoses: "On the Catatonic Attack" (1920), "The Course of the Libidinal Conflict in a Case of Schizophrenia" (1921), and "States of Depersonalization in the Light of the Libido Theory" (1924). In the "Catatonic Attack," it is especially fascinating to follow the dissection of the case material and the reconstruction of an unbroken line through the sequence of libidinal phases backward to cannibalism and to the unity with the mother in the womb fantasy. In this essay there also is the characterization of the delusional system as an attempt "to cathect anew the objects of the outside world with the overflow of narcissistic libido," and of the manner in which parts of the patient's own body represent themselves to the ego as objects. Since, in this stage of the illness, "the verbal and concrete ideas" are only loosely connected, and the attempts to regain the objects are enacted on the verbal ideas, the relations to the external world are expressed in a primitive, concrete language which Nunberg characterizes as "organ speech."

In "States of Depersonalization," a convincing link is made between the common phenomenon of "estrangement" and its pathological exaggeration in the feeling of depersonalization, the former being no more than an initial phase of repression. There also is, I believe, a link here to the much-discussed problem of "boredom" in its everyday as well as its symptomatic form. If depersonalization equals the loss of libido, boredom may equal a state where the libido is out of reach, withdrawn owing to repression, but in this case from the ego interests rather than the object world.

The trains of thought contained in "States of Depersonalization" were developed further by Nunberg at a later date. In his *Principles of Psychoanalysis* (1932) we find him concerned with the fact that in depersonalization the libidinal cathexis is withdrawn from the ego's organs of perception as well as from its thoughts and feelings, or is diminished in these respects. He concludes from this that in order for the ego to function correctly, these organs, thoughts, and feelings must be cathected either with direct libido or with indirect, sublimated libido, but that this alone is not sufficient; for the perceptions of the ego to become fully real, they have to receive the sanction of the superego (society). In other words: the recognition of reality—improbable as this may seem—is also dependent on the superego or morality. To quote a passage from the *Principles*: "That may perhaps explain in part why denying reality, not telling the truth, is considered immoral."

So far as *clashes within the id* are concerned, "Problems of Bisexuality" (1947) and *Curiosity* (1961) are of the greatest clinical importance, the former illustrating the conflict between masculine and feminine strivings via the male's attitude toward circumcision.

The *superego* comes into the orbit of Nunberg's writings in "The Sense of Guilt and the Need for Punishment" (1926) and in "The Feeling of Guilt" (1934).

But in spite of this impartiality of interest displayed, Nunberg will find himself quoted most frequently in connection with his "The Synthetic Function of the Ego"

(1930), an exciting paper which inevitably arouses the envy of many other authors on the subject of ego psychology. In it, the role and functioning of the *ego* are described in terms which, in their lucidity, come second only to Freud's description of the ego's simultaneous helplessness, compliance, and mastery with regard to the external and internal world, the classical simile of "the rider and the horse." In Nunberg's words, the ego unites, binds, and creates; simplifies and generalizes; assimilates alien elements, mediates between opposing ones, reconciles opposites, sets mental functioning in train; driven by an overwhelming need for causality, it forges links between past and present events, thereby establishing a synthesis in time. He leaves no doubt that, to his mind, the synthetic function is one of the most essential agents in the upkeep of normal functioning; its breakdown or failure to develop, one of the most weighty pathogenic factors. To free the synthetic function from interference by pathology is viewed as a major therapeutic task. In this light, it becomes obvious, of course, why no synthesis needs to be introduced into the technique of psychoanalytic treatment, this being provided automatically by the restored synthetic function of the ego after the analytic process has run its course.

As regards "Ego Strength and Ego Weakness," a problem topical at the time of the Marienbad Congress, this was treated by Nunberg in 1939.

There is also no scarcity of papers dealing with the *interaction between the inner agencies*, i.e., the way in which the rational deals with the irrational side of the personality, especially where patients' reactions to analytic therapy are concerned. In this area Nunberg starts with a basic idea concerning the patient's attitude to getting well, a factor which is underestimated in its importance by many analysts today. We find it elaborated for the first time in "The Will to Recovery" (1925), where the connection is traced from conscious to unconscious fantasy and the latter's relevance for an analytic cure is demonstrated. The theme is carried further in "Problems of Therapy" (1928), "The Theory of the Therapeutic Results" (1937), "Psychological Interrelations between Physician and Patient" (1938), and "Limitations of Psychoanalytic Treatment" (1943).

It is this comprehensive grasp of the whole body of psychoanalytic theory which enabled Nunberg to write one of the few existing *textbooks* of psychoanalysis, his *Principles of Psychoanalysis: Their Application to the Neuroses*, published in 1932. Likewise, it was his *historical sense* and respect for the gradual growth of the psychoanalytic discipline which made him undertake the arduous task of editing the *Minutes of the Vienna Psychoanalytic Society*, which Paul Federn, the Society's former President, had left him as a legacy.

More significant even than the enumeration of an author's publications is a description of his methods of production and creation. This, with Nunberg, is a rare combination of detailed clinical observation and experience with carefully restrained, cautious theoretical abstraction. His clinical papers invariably yield theoretical results, while his theoretical essays are built on case histories from which they hardly detach themselves. Interpretation of clinical data is occasionally introduced by phrases which sound almost apologetic, such as "Alerted by this fragment of theory . . . ," or "If we yield to our inclination for generalization . . . ," indicating that the application of preconceived theoretical notions and the tendency to abstract and generalize are not considered assets in an analytic author.

Much could be said in praise of such restraint, if it had not already been said with greater authority in the Fore-word to Nunberg's *Principles of Psychoanalysis*. There, Freud welcomes the book as "the most complete and ac-curate presentation we have at this time of a psychoanalytic theory of neurotic processes," and characterizes the author's working method as avoiding "simplification and a glossing over," as showing a full appreciation of the rich diversity of mental happenings; above all, he praises Nunberg's spec-ulation as never running free but remaining guided by and tied to clinical experiences.

To distinguish conscientiously between facts and opin-ions, and to remain mindful of the human tendency to find facts which give backing to our opinions are not easy tasks for an analyst, and to persist in their maintenance requires discipline, restraint, caution, self-criticism, and the absence of undue optimism, all of them attitudes which are characteristic of Nunberg. He shares these with the dis-tinguished figure of Josef Breuer, who played a decisive role in the origins of psychoanalysis.

When I was recently rereading correspondence of the past, I came across the following passage in a letter written by Breuer to Wilhelm Fliess in 1895 concerning the latter's enthusiastic working association with Freud at the time: "When I formulate opinions, or embark on action, I can-not help thinking that, perhaps, in reality, the facts are quite different from what I imagine them to be. And that is why I envy you two [Fliess and Freud]. I wish that on the

highest holidays, I could feel as sure of myself and my findings as you are on every ordinary working day."

This, I felt, could have been written by Nunberg. It
made me wonder how often he feels this way about us
others, the more incautious ones.

13

Links Between Hartmann's Ego Psychology and the Child Analyst's Thinking (1966 [1964])

To speak to an audience in honor of Heinz Hartmann on the occasion of his 70th birthday is not an assignment to be taken lightly. With Hartmann himself present as a listener, obviously nothing will fulfill the purpose of a tribute except an address which approximates his own, exacting level of thinking. To the lecturer this presents the task of showing himself fully conversant with the body of theories

Lecture in honor of Heinz Hartmann's 70th birthday, New York Academy of Medicine, November 4, 1964. Reprinted from *Psychoanalysis—A General Psychology: Essays in Honor of Heinz Hartmann*, ed. R. M. Loewenstein, L. M. Newman, M. Schur, and A. J. Solnit. New York: International Universities Press, 1966, pp. 16-27.

which owe their origin to Hartmann, of proving her appreciation of them by measuring against them her own notions and opinions, for whatever these are worth, and of surveying beyond this the superior achievement of a brilliant mind trained to rigorous scientific effort.

HARTMANN'S EGO PSYCHOLOGY

Opposition and Acceptance

In their Preface to Hartmann's *Ego Psychology and Problem of Adaptation,* the editors speak of "the remarkable degree to which Hartmann's ideas have shaped, and become assimilated into current psychoanalytic thinking" (p. viii). If, thereby, they create a picture of an author's ideas being accepted easily and quickly, the impression is misleading. On the contrary: although this had no power to deter him, Hartmann's ego psychology met with an extraordinary amount of opposition in the analytic world. There were many analytic colleagues who took exception to the degree to which he turned his mind away from the problems of psychopathology to contemplate instead the possibility of securing for psychoanalysis the status of a general psychology. Others had misgivings on principle concerning the manner in which, in Hartmann's writings, theoretical thinking took precedence over the clinical concerns of the analyst in practice. But, above all, there were many who feared that the explicit introduction of an ego psychology into psychoanalysis endangered its position as a depth psychology, a discipline concerned exclusively with the activity of the instinctual drives and the functioning of the unconscious mind. Taking the stand that work on the ego was an unwarranted extension of analysis, they ignored the fact that, from its beginnings, psychoanalytic metapsychology was intended to embrace all the agencies within the mental apparatus, plus their interactions.

However this may be, it took years until, by the mere weight of his published work, opposition was silenced sufficiently to allow one after the other of his notions to become accepted, to penetrate to the knowledge of the membership at large, and to infiltrate gradually into the teaching programs of many of the official training institutes. By now, concepts such as the conflict-free sphere of the ego, primary and secondary ego autonomy, intrasystemic conflicts within the ego, the notion of energy change in sublimation, interest in the undifferentiated id-ego sphere, etc., are familiar elements in the analytic theory.

Hartmann's Theories and Child Analysis

If "the assimilation of Hartmann's ideas into current analytic thinking" applies to the analytic world in general, it does so even more in the area of child analysis. The child analyst's thinking, governed as it is by the developmental aspects of the human personality, does not thrive on the basis of drive psychology alone, but needs to range freely in the whole theoretical field of psychoanalysis, according equal significance to id, ego, and superego, to depth and surface, as Hartmann does. This creates the specific links between his work and the child analyst's thinking, which is indicated in the title.

SOME INTERRELATIONS BETWEEN
HARTMANN AND MYSELF, PAST
AND PRESENT

Since I had myself in mind in this title, as the representative of at least one brand of child analysis, and since it is my own thinking which I propose to compare with Hartmann's, some personal remarks concerning our common past will be needed here.

Heinz Hartmann and I entered the Vienna Psychoanalytic Society almost simultaneously, some forty years ago, he being analytically my slightly elder brother, or half brother, since in some respect we even shared the same father. In the field of ego psychology, too, we appeared almost at the same time, in the 1930s. I came into it, more conventionally, from the side of the ego's defensive activity against the drives; Hartmann, in a more revolutionary manner, from the new angle of ego autonomy, which until then had lain outside analytic study. This revealed itself openly for the first time in the Vienna Society in the discussion following the presentation of my first two chapters of *The Ego and the Mechanisms of Defense* in 1936. Hartmann showed himself appreciative on the whole, but he emphasized the point that to show the ego at war with the id was not the whole story; that there were many additional problems of ego growth and ego functioning which needed consideration. My views were more restricted at the time, and this was news to me which I was not yet ready to assimilate.

From that point onward we went ahead, each of us very much immersed in our special field, respecting each other, quoting each other, but not in active interchange. In production and achievement, Hartmann always remained some way ahead, owing to his genuinely scientific mind and thorough scientific training, both of which I lacked and had to acquire slowly. It was not easy for me, or for anybody at the time, to catch up with the rapid development of his systematic thinking.

Our ideas met fully and squarely for the first time in the Symposium on "The Mutual Influences in the Development of Ego and Id," held at the Amsterdam Congress, 1951, and they remained firmly linked since then. In his and my contribution presented there (see Volume IV, ch. 9) already can be found the germs and nuclei of all the topical links on which I propose to enlarge in what follows.

LINKS BETWEEN HARTMANN'S AND MY (THE CHILD ANALYST'S) THINKING

Although the connections may be infinitely more numerous when traced in detail, I single out for the present purpose seven of them which seem to me to represent basic concepts in Hartmann's scheme as well as cornerstones in my recent account of work in the Hampstead Child-Therapy Clinic. This may be an unorthodox procedure of approaching another author's work, but one which will, I hope, serve the present purpose and in turn elicit some reactions from the other side.

The Conflict-free Sphere of the Ego

Following his discussion remarks in 1936, Hartmann presented his paper on *Ego Psychology and the Problem of Adaptation* in 1937. There we find for the first time the exhortation to analysts that "we must recognize that, though the ego grows on conflicts, these are not the only roots of ego development." Obvious though this point of view seemed to him, no one found it easy at the time to turn his interest away from the internal conflicts between ego and drive activity and the symptomatology resulting from them, and to become concerned with the purely maturational and developmental side of ego growth, that is, with events which proceed silently, without clamor, outside the realm of conflict. On the other hand, since these processes determine the shape of the very ego apparatus and ego functions which are later drawn into the orbit of conflict, and which serve as tools in the ego's struggle for mastery over the id, this—as Hartmann stressed—is no less decisive for the upkeep of normality or for psychopathology than all the other items of mental functioning which traditionally come under the analyst's scrutiny.

As indicated above, the correctness of this point has been accepted in the analytic world by now, although the analysts of adults often pay no more than lip service to it. Where child analysis is concerned, on the other hand, as in our Hampstead Clinic, it has been put into action very vigorously in the Diagnostic Profile, used for the assessment of a child's development in general or his psychopathology in particular. With the Profile scheme used as a guide, the diagnostician's attention is directed as decisively to "conflict-free," autonomous ego growth, and the irregularities and failures of building up ego apparatuses and functions, as it is directed to the ego's defense organization or the vicissitudes of drive development.[1] To my mind, these sec-

[1] See Profile, Section V, B, Ego and Superego Development, (a), (b), and (c) (Volume VI, p. 142).

tions of the Profile carry out the suggestions introduced and upheld by Hartmann during the past thirty years. Whether this application to diagnosis is in fact far-reaching enough and meets his demands in full remains for him to confirm.

The Intrasystemic Approach

Moving from the concept of a conflict-free area to that of conflict, Hartmann wishes analysts to pay attention to those clashes which occur not between the mental agencies but within the particular systems. Intrasystemic conflicts had of course always been prominent in psychoanalytic theory. Within the id, they are known to be only potential ones, since drive opposites such as passive-active, feminine-masculine, love-hate, are contained without contradiction so long as they remain unconscious and turn into "conflict" only when they rise to the surface and approach the conscious ego. Within the superego, clashes have been shown to arise between conflicting identifications with and internalizations of external figures of authority, which genetically have served as its sources. But what Hartmann has in mind here are the ways in which, during its growth, the ego is torn within itself, the development of one side of it acting as an obstacle to the intactness of another side. In his "Technical Implications of Ego Psychology" (1951), for example, Hartmann emphasizes the necessity to examine "whether the autonomous ego functions are interfered with by the defensive functions."

This, to me, too, has seemed an important point for years. It is true that in clinical descriptions of analytic cases it has always been implied and that it has been alluded to under terms such as "the price paid by the ego for the up-keep of its defense organization"; the "harm done by pathology to normal functioning," as, for example, the damage done to normal motility by a hysterical paralysis, or the damage done to rational thinking by the obsessional devices. But what Hartmann and I have in mind goes beyond these facts encountered in pathology, to events which happen normally in every individual's development. As I have expressed it elsewhere (Volume VI):

> As the ego of the child grows and improves its functioning, better *awareness* of the internal and external world brings it into contact with many unpleasurable and painful aspects; the increasing dominance of the *reality principle* curtails wishful thinking; the improvement of *memory* leads to retaining not only pleasurable but frightening and painful items; the *synthetic function* prepares the ground for conflict between the inner agencies, etc. The resultant influx of unpleasure and anxiety is more than the human being can bear without relief; consequently it is warded off by the defense mechanisms which come into action to protect the ego.
>
> Thus, *denial* interferes with accuracy in the perception of the outer world by excluding the unpleasurable. *Repression* does the same for the inner world by withdrawing conscious cathexis from unpleasurable items. *Reaction formations* replace the unpleasurable and unwelcome by the opposite. All three mechanisms interfere with memory, i.e., with its impartial functioning, regardless of pleasure and unpleasure. *Projection* runs counter to the synthetic function by eliminating anxiety-arousing elements from the image of the personality and attributing them to the object world.
>
> In short, while the forces of maturation and adaptation strive toward the increasing, reality-governed efficiency in all ego functioning, the defense against unpleasure works

in the opposite direction and, in its turn, invalidates the ego functions [p. 104f].[2]

Other Intrasystemic Aspects

In the same paper, "Technical Implications of Ego Psychology," Hartmann speaks of "the relative preponderance of certain ego functions over others," and in his "Psychoanalysis and Developmental Psychology" (1950a) he advocates that it should "be feasible and useful to replace the global . . . terms like 'precocious' or 'retarded' ego development by more detailed statements specifying what ego functions have actually undergone a precocious or retarded development in relation to the drives and in relation to one another" (p. 107).

In fact, for the accurate assessment of any child's developmental status, no point can be of greater assistance than this particular one which complements what has always happened in analytic diagnosis with regard to the sequence of libidinal, later also of aggressive, stages. So far as I am concerned, I have tried to take care of this by establishing the concept of *developmental lines*, contributed to both from the side of id and of ego development; these developmental lines lead from the child's state of immaturity to the gradual setting up of a mature personality and are, in fact, the result of interaction between maturation, adaptation, and structuralization. While what enters into this combination from the side of the drives is better known to us at present, the obvious need to fill in the missing data on the side of the ego spurs us on to greater efforts in exploring

[2] See also Volume IV, ch. 1. In the Profile this point of Hartmann's is taken care of in section B (d) (Volume VI, p. 143).

those aspects of ego growth which Hartmann has in mind.

The disharmony and disequilibrium between the lines of development, in their turn, serve to highlight precocity or retardation of specific ego functions as well as "the relative preponderance of certain ego functions over others," in Hartmann's sense.

"The Sign and Signal Function of Behavior"

With regard to the observation of behavior for the purpose of assessments of development, it gives me particular pleasure to find in Hartmann's attitude that of a fellow rebel. He writes in "Psychoanalysis and Developmental Psychology" (1950a) as follows: "We come to the conclusion that psychoanalytic psychology is not limited to what can be gained through the use of the psychoanalytic method" (p. 103). And further: "Such [developmental] studies will of necessity lead to a growing awareness of the sign- or signal-function which behavior details may have for the observer, that is, to a better or more systematic understanding of how data of direct observation can be used as indicators of structurally central and partly unconscious developments —in a sense that by far transcends the possibilities of sign interpretation acessible to the various methods of testing" (p. 102).

The suggestion made here by Hartmann—that development, finished character structures, and even pathological formations can be assessed outside of the analytic session— runs of course counter to the beliefs of many analysts who wish to rely exclusively on the material produced by their patients via the analytic method. On the other hand, it is a point to which I subscribe fully (Volume VI, Chapter 1).

I have also tried to demonstrate in detail that in the historical development of psychoanalysis such complete restriction of observation to the privacy of the analytic setting is a fiction rather than reality; that derivatives of the unconscious, observed in normal people not under analysis, were considered a legitimate source of information at all times, viz., faulty and symptomatic actions, daydreams, children's dreams (see Freud, 1900, 1901); that, at a later date, the same became true of the revealing functions of certain characters.[3]

Personally, I can see no difficulty in extending this conviction of certain fixed relationships existing between surface appearance and id content from the mental phenomena named above to particular items of behavior, especially of children, as they can be observed in the areas of play; in hobbies; in the attitude to illness, food, clothing, etc. I believe, what deters the majority of analysts from accepting this suggestion is not so much a disbelief in the validity of this material, but a reminder of certain phases in the history of psychoanalysis when such items were used profusely and disadvantageously for the purpose of symbolic interpretation within analysis, which is a technical mistake, of course.

That the intellectual ego functions as such can be assessed in surface observation, i.e., testing, naturally needs no further proof.

---

[3] As emphasized by S. Freud (1933), concerning the obsessional character, with the expectation ". . . that other character traits as well will turn out similarly to be precipitates of reaction-formations related to particular pregenital libidinal structures" (p. 102).

Problems of the Infantile Neurosis

Nowhere, of course, does Hartmann come nearer to the concerns of the child analyst than in his paper on the "Problems of Infantile Neurosis" (1954).

He asserts that "at present we have more questions than answers" and that "what Freud said about infantile neurosis long ago remains true today. But it is also obvious that in the course of the development of analysis reformulations are inevitable"; that it is "actually not easy to say what we call an infantile neurosis." He also speaks of neurotic problems in children "limited to a single functional disturbance" and of the fact that "the way from conflict to symptom is often shorter than in adult neurosis" (p. 208f.).

The problems alluded to here by Hartmann are precisely those which engage our interest in the Hampstead Clinic and which have given rise to some of our publications.[4] We agree with Hartmann that the term "infantile neurosis" has been overused, and extended to cover a large variety of disturbances which do not come under the heading of neuroses since they are either not the result of conflict at all or, in any case, not of the type of internal conflict where danger comes to a head during the oedipus complex, regression takes place from there to earlier, prephallic fixation points, and a pathogenic conflict arises between these reawakened pregenital strivings and the ego—conflicts which are solved by compromise, i.e., by symptom formation. Far from corresponding to this classical definition of the infantile neurosis, many of the childhood disturbances seen in the Clinic are (nonorganic) disturbances of vital body needs ("limited to

[4] See, for example, Volume VI, Chapter 5, and Nagera (1966b).

one functional disturbance," in Hartmann's terms); or they represent excessive delays in acquiring vital ego functions; or primary disturbances of narcissism (Sandler, 1966) or of object relatedness; or lack of ego control or faulty superego development or both. We subscribe to the same view as Hartmann, that some of the quasi-pathological formulations "represent the best possible solution of a given infantile conflict," and we agree wholeheartedly with him that the whole subject of diagnostic categorization needs reformulation so far as childhood pathology is concerned.

One of our suggestions in this direction is to clear the field by establishing as a separate diagnostic category the so-called *developmental disturbances*, namely, disorders which arise owing to the particular external and internal strains and stresses, dangers and anxieties connected with particular developmental phases, and which are transitory in the sense that they fade away with the passing of the developmental level on which they have emerged. As shown by Nagera (1966b), it is a long way from this type of childhood problem to the infantile neuroses proper, and the gap can be filled by a whole hierarchy of other forms of infantile pathology.

Hartmann shows himself concerned further with "the simple clinical question of what the actual correlations between childhood neurosis and form and intensity of adult neurosis are" (p. 209f.), and he quotes the Wolf Man case as one of the rare opportunities where such a correlation can be found in the literature. Simple as the question may be, the answer is not easy to give, and at present no more can be offered than a few tentative ideas. While we know for certain that every adult neurosis is based on an infantile one, it has been demonstrated by experience that this state-

ment is not reversible: not every infantile neurosis is followed by an adult neurosis. Moreover, in childhood there
are many more dissocial individuals, exhibitionists, fetishists,
and transvestites than there are adult delinquents or perverts, notwithstanding the fact that adult delinquency,
criminality, and perversion invariably begin in early life.
Hartmann is right in asserting that "more systematic study"
of these problems is needed before we can predict with any
degree of certainty what will be the further fate of an infantile neurosis or any other childhood disorder: whether,
as phase-determined, it will be "outgrown"; whether it will
persist unaltered into adulthood, as some of the perversions
do; or whether it will change form, as it happens from the
dissocial to the compulsive, or the phobic-hysteric to the
obsessional, or from the obsessional to the schizophrenic.

The Problem of Morality

As regards the problem of morality, my developmental
study of the attainment of law abidingness in individual life
does not in any way come up to Hartmann's closely argued,
beautiful, objective essay on the whole relationship between
psychoanalysis and moral values (1960). But, at least, as it
seems to me, I have managed to fulfill Hartmann's demands
in one particular respect, namely, to trace how, to use his
terminology, "the various ego functions and acquisitions
enter into the final result as independent variables." Like
Hartmann, I have been impressed by the state of affairs
which exists in this respect. Although, intrinsically, ego
functions such as memory, secondary process thinking, reality testing, integration, control of morality have neither
a moral connotation nor the opposite, social behavior and

law abidingness cannot come about without them, nor can they without ego mechanisms such as imitation, identification, introjection. It is a fascinating developmental study in itself to see each ego attribute, as it appears during the individual's growth, contribute to the unfolding of the socially adapted, moral personality. Memory is indispensable for the individual's acting on experience and foresight; reason and logic for understanding cause and effect in relation to behavior; ego control of motility for preventing action on impulse; identification and introjection for internalizing the external social norms, etc.

I am well aware that this does not cover the problem of morality, nor does it touch on the value issues, as they are raised by Hartmann. My exposition merely serves to demonstrate the double pull within the personality, the various ego characteristics helping the individual toward morality while the id strivings exert their urge in the opposite direction.

The Concept of Health

Finally, Hartmann and I come very close together in our approach to the concept of health, which, like the study of normality, is a neglected area in the analytic literature.

We agree with each other in *not* conceiving of psychic health in terms of the *opposite of neurosis*, since phenomena such as conflict, defense, compromise formations are necessary for both, and are merely quantitatively and not qualitatively different in the mentally ill and mentally healthy.

We also agree that mental health cannot be characterized by the absence of *suffering*. Hartmann (1939b) expresses

this by writing "that a limited amount of suffering and illness forms an integral part of the scheme of health" (p. 7).
For me it is an important point that, regarding children,
the presence of suffering is no reliable indicator for the
presence of pathology; that, on the contrary, mental distress
has to be accepted as a normal by-product of the child's
dependency, his exposure to frustrations, and the inevitable
strains and stresses of development; more than this: that
the absence of suffering in an individual child may be an
ominous sign of ill-health, pointing to organic damage,
mental backwardness, or extreme passivity.

So far as the *location and maintenance* of mental health
are concerned, Hartmann points above all to the intactness
of the synthetic and adaptive functions of the ego. I assess
in a more global way the intactness of the whole trend of
progressive id-ego development, asserting that children in
whom these progressive tendencies outweigh the regressive
ones are more safely anchored in health, and are helped to
maintain health by the pleasure gains which they experience during maturation, development, and adaptation.

There is no doubt that we both regard personal characteristics such as frustration tolerance, anxiety tolerance, and
a high potential for sublimation and neutralization of drives
as substantial aids in maintaining the status of health.

Altogether, I cannot help feeling that it is in this particular area of the concept of mental health where the links
between Hartmann's and my thinking become most obvious. While other psychoanalytic authors emphasize what
ego and superego do to make us neurotic, Hartmann and I
both have given added weight to that side of the analytic
theory which convincingly shows the immense efforts made
by the ego and superego to keep us healthy.

CONCLUSION

One concluding remark: there were occasions in the past when Hartmann used to refer to me as his "silent critic." Obviously, he misunderstood my attitude since, though I have been silent, while waiting for increased understanding, I was never critical. I hope I have convinced him now, at this late date, that far from being a silent critic, I am an eloquent supporter of his work.

14

Comments on Psychic Trauma
(1967 [1964])

I

GENERAL REMARKS

Much important ground has been covered by the preceding papers and statements and by the illuminating summary given by Robert Waelder. Accordingly, in what follows,

This paper was presented at the Symposium on Infantile Trauma, sponsored by The Psychoanalytic Research and Development Fund, held in New York on April 3-5, 1964.

The sections here labeled "I. General Remarks" and "III. Final Summary" were first published in *Psychic Trauma*, ed. Sidney S. Furst. New York & London: Basic Books, 1967, pp. 235-245. Section II, "Discussion Remarks," is here published for the first time.

The other contributors to this symposium were Sidney S. Furst, Leo Rangell, Peter B. Neubauer, Phyllis Greenacre, Marianne Kris, Joseph Sandler, Albert J. Solnit, and Robert Waelder (see Furst, 1967).

I extract from these merely what seem to me the most relevant aspects for further constructive thinking on the subject.

As all the other members of the Symposium have done previously, I welcome this opportunity to inquire more closely into the current usage of the term "trauma," and perhaps to rescue it from the widening and overuse which are the present-day fate of many other technical terms in psychoanalysis and in the course of time lead inevitably to a blurring of meaning and finally to the abandonment and loss of valuable concepts. We are in the position of witnessing this typical process with regard to the definition of trauma, which extends at present from the original notion of the break through the stimulus barrier at one extreme end to the notions of the accumulative, the strain, the retrospective, the screen trauma, until it becomes difficult at the other extreme end to differentiate between adverse, pathogenic influences in general and trauma in particular.

In picking my own path within this bewildering maze of ideas, I turn to four aspects of the problem and offer these for further consideration in the discussion.

Concerning the Break Through the Protective Shield or Stimulus Barrier

As Peter Neubauer has done, I start out from Freud's statement (1926a) that the essence of a traumatic situation is an experience of helplessness on the part of the ego in the face of accumulation of excitation, whether of external or internal origin. This formulation seems to me essential since, on the one hand, it designated the ego as the central victim in the traumatic event; and, on the other hand, it implies that there exist not one stimulus barrier (against environmental stimuli) but two protective shields against two types of dangers threatening from the inner as well as from the outer world. These include, of course, those occasions when otherwise harmless external happenings are given threatening meaning on the basis of existing internal constellations.

On the strength of this view, the entire defense organization of the ego is endowed with the characteristics of a protective shield and drawn into the orbit of potential traumatic onslaught. Any event for which an individual's defensive measures are not sufficiently competent becomes potentially a traumatic one.

It is true, and has been pointed out by others, that for this particular view of trauma two characteristics of the event are essential requirements: (1) its suddenness and unexpectedness which do not allow for shifts, rearrangements, or other defensive maneuvers; and (2) some visible and immediate aftereffect of the event as a tangible sign of the disruption of the ego equilibrium which has taken place (Greenacre, Waelder). It is also true that this restricted notion leaves no room for the retrospective and screen trauma, while strain and accumulation appear in this light as preparatory happenings leading up to but not representing the traumatic event as such.

Concerning the Level of Individual Tolerance for Excitation (the Economic Aspect of Trauma)

INDIVIDUAL DIFFERENCES

I share the view of previous speakers, of course, that individuals differ widely from each other as to the degree of external and internal stimulation with which they can cope habitually without being endangered. We recognize basic, i.e., constitutional, differences in this respect and add to them those differences in tolerance or intolerance for unpleasure, anxiety, or danger which are acquired by painful experience, i.e., by sensitization. Of the greatest significance in this respect seems to me Phyllis Greenacre's statement that no truly traumatic event is ever wholly digested, that increased vulnerability is left inevitably, and that the individual concerned is prone to break down at some later date, even if this hazard is restricted to those occasions when he is faced not only with a quantitative but also with a qualitative repetition or near repetition of the original injury.

DIFFERENCES AT DIFFERENT AGES

I also agree wholly with Leo Rangell who stresses that "the economic factors themselves are subject to the genetic developmental process and undergo phase-specific modifications with development and maturation . . . throughout the entire life cycle." We know that tolerance for the influx of upsetting external stimuli and for internal sensations of unpleasure through frustration, deprivation, etc., increases in step with the gradual maturing and perfecting of ego apparatuses and functions; also, that the individual is most vulnerable after birth and in infancy, i.e., before the ego has been crystallized out of the undifferentiated substratum of the organism. During this period the mother in her role as auxiliary ego is the only protective shield available to the infant, and this leaves him at the mercy of injury by so-called "cumulative trauma" (Masud Khan, 1963), whenever the mother-infant relationship does not function smoothly.

Further, it is only logical that the young child's task of building up the stimulus barrier and a defense organization is made immeasurably more difficult if traumatic experiences have to be endured during the critical period of maturation and development, just as the supporting walls of a house are more open to damage during building operations than after completion. Phyllis Greenacre's view of the extreme damage done to the organism by overexcitation in the whole pregenital period fits into this scheme of thinking.

Furthermore, Leo Rangell reminded us that what changes from one age period to the next is not only the toleration of stimulation but also the need for it, in the sense that amounts which are adequate for old age constitute a traumatically low supply in childhood and adolescence, a point to be taken into consideration under the next aspect.

ADAPTATION TO STIMULATION AND FLUCTUATION OF TOLERANCE LEVELS

So far it has not been brought forward in discussion that we can also observe alterations in tolerance levels which are due neither to individual nor to age differences but are connected with characteristics of the external (often communal) situation. An individual's adaptation to his environmental circumstances includes, of course, adaptation to the strains and dangers inherent in them, whether the life conditions are those of the adventurous explorer, the soldier or sailor, the civilian in a bombed city or during an epidemic, the inmate of a concentration camp, the member of former generations, for example, in the Middle Ages, during the Thirty Year War in Central Europe, etc. (Freud). It is unknown to us by what means people succeed under such conditions in raising their stimulus barrier, i.e., to lull or harden their sensitivities as a safeguard against breakdown. What we know, on the other hand, is that it is easy to commit errors of judgment when judging somebody's tolerance for excitation from the vantage point of a totally different external situation where stimulus barriers stand at a different level. This happened during the war when Americans, from the greater safety of their home scene, thought of their British friends under bombing as exposed to continuous traumatization, or as "heroic," while in Britain, at this time, stimulus barriers had been raised to include the danger as a familiar, nontraumatic item. On the other hand, changes of this kind are not permanent acquisitions. With the return of peacetime conditions, these same individuals, when looking back on their war years, see themselves as they were seen from abroad at the time—as victims of intolerable, potentially traumatic circumstances.

Similar errors of judgment or misunderstandings occur where human beings live closely together who do not share the same level of excitation tolerance. Not only do they suffer through being exposed to quantities of stimuli which do not correspond with their own needs or capacities for assimilation, as shown by Rangell, but they are also out of harmony with each other, as we can frequently observe in marriages between people of hysterical and obsessional personalities. The obsessional fails to understand how the hysteric tolerates the constant emotional turmoil which, for him, would prove traumatic, while the hysteric has no sympathy with the degree of protective defense which, for the obsessional character, is essential for comfort.

In the upbringing of children, where frustration, criticism, and punishment are concerned, it is well known that the individual child tends to adapt to the level of parental handling and reacts traumatically only to the unexpected, i.e., the unfamiliar. A harsh scolding or slaps by a habitually tolerant parent may have a devastating, "traumatic" effect on a child, while the same treatment is assimilated in a much less dramatic manner by the children of harsh and exacting parents. The phenomenon met here obviously is the direct opposite of the much-discussed sensitization to traumatization. Looking at Solnit's patient, Margaret, in this light, we may wonder why she reacted so traumatically to the threat of abandonment and had failed to raise her stimulus barrier despite constant exposure to a nagging and inconsiderate mother.

Provocation of Trauma

That the ego's defensive system acts as protection against traumatization becomes evident whenever an individual is prevented from using a habitual defense in a situation which represents a specific danger for him. This can be seen most clearly in cases of denial or of phobic avoidance, both of which are open to interference by external agencies (in contrast to regression, repression, reaction formation, turning passive into active, turning against the self, etc., which are removed from outside influence). The phobic patient who is made to meet the object of his anxiety (instead of avoiding it) is thereby forced undefended into a traumatic situation and breaks down in panic; so does the individual who has warded off a painful reality fact by denial (impending blindness, cancer, threatening object loss) and is forced to take cognizance of it against his own intentions.

Although we do not experiment with human beings in situations of such magnitude, there are laboratory settings outside the human range which are relevant in this respect. You may remember the experimentation done with cats and monkeys reported on by Masserman in which the animals were rendered "neurotic," allegedly by being exposed to the choice between avoiding a painful stimulus and attaining a wished-for one. To my mind, the reason for this was different. It seemed to me that, exposed to the painful stimulus, the monkey had at its disposal only one built-in response, i.e., the defense of flight. Since this could not be carried out in the laboratory conditions that nailed him to the spot, the animal became confused, panicky, and—traumatized.

Concerning Qualitative Considerations

The problem of quality as opposed to quantity of excitation has been discussed under the aspect of sensitization to trauma by Greenacre, Rangell, Solnit, and Waelder.

As stated by Greenacre, no previous trauma, however well it apparently has been overcome, will remain dormant if touched on by occurrences of the same psychic quality. This creates the obligation to consider traumatic events from their qualitative aspect and, if possible, to establish a hierarchy among them.

To begin with external traumatic influences, what is inflicted on human beings from outside, in a shape too upsetting to be coped with, may be the result of natural forces beyond human control or the result of *accidents, illness, frustrations, deprivations,* etc.; or it may be inflicted on them intentionally in the form of *attack, insult,* or *punishment.*

Such external traumata are turned into internal ones if they touch on, or coincide with, or symbolize the fulfillment either of deep-seated anxieties or of wish fantasies. In the first instance, the traumatic event is experienced as *annihilation* (in extreme danger to life), as *abandonment* by the object (as in the case of Margaret), as *castration* (operations, threat of blindness). In the latter case, the wishes fulfilled (i.e., overfulfilled) by the trauma may be aggressive ones (such as *death wishes* against siblings or parents) or sexual ones *(seductions)*, and these again may be ego syntonic or dystonic, phase adequate or phase inappropriate. When the traumatic event fulfills a phase-inappropriate wish, the result is disruption of the developmental sequence (Greenacre); when it fulfills ego-dystonic wishes, the results are outbreaks of panic, their prototype in normal life being anxiety dreams, nightmares, etc.

Whether traumata of one kind sensitize an individual to repetitions of events of the same specific quality only, or to traumatization in general, remains an open question. So does the problem whether inner events as such can cause trauma (Rangell), without the upset being triggered off by external happenings.

Finally, I cannot help commenting on the concept of a "constructive trauma" alluded to by Robert Waelder, which I find difficult to assimilate. We may compare it with the event of an earthquake which shatters a city. If this city is built up again afterward on improved lines, this is doubtless a successful reconstruction. But, to my mind, the notion of constructiveness attaches to the later efforts, not to the event itself, which remains shattering, i.e., destructive. This leads into the problem of recovery after trauma, which I shall deal with in my final remarks (see Section III).

II

DISCUSSION REMARKS[1]

Traumatization in the Blind

Blindness presents us with the clinical picture of an abnormal condition that is present from the beginning of life and exists for a considerable period of time as a nontraumatic one. It acquires traumatic quality only when two different developmental stages are reached: on the side of the ego, various functions need to mature sufficiently to make the child aware of the lack of sight and the implied difference from normal people; on the side of the drives, the phallic stage has to be reached to turn this awareness into the semblance of a castration shock. When both advances occur simultaneously, awareness of the visual defect may become a traumatic experience. For the therapeutic handling of the situation, we may extract from this the hint that every effort should be made to assist the blind child's ego in assimilating the fact of blindness before the phallic stage has come into being.

The Concept of Trauma and the Result of the Traumatic Event

To return to the two different processes described earlier by Robert Waelder under the terms "evolution" and "revolu-

[1] The remarks contained in this section were all made in response to questions and statements by the other participants.

tion": perhaps we can include under evolution those happenings within the mental apparatus which occur under the aegis of the ego, while revolution designates a state in which the ego in its role as mediator is overthrown and put out of action.

What happens after this moment—the traumatic one—deserves separate consideration. What we can introduce here is the concept of recovery from trauma. Commensurate with the injury suffered by the ego, the time lag until reinstatement of ego activity is of varying length, and the questions which arise are not only when recovery takes place, but whether it takes place at all, in what form, on what basis; whether the individual's state after recovery is regressed or, perhaps, advanced in comparison with the pretraumatic state, etc.

The period between trauma and recovery has been described by Leo Rangell as a state of helplessness. I should like to stress here that this helplessness should not be considered an ego state, but a state of disorientation and powerlessness in which the organism finds itself when it is deprived of ego mediation. As Phyllis Greenacre has shown, the organism then falls back on pre-ego mechanisms, since the ego has temporarily become unable to fulfill its task.

Logically, this leads to the conclusion that, instead of being extended as it is at present, the concept of trauma should profitably be restricted to those stages in human life when structuralization has taken place and ego mediation is the normal order of the day. While the infant is an undifferentiated being, he experiences distress, not trauma in the strict sense of the word. But this distress of the infant is probably identical with the older being's helplessness before recovery from trauma. What the two have in common is the absence of a functioning ego.

External and Internal Causes of Trauma

[In response to Robert Waelder, who emphasized the difficulties of reconstructing external events and sorting out what factors triggered, e.g., a heart attack.]

This is no more than our familiar problem of the complementary series. The question can be reformulated as follows: Are there any external events which will cause pathology without help from internal ones; or any internal events which will do so without external provocation? There may be at the extreme ends of the series events of such magnitude that they can cause pathology on their own, but we have no certainty about this.

In our clinic, we are at present puzzled by the case of a girl of thirteen, who was sexually abused by her father at age five. The father came before the court and received a long prison sentence. While he was away, the child developed well, only to become disturbed when the father, obviously a paranoiac, came out of prison and took up contact with her again. She knows that her father went to prison for some offense committed against her, "but I don't know what, and they don't tell me what." It is difficult to decide on the basis of the present picture whether the symptoms she is developing now—such as school failure, etc.—are the direct outcome of the past event, which by rights should have been a traumatic one, or whether they are merely the result of the mystery which she resents, vague guilt feelings about her own role in the father's imprisonment, the advent of adolescence with the accompanying heightened sensitivity toward sexual matters, etc. Although the seduction itself is without question a massive external event, it seems impossible to separate it off from the internal repercussions so far as pathogenesis is concerned.

Neglected Children

In my opinion, these are severely deprived children[2] who, owing to the absence of opportunity and response from the object world, have failed to develop normal object relationships in their infancy, i.e., children in whom very important affective potentialities have remained untapped. When an object is offered at last, the children respond in ways which belong to an earlier developmental period. I cannot see any similarity to a trauma in this.

The deprivation itself may have been traumatic in the sense used by Phyllis Greenacre, but do we really wish to widen the concept to include this?

In the children described by Peter Neubauer, the primary damage is to the libido, not the ego. Nevertheless, when the child reacts with early libidinal attitudes, these are accompanied by regression to early ego responses. These latter resemble the regressions which take place after the trauma, but this resemblance is superficial and does not turn the event itself into a trauma.

Ways of Coping with Traumatic Events

In 1956, Erna Furman published the case of a child who to all intents and purposes gave the impression of a severely

[2] [Peter Neubauer described children who lacked mothering during their first two years.]

retarded, mentally deficient child but whose analysis revealed that she was a seduced child. From the traumatic moment of seduction onward, the child had ceased to develop either libidinally or on the ego side, and nothing had happened further except endless disguised repetitions of the event itself, in the classical manner of a traumatic neurosis.

Mary Bergen (1958) published a case report on the effect of severe trauma on a four-year-old child. In this case we expected the event to be even more traumatic than it proved to be.

Actually, the child was faced with two facts, both equally difficult to assimilate: that her mother had been killed and that her much-loved father was a murderer. She and her siblings were permitted to visit the father in the mental institution where he was confined, and they showed no fear or horror of him, sat on his lap, fondled him, etc. Nevertheless, one had to foresee that, at some later date, the realization of the father's deed might acquire traumatic impact. At the time, this was not in evidence.

What had had traumatic impact was the mother's shouting to the child "Get out" just before she was killed—a fact we could deduce from the child's transference behavior. She made an excellent transference to her therapist and repeated in this relationship all the difficulties she had experienced with her mother, her jealousies, disobediences, etc. This included the problem of leaving at the end of her session. Later, at a high point of her positive transference, she suddenly showed herself ready to make what for her was the major sacrifice by asserting passionately: "And I shall always leave when you tell me to." We took this as proof that to "go away," "get out," was the central point of the tragic experience for her.

This child, as many of our bombed-out war children did, repeated her experience in play, whereas the children who are fully traumatized are blocked in play and instead relive the event in the place of realistic behavior.

I agree fully with Phyllis Greenacre that no experience of the kind suffered by this child (and even experiences of lesser magnitude) can be assimilated without leaving a scar, whether visibly or otherwise: and there is no scar in mental life which cannot reopen under specific conditions. If this happens, the whole structure of the personality is shaken to the core.

The Essence of Traumatization

It is true that the notion of a stimulus barrier is a metaphor, but the pathological processes which occur as the result of a breakthrough are very real indeed. That the ego is put out of action is a fact and in this lies, to my mind, the essence of the trauma. A child may meet a major detrimental experience without being traumatized, i.e., may cope with it with the help of one or the other of his ego mechanisms. When this happens, we should not speak of traumatization.

I quote in this connection from another case of our wartime experience. A boy of three and a half had lost his father, who was killed in an air raid. For a number of days the distracted mother went from one warden's post to another to trace him, dragging the child along with her. Finally, when his body was found and identified, she suffered a psychotic breakdown and was sent to a mental institution where she remained.

The boy arrived in our Residential Nursery, apparently normal, and shared life and play with the other children. He gave no sign of the experience he had gone through, could not be made to verbalize it, to re-enact it in play, etc. The only symptom which appeared was a tendency to be hypochondriacally concerned about himself. He was afraid of catching cold and wrapped himself up in overcoat and scarf, no matter how warm the weather was. If asked to unwrap himself, he simply refused with the explanation: "My Mummy would not want me to get cold." Obviously, he used the ego mechanism of identifying with the absent mother, and he mothered himself.

For six months he lived thus, outwardly normal, but internally as mother and child rolled into one. Then, on the occasion of a slight intercurrent illness, when he was comfortably installed in the sickroom under the care of the sick nurse, he began to play the bombing with the help of small toys given to him on a tray. Gradually, the events were readmitted to consciousness—the death of the father, the disappearance of the mother, who, in his understanding, had joined the dead father. He then could verbalize what, up to that time, had been contained in the hypochondriacal symptom.

The question arising here is whether this child had been traumatized in the true sense of the word. Ordinarily speaking, we would be inclined to say so. Seen metapsychologically, there is no doubt that his ego remained in action and that an ego mechanism (identification) was used to cope with the experience.

We met our little boy again after an interval of almost twenty years. Brought up, after leaving our Nursery, by his grandparents in Ireland, he had turned into a big, strapping guardsman in whom no one could have recognized the formerly delicate child.

Nevertheless, it is easy to imagine that he would not be immune to breakdown, given a war and bombing experience which approximates his father's fate or, perhaps, the incidence of mental illness and object loss of a wife which repeats his mother's illness and desertion of him.

Repetition

With regard to "repetitive working over," we should differentiate between two types of repetition. One is an ego mechanism, repeating an experience with variations suitable for its assimilation, such as turning a passive experience into an active one. The other is a pre-ego process, i.e., the repetition compulsion pure and simple.

III

FINAL SUMMARY

I would like to cast my final statement in a personal form, summarizing under a small number of headings the gains which I derived from our discussion of trauma.

Definition of the Concept of Trauma

Like everybody else, I have tended to use the term "trauma" rather loosely up to now, but I shall find it easier to avoid this in the future. Whenever I am tempted to call an event in a child's or adult's life "traumatic," I shall ask myself some further questions. Do I mean that the event was upsetting; that it was significant for altering the course of further development; that it was pathogenic? Or do I really mean traumatic in the strict sense of the word, i.e., shattering, devastating, causing internal disruption by putting ego functioning and ego mediation out of action?

Evidence of Trauma

If the last-named eventuality is the one I have in mind, some further questions become relevant, namely, those as to the evidence contained in the clinical material. What I would consider as evidence for the occurrence of a traumatic event is, as an immediate reaction to it, a state of paralysis of action; of numbness of feeling; in the case of a child, a temper tantrum, physical responses via the vegetative nervous system taking the place of psychic reactions. What all these have in common is that they are substandard from the point of view of the ego, and therefore signify that ego functioning has been put out of action and that the organism has been forced back to the use of archaic, pre-ego modes of functioning.

Characterization of the Ego Injury

If evidence for one or several of these reactions is sufficient and establishes, to my mind, the incidence of trauma, some further points need to be clarified. From what direction was the attack launched to which the ego fell victim? Did the overwhelming threat arise from the external world in the first instance or was there some constellation in the internal world with which the ego found itself unable to cope, to the extent of breaking down completely? Was it only the internal happenings which lent meaning to the external

ones, or vice versa? It is of the utmost importance, theoretically, to apportion pathogenic responsibility to the
right quarters, but, clinically, no other demand is as difficult to fulfill.

Problems of Quality

Next, when assessing the internal meaning of the traumatic
event, I shall remember not to confuse my own with the
victim's appraisal of the happening. The trauma may be
derived from a deprivation, an injury, accident, attack, or
from a deliberate punishment inflicted by the environment.
Internally, it may be understood as the realization of a
fantastic fear or as the excessive fulfillment of a wishful
fantasy, the latter being either ego syntonic or dystonic,
phase adequate or phase inappropriate. I should not expect
this internal meaning to reveal itself except during the
process of analysis.

Range of Traumatic Result

I shall wish to determine further the extent to which the
ego has been put out of action by the traumatic event, i.e.,
the duration of disturbance and its range. Is dysfunction
only partial or wholesale? Are there portions of ego functioning left intact and which are these portions? Above all,
are some defenses left working or, perhaps, is the whole
defense organization merely reduced to a more primitive
level? Such regressions should not be confused with a total
suspension of ego functioning and speak against the occurrence of trauma in the strictest sense of the word.

Recovery from Trauma

A further important aspect to consider is the mode of recovery from a traumatic event, i.e., the eventual reinstatement of ego functioning following its suspension. I shall look at the clinical evidence to answer points such as the following: whether recovery is instantaneous, fast, slow, or, most important of all, whether it is occurring at all; by what means it is brought about, and whether the transition from pre-ego to ego functioning (for example, from the repetition compulsion to denial or from the passive into active mechanism) is a sudden or a gradual one. I shall find it difficult, probably, in many instances, to distinguish between residual ego functioning and the recovery of function, which may look identical insofar as the clinical material is concerned.

The Postrecovery State

It will be my next task to compare the patient's (child's or adult's) state after recovery with the level of personality development which had existed before the incidence of trauma. Especially in the case of children, these questions have to be answered: Is recovery complete so far as the developmental level is concerned? Is ego functioning taken up again at a regressed level, or do the traumatic results have to be considered as "constructive," in the sense that, during the period of ego suspension, developmental advances have been made, as they sometimes also occur during sleep, illness, etc.? In other words, how far has ego activity been interrupted, harmed, or aided by the trauma?

Considerations of Development

Again, in the case of children, it will be necessary to relate the traumatic event to the whole of the developmental process and to determine how far maturation and forward development as such have been affected in their course, i.e., arrested, distorted, deflected from the usual chronological sequence of progressive levels, stages, and phases on the drive and ego sides. It will be more prudent in this respect not to count on a straightforward correlation between the economic magnitude of trauma and a correspondingly severe disruption of development.

Diagnostic Considerations

With regard to diagnostic categorization, care has to be taken not to confuse the traumatic event with its potential result, i.e., the traumatic neurosis. For my own use I am determined to reserve the term "traumatic neurosis" for those cases where all the pathology, or at least the bulk of it, has to be considered the direct consequence of the traumatic event and corresponds to attempts to assimilate it. In clinical practice, we shall not be surprised to find that such pure cases are much rarer than those mixed states where the traumatic event becomes pathogenic mainly through triggering off an ordinary neurotic conflict or neurosis that has lain dormant.

15

Obsessional Neurosis

A Summary of Psychoanalytic Views
(1966 [1965])

Despite the help in summarizing given to me by my three colleagues, K. T. Calder, P. G. Myerson, and S. Ritvo, the task of surveying the Congress's views on obsessional neurosis remains a formidable one. Above all, it is not one which can be compressed into a short time, and for this I ask the indulgence of an audience already tired out by listening.

In selecting obsessional neurosis as the main topic of

Presented as a summary of psychoanalytic views at the conclusion of the 24th Congress of the International Psycho-Analytical Association, Amsterdam, Holland, July 30, 1965. First published in the *International Journal of Psycho-Analysis*, 47:116-122, 1966.

the Congress, the Program Committee, knowingly or un-knowingly, seems to have been guided by two sentences taken from Freud's "Notes upon a Case of Obsessional Neurosis" (1909b). One, that he was puzzled why it is so difficult to understand obsessional neurosis when, after all, the thought processes in it are so near to ours and the mys-terious transition from mind to body, met with in hysteria, is not present. Second, that in this respect the concerted effort of a group of people may succeed where the single individual fails.

As regards the first point, some guidance has already been offered to us by one of the papers contributed to the Con-gress: namely, that obsessional neurosis is hard to unravel not in spite of, but because of, the pathology being located in the thought processes themselves, thereby attacking the patient's very means of communicating with us as well as our ability to identify with him and the aberrations of his logic and reasoning. As regards the second point, it is left to our interpretation whether what Freud had in mind was concentrated work on obsessional neurosis by many analysts individually, or the deliberate effort in group discussion and interchange of opinion, as we have witnessed it during this Congress, an effort the result of which we are now en-couraged to assess.[1]

THE CONCEPT OF OBSESSIONAL NEUROSIS AS BROUGHT TO THE CONGRESS

I assume that all members of the Congress brought with them to Amsterdam their own definition of the structure

[1] For the relevant Congress papers and discussions dealing with obsessional neurosis, see *Int. J. Psycho-Anal.*, 47:123-217, 1966.

of an obsessional neurosis and that they listened to the proceedings with the questions in mind how far this personal conception needed amendment, i.e., to be made more precise; to be extended on the basis of more clinical material; or to be adjusted to accommodate advances in factual knowledge and new theories.

Speaking, thus, as the average individual Congress member, I review in what follows my own picture of obsessional neurosis.

As regards its *range*, in consensus with general opinion, I have always viewed it as a specific kind of mental constellation, extending from the ego syntonic and near normal—during development, in character formation—to the status of an extremely severe neurotic disturbance, bordering occasionally on the schizoid and schizophrenic proper. While, at the former end of the series, the obsessional manifestations prove stabilizing for personality formation, at the extreme latter end they are devastatingly crippling and equally harmful for the internal equilibrium and the external adaptation of the individual.

As regards the *quality of the id content* warded off in obsessional neurosis, my case material never led me to doubt that these are the impulses of the pregenital (i.e., prephallic) anal-sadistic stage.

As regards the *ego devices* used for the purpose of warding off from consciousness, what I am familiar with are the following in varying combinations: denial, repression, regression, reaction formation, isolation, undoing, magical thinking, doubting, indecision, intellectualization, rationalization—altogether a formidable array, all of them, with the exception of regression, operating strictly within the area of the thought processes.

As regards the *external clinical picture*, I find this determined above all by the prominence of the reaction formations which provide the impression of stability and immutability; by the intensity of the countercathexes which provides the mental strain; and by the profusion of intellectualizations, i.e., the attempt to bind id energies through secondary process thinking. It is the last-named factor which ties the occurrence of obsessional neuroses to a particular level of ego development before which other than obsessional solutions of conflict have to be resorted to.

That there is no obsessional neurosis in which reaction formations and intellectualization do not play a large part also helps me to differentiate between obsessions proper and some other manifestations which appear similar on the surface and, for this reason, are often confused with them. What I have in mind here are, for one, the repetitive tendencies as they are found in the very young, normally, and in mental defectives, abnormally; they are pre-ego mechanisms arising from the repetition compulsion and have nothing in common with obsession except their monotony. Secondly, what is often wrongly classified as obsessive are the urges which govern the behavior of addicts, psychopaths, many delinquents, etc.; but, far from being compulsive, i.e., reactive, defensive, these are merely compelling, due to the full force of an id urge, not of an ego device behind them.

As to the *conditions which are favorable* for the formation of an obsessional neurosis, my views of them coincide with the ideas to be found in the analytic literature. There is the suggestion that obsessional defense sets in if the ego matures more quickly than the drives, i.e., in those instances where the anal-sadistic trends come to their height when

ego and superego are already too far advanced to be able to tolerate them. There also is the typical, and widely accepted, precondition that obsessions arise when the individual regresses libidinally from the phallic to the anal-sadistic level while ego and superego retain their moral and aesthetic standards.

Obsessional outcomes are also promoted by a constitutional increase in the intensity of the anal-sadistic tendencies, or a constitutional preference for the use of defense mechanisms such as reaction formation, intellectualization, isolation, etc. Both are found in the children of severely obsessional parents, probably as the result of inheritance combined with parental handling. Traumatic happenings during the anal phase, such as seductions or undue interference by excessively early and strict bowel training, also exert their influence in the same direction.

Finally, to cover all the facts known to us, any satisfactory conception of obsessional neurosis has to go beyond the aspect of intersystemic conflict between id, ego, and superego, and take into account *the intrasystemic contradictions* within the id such as they exist between love-hate, passivity-activity, femininity-masculinity. It is true, of course, that these are present in everybody as the ambivalence and bisexuality inherent in human nature. But, normally, ambivalence is taken care of by fusion between libido and aggression; and bisexuality, by the synthetic function, which deals with opposing strivings as soon as they arise from the unconscious and approach the conscious surface of the mind. Both these functions seem to fail in individuals who are destined to become obsessional; or, to express it better, it is above all the failure of fusion and synthesis which determines the occurrence of an obsessional neurosis. Why

this happens is still an open question, although some possible answers are hinted at in the literature: when excessive amounts of aggression are turned inward against the self, the individual becomes torn within himself and develops a preference for inner strife as opposed to striving for inner harmony. This increases normal ambivalence, and ambivalent strivings are used for the purpose of perpetuating inner conflicts. For the obsessional, then, it is as natural to be at cross-purposes with himself as he invariably is at cross-purposes with his objects. Aggressive argumentation and hostile attitudes to the environment run parallel with the torturing relationships which exist between his inner agencies.

The *variations in the symptomatology* of obsessional neurosis seem to me accounted for by the many elements which enter into its causation such as the prominence of either the sadistic or the anal tendencies in the id; the excessive use of any one or of several of the relevant defense mechanisms; the different rate of growth in id and ego; the prominence of either mother or father as the main target of the child's death wishes; the interaction between intersystemic and intrasystemic conflicts, etc. There are so many elements, and the possible combinations between them are so endless, that it needs not an analyst's but a mathematician's mind to calculate their number.

QUESTIONS BROUGHT TO THE CONGRESS

Doubtless, the average member of the Congress also brought with him an array of open questions, hoping to find answers to them.

As it emerged in the discussions, we seem to know more

about obsessional neurosis as a completed mental structure and about its impact on character and personality than we know about either its prestages or its future fate. Accordingly, the queries turned very noticeably in two directions: the past and the future of the obsessional neurosis.

The Past

The question was raised repeatedly *how early* we can detect the signs indicating that a particular individual is predestined to develop an obsessional neurosis.

Can it already be seen in the *oral phase*, or, at any rate, before anal sadism has achieved phase dominance?

If this can be done, in *which areas* of the infant's personality should we expect to find the clues?

Will the success or failure of the *mother-infant* relationship be a decisive factor?

Or is it the type and rate of *ego* development by which the issue is decided?

In other words, is there a *recognizable matrix* within which the ground is prepared for obsessional development?

The Future

Is the adult obsessional neurosis always *preceded* by an infantile one?

If not, which other type of neurotic disturbance is its most frequent *forerunner?*

Or vice versa: is an infantile obsessional neurosis always *followed* by an adult one?

If not, what is its further fate?

Does experience indicate that an infantile obsessional neurosis can be *outgrown?*

If not, what are the most frequent developments in later life, *neurotic* or *psychotic?*

In short, the whole "natural history" of obsessional neurosis, past, present, and future, was brought into discussion during the Congress, at one time or another.

MATERIAL OFFERED TO THE CONGRESS

For the elucidation of the foregoing problems, we were offered two patients and, concerning them three case histories, namely, the Rat Man, analyzed by Freud, and Frankie treated first by Berta Bornstein and subsequently by Samuel Ritvo, the latter presenting the "Correlation of a Childhood and Adult Neurosis," the main theme of the Congress program. We owe thanks to Berta Bornstein as well as Ritvo for allowing their material to be discussed freely, from all viewpoints, and searched for significant clues in all directions.

That one of the case histories under scrutiny concerned a child was profitable, of course, but also led to some complications.

In discussing the diagnosis of Frankie's infantile disturbance and the changeover in his symptomatology from phobic to obsessional, the Congress, I felt, did not acknowledge sufficiently the difference between children and adults so far as diagnostic categorization is concerned. As expressed later by some authors, the current psychiatric diagnoses do not fit our adult analytic patients. I should like to add that they fit our child cases even less and that the need for their reformulation is urgent to avoid misunderstandings as they occurred in discussing Frankie.

While the adult patient is a person in his own right, his self divided off from the object world and structured inwardly, and while his pathology is more or less static, nothing of this is true for the child. The younger he is, the more undifferentiated is his personality; his self, or later at least his superego, merges with the objects; his body merges with his mind; his affects, with his intellect. His defense organization is incomplete and his pathology fluid, open to developmental alterations. While passing from one stage to another, he also passes through crises, upheavals, chaotic states, for which transient solutions are adopted.

As regards Frankie's change from a predominantly phobic child into a predominantly obsessional adolescent, it did not seem profitable to me that the Congress looked for reasons to the technical handling of the case, or discussed the alternative whether this change was due either to drive regression (from phallic-genital to anal) or to ego progression (from bodily to purely mental mechanisms). To me it seemed obvious that his symptomatology had to undergo changes since he was certainly not ill enough, and also helped analytically enough, not to be at a standstill between age seven and twenty-one. His object world had changed progressively, the mother being replaced by a young female. His drives had changed level, the genital dangers and concerns being added to the previous phallic ones. Since, according to the severity of his infantile disturbance, he remained in precarious mental balance, the adult pathology was determined neither by the child analyst's influence nor by an either-or of progression versus regression, but was determined by a combination of his progressively intellectual defense organization with a regressive inability to tolerate and maintain genitality and object love.

Much valuable Congress time was spent on this discussion.

For the rest, the material offered proved excellent as a clinical basis for much theoretical speculation. From this it seems possible to me to abstract some distinct topics and to outline some contributions made to them by the Congress.

CONGRESS TOPICS

The Matrix of the Obsessional Neurosis

To pursue every mental disorder back to its earliest indications in individual life is considered the duty of every analyst and, as such, has loomed large in many of the Congress papers.

In 1909, when Freud published his "Notes upon a Case of Obsessional Neurosis," it was a pioneering achievement to look behind the apparent pathogenic importance of recent events, such as the father's death, difficulties in love affairs, etc., and to unearth the upsetting events of the anal-sadistic stage as preceding them. Today, with much analytic interest concentrated on the first year of life, the anal period as the beginning of pathology seems disappointingly late to many authors. Hence, every attempt was made to antedate the onset of obsessional neuroses.

In fact, almost every element of early infantile life was brought forward in this respect, and especially the events within the early mother-infant relationship were named as relevant pathogenic factors. Weight was given to the consequences of the mother's failure to cathect the infant or the infant's failure to relate to her; to the mother's influence on normal body-mind interaction; her failure to act as

comforter and protector against anxiety; her assistance or lack of it in the infant's task of joining up part objects and establishing whole object relationships; her role in determining the later difference between the neurotic and the schizoid type of obsessional neurotics, the former operating within the area of object love, the latter falling back on more primitive narcissistic positions. Equal weight was given by other authors to the experience of object loss, and this particular factor was also transposed back and inserted into the history of the Rat Man via the early death of his beloved sister.

Important as all these points are in general, it must have struck many listeners, as it struck me, that here the Congress failed to distinguish adequately between the specific and the nonspecific, since only some of the suggestions quoted represent elements of the first kind. Lack of a healthy earliest relationship to the mother has its consequences, certainly, for the infant's interest in and cathexis of the environment; leads to delayed or defective unfolding of many ego functions; damages the building up of a defense organization, of drive and anxiety control. But, and this seems to me a compelling argument, the resulting faulty personality development can serve equally well as a basis for any other neurotic or psychotic disorder or disturbance of adaptation. If we want to restrict ourselves to those factors in the mother-child relationship which are truly specific for obsessional neurosis, then we are left with only a few, such as damage done to the synthetic function; to the capacity for fusion of love and hate; to the ability of maintaining object love as contrasted with self-love. Furthermore, where early object loss is concerned, we have to think in less global terms. Losing a love object in early life

(through rejection, withdrawal, neglect, separation, death) is an experience which can initiate a variety of disturbances. What is significant for obsessional neurosis is not the event as such but the child's belief that it is the result of his own death wishes and the feelings of guilt attached to this interpretation.

We should also take into account that an excellent early relationship to the mother may promote rapid ego growth and, instead of safeguarding the individual, this may be instrumental in creating the very precocity of superego functions which we have met as one of the preconditions of obsessional neurosis.

The Instinctual Background of Obsessional Neurosis

Not all the contributors to the topic were ready to accept the classical view that it is the id content of the anal-sadistic phase which is warded off by means of the obsessional symptomatology; and some rival claims were raised, especially for the tendencies toward oral incorporation of the object and for voyeurism. There was even one attempt to disconnect obsessional neurosis altogether from any specific instinctual content and to consider its symptomatology instead as wholly determined by the ego mechanisms which are characteristic of it, whatever the nature of the warded-off material. What speaks against this opinion is the fact that in clinical work we always uncover anal-sadistic material when we undo defenses such as reaction formations, isolation, undoing, i.e., the obsessional ones *par excellence*, while other id material is found to have been dealt with by other mechanisms and to produce different symptoms.

What I missed in this particular area of the discussion

was a more detailed investigation into the events and trends of the anal-sadistic phase itself. Little was said about the distinction between anal passivity and anal aggression as the source of danger, although the difference between these two eventualities is decisive for the type of obsessional symptomatology which is produced. Neither was there mention of how difficult it is to decide in the analysis of an obsessional patient whether his excessive anal passivity is a direct instinctual expression or a reaction against his anal sadism, or, vice versa, whether his aggression is a direct id urge or reactively heightened to ward off passive fantasies. Another aspect hardly touched on was the economic one, i.e., the question of relative quantity in the instinctual endowment of obsessional individuals.

On the other hand, differences were brought out sharply and argued closely with regard to the role of drive regression. For all authors operating within the classical theory, the step backward from the phallic-oedipal level to anal sadism is a *sine qua non* for the formation of an obsessional neurosis. For many others, this seems to be an expandable pathogenic factor.

A Possible Link between Matrix and Anal Sadism

Personally, I could not help waiting for the mention of a specific factor which might bridge the gap between the relevance of the early mother-infant relationship and that of the later anal-sadistic stage. I had met with this in a case and wondered whether other analysts had had similar experiences.

In the instance I have in mind, a boy in his anal phase (two to three years) exasperated his mother by being a per-

sistent soiler. Resisting all her efforts to make him defecate at the appointed time and place, he dirtied himself all over as soon as he was left on his own. This remained unexplained until, one day, he was actually overheard to talk to his excrement and call on it to come and keep him company. It then emerged that he had been exposed to traumatic separations from his mother in his first year, had suffered neglect from caretaking strangers, bewildering changes of environment, etc., and that, in the course of these events his libido had withdrawn from the object world and turned to the body product, thereby producing this particular exacerbation of anal concerns.[2]

Links of this kind between failure in object relations and heightened anality may be more common than we realize. If that should be the case, the repercussions for later defense against anality may be significant. However that may be, no instance of this type was mentioned at the Congress.

The Ego in Obsessional Neurosis

According to the trends of the time, the contributions to this topic were numerous and left few areas unexplored.

One innovation, brought more or less independently by a number of authors, was the notion of a general cognitive and perceptive style of the ego. This implies an extension of the concepts of defensive devices, defense mechanisms, defense organization, to include besides the ego's dealings with danger, anxiety, affects, etc., its everyday functioning as well, such as perceiving, thinking, abstracting, conceptualizing. An ego style, in this sense, is linked with the

[2] [This case has also been referred to in Volume IV, ch. 16, and this volume, ch. 17.]

concept of defense but by no means identical with it. It represents an attempt to embrace the area of conflict as well as the conflict-free area of secondary process functioning.

The authors claim that some of these "ego styles" are more relevant for the obsessional type of defense than others. Since they assume that ego styles are adopted fairly early in infantile life, and remain permanent, they conclude that detailed examination of ego functioning in this respect may enable the observer to predict the individual's later choice of neurosis.

With regard to early and transient obsessional symptomatology, stress was laid by some authors on its signal function for the ego's affect and energy control, as opposed to the later function of obsessional symptoms as static and limiting compromise formations.

No new defense mechanisms were added to those with which we are familiar.

Mutual Influences between Id and Ego in Obsessional Neurosis

Although the interactions between id and ego are central to the problem of obsessional neurosis, only two of the main topics are singled out here as having played a prominent part in individual papers and group discussions.

THE RELATIONS BETWEEN DRIVE AND DEFENSE

Several possibilities were offered to the audience in this respect:

(a) For warding off id content, the ego is limited to employing the mechanisms available to it according to its level of development. This is a chronological view according to which early instinctual trends are dealt with inevitably by the most primitive early defense mechanisms, and drive and defense are interlinked according to the time of their emergence.

(b) Instinctual level and ego defense level do not always coincide owing to id and ego progressing occasionally at different speeds. Accordingly, for example, obsessional defenses may appear in the ego before the individual has reached the anal phase.

(c) Every instinctual trend evokes a defense mechanism specific to it, and defenses change for developmental reasons in conformity with changes of the id content.

(d) At an early date, under the influence of the id, the ego develops a style which from then onward remains permanent, irrespective of developmental changes.

It must have been obvious to the audience that some of these theoretical suggestions are incompatible with each other and that a choice will have to be made between them on the basis of further clinical observations.

THE RELATIONS BETWEEN DRIVE REGRESSION AND
EGO REGRESSION IN OBSESSIONAL NEUROSIS

Those authors who regard regression as an indispensable element in the buildup of an obsessional neurosis brought forward a number of valuable suggestions, amendments, and additions to existing theory, such as the following:

(a) The term regression with regard to its occurrence in the obsessional neurosis should not be used in a global way, but a careful distinction should be made between regression on the instinctual side and on the ego side, including the interactions between them.

(b) If drive regression is followed by ego regression, a

distinction should be made between structural regression, (i.e., lowering of standards, demands, etc.) and functional regression (i.e., return to magical, wishful, primary process thinking, lessening of reality testing, of the synthetic function, etc.).

(c) Regression in id or ego should be considered from the aspects of depth, spread, irreversibility, etc.

Obsessional Neurosis versus Phobia

Based on the case of Frankie, great interest was expressed in the change of pathology from a phobic to a predominantly obsessional illness. The phenomenon was discussed from a number of angles, such as the following:

(a) as a step from defense by motor action and body language to defense by thought manipulation, possibly representing an advance in ego maturation;

(b) as a general phenomenon within the body-mind problem: while in hysteria the body behaves as if on its own, the mind does the same in the obsessional neurosis;

(c) from the aspect of countercathexis: while, in a phobia, representation of danger may be compressed successfully into a single material object, locus, etc., which is then avoided, obsessional symptoms have the tendency to spread and a greater and more constant expenditure of countercathexis is needed to hold them in check;

(d) from the aspect of analytic therapy: during the analysis of adult obsessionals, earlier phobic states reappear slowly, which is a favorable prognostic sign. In child analysis, on the other hand, where obsessional defense may dissolve quickly, uncontrolled impulsive behavior appears instead, a difference which is, so far, unexplained.

Attempts at Avoiding Obsessional Pathology

During the discussion of the Frankie case, certain elements were mentioned as part of his obsessional neurosis which, I believe, permit a different classification.

His "could not care less" attitude, his depersonalization of the analyst, his insolence in the transference are, to my mind, items of pathological behavior aimed at playing down his own feelings as well as devaluating the object world. They are on a par with the "computer ideal" of some individuals, i.e., the conception of themselves as a mind without body, or an intellect without feelings. Such attitudes are defensive, not in the sense of warding off or immobilizing a particular instinctual trend, but more generally in the sense of trying to do away with sources of danger altogether. When they are successful, the need for further defense activity is eliminated at the expense of a character or behavior change, and no obsessional neurosis proper is organized.

The well-known sexualization and consequent play with anxiety serve the same purpose. If a potential danger situation is turned into a source of masochistic pleasure, no further symptom formation is necessary.

Beneficial and Harmful Effects, Successes, Failures, and Limits of Obsessional Neurosis

It remains to summarize the opinions expressed concerning the impact of obsessional development on personality growth, on character formation, and, more generally, on the maintenance or loss of mental equilibrium.

Repeated mention was made of the *beneficial* aspect of

the defenses characteristic of obsessional neurosis, namely, of their serving as safeguards against impulsive behavior, delinquency or schizophrenic breakdown—in short, of their stabilizing effect. Under the same heading, obsessional symptomatology was described as halting regression from proceeding to levels earlier than the anal phase, and thereby preventing further spread of pathology.

In connection with the Rat Man and Frankie, their *harmful* effect on ego activity and the distorting effect on the personality as a whole were discussed.

Frankie was also used as an example to demonstrate the partial *failure* of obsessional defense, his doubts about his intellectual capacity being regarded as a return of the repressed castration fantasies, as well as, in general, the return of the warded-off self-awareness of defect. Similar doubts of obsessional patients about their own intactness, whether intellectual, emotional, aesthetic or moral, are well known and, I believe, always indicate that the obsessional symptoms have failed, partially at least, to accomplish their objective.

Finally, the *limits* of obsessional neurosis were outlined clearly. As shown in Frankie's case, death wishes against love objects, fantasies of drowning in a sea of defecation, passive feminine trends, etc., are held in check successfully by denial, repression, reaction formation, intellectualization, etc.—in short, by an obsessional neurosis. On the other hand, tendencies toward merging with the object, primary identification, loss of personal identity are beyond the scope of the obsessional devices. Since they demand stronger measures such as splitting of the ego, projection, etc., they expose the patient to the danger of paranoid or perverse solutions.

CONCLUSION

The Program Committee's endeavor to crystallize the interest of Congress members around a main topic seems successful on the whole. To say the least, it has presented us with a vivid picture of analytic problem solving, with its painstaking back and forth between observation of clinical data, abstraction and generalization, and reapplication of theoretical thinking to the further elucidation of our patients' material.

Part III

This section contains papers addressed primarily to non-analytic audiences. It corresponds to Part II in Volume IV.

Unlike the practice in other sections and in Volume IV, the chronological order of presentation has here not been strictly adhered to. Rather, the papers addressed to the same professional or lay audience are grouped together.

Editor's note

Part III

16

Psychoanalytic Knowledge
Applied to the Rearing
of Children
(1956)

Psychoanalysis discovered early that the human personality
develops under the impact of two forces which clash with
each other, one represented by the innate instinctual drives,
the other by the demands which the environment makes
on the individual. The results, as we know, are only too
often intense unhappiness, neurotic symptomatology or
mental illness of some form or other.

While we are unable to alter the innate givens of a hu-

Based on a lecture entitled "Emotional Factors in Education,"
which was presented to the faculty and students of Western Reserve University Medical School, Cleveland, in September, 1956.
It is published here for the first time.

man being, we may be in the position to relieve some of
the external pressures which interact with them. What is
needed for such a task is insight into the potential harm
done to young children during the critical years of their
development by the manner in which their needs, drives,
wishes, and emotional dependencies are met.

It is not unreasonable on the part of parents and educators to expect such enlightenment from psychoanalysis.
After all, it was psychoanalytic study which pinpointed the
conflicts that disrupt the harmony of the personality and
give rise to neurotic symptom formation, the delinquencies,
perversions, character deformations, etc.

Unfortunately, the pathways leading from insight into
the etiology of psychological disorders to their prevention
are not straightforward ones. There is a multitude of external and internal factors which combine their influence
to cause mental suffering; with the best will in the world,
not all of them can be eliminated from the child's life.
Some are anchored in the very traditions of the society in
which the child grows up, are part and parcel of it, and as
such immovable. Some, though harmful from certain aspects, are beneficial from others and therefore indispensable for normal life. Some are the result of development itself, i.e., inextricably tied up with the complexity of the
child's growing personality, his moral demands on himself,
his attempts at adaptation to the environment. In fact,
nothing that we learn in this respect from psychoanalysis
entitles us to expect more than a reduction in the number
of these pathogenic agents.

But in spite of this cautious attitude toward the prevention of mental illness, we analysts have not always succeeded in preventing the lay public from building unrea-

sonably high hopes on the application of psychoanalytic findings to the upbringing of children. What the public expected was no less than a revolutionary but systematic, well-integrated guide to the rearing of a new, healthier, and happier generation. What they received, in fact, were isolated, hard-won insights, highlighting sometimes one, sometimes another area of the child's mind, frequently transmitted without the relevant guidance to their proper application. These resulted, it is true, in some significant successes, but not without an almost equal number of significant failures and disappointments.

Taken as a whole, the gradual filtering through of knowledge from the psychoanalytic to the educational field can be seen in a chronological sequence. In what follows, I describe it as such, although this slightly falsifies the events. In actual fact, the phases which I separate from each other for the purpose of clarification overlapped with each other in many instances.

PHASE 1: THE SEXUAL ENLIGHTENMENT OF CHILDREN

The first psychoanalytic discovery which had far-reaching effects on the upbringing of children concerned the fact that sexual life begins not at puberty but at birth, with a preparatory period that extends from infancy over the intervening years of childhood, until preadolescence and finally adolescence are reached. During this time, sexual sensations are centered around various body parts such as mouth and anus, with the sex organs themselves (the phallus) not assuming major importance before the end of the first period of childhood (approximately three to five years of age), when attitudes such as sexual curiosity, the wish to look and to be looked at also become part of the child's sex life. Psychoanalysis has further maintained that the child's relationship to his parents is far from "innocent," and that between his first and fifth year of life every child passes through various stages of a most intense love life accompanied by sexual desires and sensations.

This psychoanalytic theory of infantile sexuality was rejected at the time by many people who merely blamed analysis for drawing attention to nonexisting or, at best, unwanted facts. At the same time there were many others who were made thoughtful by it. If the discovery of analysis was to be taken seriously, it implied that until then children had been misjudged in many ways. They had been blamed for being naughty, pathological or depraved for merely following trends which were inherent in their nature. Further, if they had a sex life of their own, and if curiosity about sexual matters formed an integral part of it, instead of being the result of seduction by unsuitable companions, a sign of precocity, etc., how could the withholding of sexual information be justified by parents or teachers in the long run?

After an interval filled with considerable doubt, uncertainty, and discussion of such questions, the new knowledge suddenly reached the public in a massive way, finding expression in the well-known slogan of the demand for the *sexual enlightenment* of children. Modern-minded parents began to inform their children about the difference between the sexes, the mystery of birth, the more courageous ones even including knowledge about sexual intercourse and the role of the father in procreation. Schools followed suit very gradually and hesitantly, over periods of many years. It was not easy for them to introduce a subject which had been banned and under the threat of heavy penalties.

Nor did the application of the new knowledge end with the mere impartment of sexual knowledge to children. What altered simultaneously was the right granted to the child to *act* on his sexual impulses, at least within limits. Pleasure gain from the individual's own body, such as thumb sucking in infancy, phallic masturbation in the following years, now became permitted. A new toleration was extended to the anal pleasures: children were trained for bladder and bowel control at later dates and with less rigidity.

It may be instructive to attempt a summing up of the gains and also of the disappointments encountered in this phase. There is little doubt that there were gains and that these showed quite markedly in the altered relationships between parents and children. Since the children no longer needed to hide their impulses and their desires, they became more honest toward their parents; vice versa, since the parents had less reason to hide their own life from their children, they became more honest in their turn. Consequently, the whole question of honesty and lying, which had loomed so large in the educational experiences of the past century, gradually began to recede from the foreground of the picture.

It came as a surprise that the efforts at sexual enlightenment itself were not equally successful. Children who were told the "facts of life" in all honesty often complained afterward that they had been kept in ignorance of them. Somehow they seemed incapable of integrating the new, adult, knowledge with their infantile beliefs. In any case, on the basis of their own sexual experiences, they persisted in believing in theories of their own: that children are born through the mouth or anus; that all children are born as boys, the girls being deprived of the penis as punishment for some misdeed; that what happens between the parents is not sex and love but violence in which either father or mother can come to grief. In this manner, their own *infantile sexual theories* clashed with the objective facts offered to them and, more often than not, retained the upper hand.

But the main disappointment which this phase brought with it lay in another direction. The hope that this first step would diminish either human unhappiness or the incidence of neurosis did not materialize. We can only say that it was still early; that the insight applied so far was a single one; moreover, that it was torn out of its context; and that it is more profitable to wait for further advances before passing judgment on it.

PHASE 2: RECOGNITION OF THE ROLE OF CONFLICT, CONSCIENCE, AND ANXIETY: LIMITING OF PARENTAL AUTHORITY

There are several reasons why, in spite of parental efforts, it remained the fate of the infantile sexual urges to be frustrated. It is not only that they are so crude, primitive, and violent that, by definition, they have to be relegated to fantasy and cannot be lived out in real life. It is more than that: they are contradictory by nature and, according to the immaturity of the child's psychic apparatus, not coordinated with each other. The father, for example, who is the boy's hated rival in the context of the oedipus complex is simultaneously the object of his love and the model for his identification. Both parents are loved when they fulfill the child's wishes and hated when they frustrate them. Consequently, love and hate, the wishes to harm and kill and to possess and keep the parents vie with each other, none of them preventing the existence of their counterparts. What is relevant here is the unsolved *ambivalence* of infantile wishes.

There is a further factor which had not been taken into account. As the child develops from one level of instinctual life to another, the impulses of the past phase become repugnant to him. Children do not admire, they usually despise the image of themselves at an earlier date. No one, for example, is more intolerant of dirty toilet habits or bad table manners than the child who has already become clean. These internal prohibitions lead to repressions, i.e., to the normal forgetting of the whole period of early childhood, to its becoming unconscious.

The analytic finding that people do not fall ill as a consequence of external prohibitions but by their internalization in the form of a personal conscience had important consequences for the upbringing of children. Parents were impressed by the discovery that their children's superego (their conscience) was built up in imitation of themselves, i.e., by identification with and internalization of their own authoritative commands. They concluded that there was only one way to prevent this from happening, and thereby to prevent the growing child from criticizing, inhibiting, and guiltily torturing himself: namely, by limiting or abrogating altogether their own authority. There was an era when some parents went as far as avoiding for their children the use of the words father and mother (or their equivalents); if children were encouraged to call their parents by their first names, this was meant to signify that parents and children, adults and minors were equals, and that the latter had nothing to learn or to fear from the former.

There were gains and losses in this phase as well. Unmistakably, some of the plights of children were mitigated. Parents were less dominating and less frightening, with a new possibility for comradeship springing up within the family. Nevertheless, children also felt a lack. The change left an unfilled gap in the place from which help, guidance, and direction had emanated before. This "reformed" method of upbringing, in the last resort, was built on wrong premises, i.e., on neglect of the fact that the child's personality structure is immature, that his control over his impulses is unreliable, his orientation in and adaptation to external reality in their beginnings only, and that, consequently, there is in the child a great need for strong external support to combat his own helplessness.

There was also another, still graver mistake made in the application of the analytic theories concerning the pathogenic role of anxiety. It is true that fear of the parents, i.e., fear of external powers, leads to the first restrictions which the child has to impose on the satisfaction of his instinctual wishes. It is equally true that, in the long run, these restrictions are incorporated in the individual's superego and that every infringement of them leads to anxiety feelings, i.e., guilt, which plays a major part in instigating neurotic character formation or symptomatology. The way in which the parents behave has a great deal to do with the amount of fear, anxiety, and guilt which is generated. But there is also a third form of anxiety which is more removed from the sphere of parental influence.

Psychoanalysis teaches that the intactness of an individual's ego depends on the latter's control over the impulses and the intactness of its defense organization which keeps the barriers against the id secure and guards against any major irruptions of uncensored instinctual elements. The growing child who is in the process of building up his ego strength is, with justification, fearful of having his efforts undermined by impulses which flood him from the deeper layers of the mind, and looks instinctively for help given by external authorities.

Where this is not forthcoming, he experiences the most devastating anxiety of all, a fear of the loss of his own integrity and identity, an anxiety which becomes visible only after the first two types (fear and guilt) have been removed from the scene. This may solve the riddle why children who are brought up with extreme leniency and permissiveness are not happier than others; why, on the contrary, they are only too frequently restless, irritable, given to extreme temper tantrums, and under the domination of a nondirected, more or less free-floating anxiety.

PHASE 3: FREEDOM FOR AGGRESSION

Whereas the disappointments of the foregoing phase checked the enthusiasm of parents to a certain degree, a further development in the psychoanalytic theories brought with it a revival of it. What I have in mind is the aggressive instinct being given equal place with sexuality as a determining force in the development of the human personality. Psychoanalytic teaching implied that the aggressive drive is more than a reaction to frustration, that it is comparable to the sexual one, inherent in human nature, exists and seeks expression from the beginning of life, and goes through its own developmental phases. If checked and prohibited too extensively, either by external or internal prohibitions, it produces similar pathological results. One of them, and an especially dreaded one, is represented by the possibility that aggression, rather than being employed toward the outer world, may be turned inward, against the individual's own body or developing self and produce either psychosomatic disease or an overstrict superego leading to obsessional neurosis, depression, etc.

Perhaps it should have been expected by us analysts that this was a dangerous piece of knowledge to leak out to parents and those engaged in the upbringing of young children. However that may be, it led to the new slogan *freedom for aggression*, on which the most unreasonable hopes were built by its advocates. Freedom for aggression, granted first by the parents, secondly by the child's own conscience, was expected to remove all the remaining remnants of unhappiness and disharmony.

While children became somewhat happier at this juncture, their parents became definitely more unhappy. Children with their aggression and destructiveness let loose were less lovable as human beings than they had been before and they taxed the parents' forbearance to the utmost. Equally, they taxed the forbearance of their own superego where this had already come into operation.

Again, it took some time to sort out the grain of truth from the mass of errors which had been committed during this particular phase. What is true is that the wholesale condemnation of aggression and its repression lead to pathological results since they deprive the human personality of a valuable and efficient element which can be employed constructively. However, the avoidance of wholesale condemnation need not lead to wholesale approval. Here, the true task of applying new knowledge is to find a way of instituting controls of the drive without rendering it more dangerous by condemnation.

PHASE 4: THE MOTHER-INFANT RELATIONSHIP

In more recent years the upbringing of children came strongly under the influence of a new trend in psychoanalytic work. Many contemporary analytic authors and researchers deflected their attention from the conflicts between the agencies of the personality (id, ego, and superego), i.e., from the internal struggle within the structured human being, to the very beginning of life when the rudiments of personality development are laid down. These studies of the *first year of life*, when applied to the reality of the infant, seemed to hold out a better prospect for the prevention of later mental upset and illness.

Inevitably these studies focused on the first interplay between the infant and the mother (or her substitute) who takes care of him and ensures his survival. It depends on the relationship which develops between this couple whether the infant's needs, bodily and instinctual, will find frustration or fulfillment and to what extent; whether pleasure or unpleasure will be the main experiences in his life; whether, for purposes of gratification, the infant's attention will be deflected gradually from his own body and emerging self and be directed toward the person who provides for him and who simultaneously is for him the first representative of the outside world; whether, finally, the first stages of merging with the mother and of loving her for purely selfish reasons give way to what we recognize as the mature way of loving an object as a person in her own right.

Psychoanalysts have studied many cases where the capacity for forming normal object relationships has been left undeveloped or has been destroyed during the earliest periods of life either through the absence of an adequate mother figure or by her unresponsiveness, her periodic absences, her illness, loss, etc. Such infants, instead of developing normally, tend to withdraw; they remain uninterested, self-centered; they become "depressed"; they fail to develop either physically or intellectually, or both. It is suspected that a number of defects, such as mental or emotional retardation, can be traced back to severe early deprivations of this kind.[1]

Here, then, was a piece of analytic information which seemed ideally suited for application to the field of child rearing. Not only were mothers encouraged by it to give a freer rein to their naturally affectionate and protective feelings toward the infant without having to fear that they might be accused of "spoiling" him; it also alerted people to the dangers of enforced separations, of inconstancy in caretaking personnel, of hospitalizations, of institutional upbringing where constant mother figures are missing. All of these insights led to important beneficial changes in the handling of young children.

On the other hand, there were also the inevitable misunderstandings, misapplications, and exaggerations. Since the mother had been singled out as the most important person in the infant's life, what was attributed to her were not only beneficial but also adverse influences. This was the era

[1] For a further discussion of this point, see ch. 18 in this volume.

when the mothers were held responsible for all abnormalities in the child's development, psychosomatic illnesses as well as character deformations and autistic and psychotic states. This led to another slogan, that of the "rejecting mother" who harms the whole future of her child by not giving him the comfort, love, and satisfaction to which he is entitled. Although in some cases such accusations may be justified, there are many others where they are unwarranted.[2]

There is still another discrepancy between the truth of the analytic findings and what the public made of them. It is perfectly true that the first relationship of the infant to his mother becomes the basis of his capacity to form further attachments and that it also serves as a prototype for them. But this capacity, important as it is, is not in itself a guarantee of future mental health. There is much that can happen within the mother-infant relationship. It can be excessive, for example, and by means of its very strength prevent the child's further advance. The infant may become so dependent on unceasing love and comfort being given, that the step to the acceptance of frustrations and independent development becomes more difficult to take; or that a point is created on which large amounts of the child's libido remain fixated. There are also difficulties which may arise within the framework of the child's ambivalence since it is more difficult to feel aggressive toward an all-loving, nonfrustrating mother; or, within the framework of the oedipus complex, for the girl to take the necessary step away from her to loving the father.

There is also much that can happen to a child after in-

[2] For a detailed discussion of the concept of the "rejecting mother," see Volume IV, ch. 29.

fancy is past such as traumatic events, losses, seductions, upheavals in the family structure. All of these will have their repercussions on the future and on the individual's mental health, even though it may be true that the type of mental illness will not be quite so severe and the disintegration of the personality not quite so complete where a firmer basis has been laid down in the first year of life.

THE CURRENT SCENE: THE MOTHER AS AUXILIARY EGO

In fact, some of the errors committed in phase 4 were corrected again by applying some current analytic researches which offered a more balanced view. We profit if we do not encourage the public to be content with isolated bits of information, relating either to the instinctual processes in the id, or to the forces of the superego, or to the importance of the libidinal or aggressive strivings, but if we insist on relating any one part of the personality to the others, as well as relating any one level of development and achievement in the child's life to the levels which have gone before or will come after.

Taking this view, we cannot fail to ask ourselves what, in fact, is the aim of education. We do not aim to reach the processes within the id, since we recognize them as unreachable and ungovernable while they are in that realm. The sexual and aggressive instinctual drives follow a prescribed course of development on which we have singularly little influence. We do aim at reaching and influencing the child's superego, although the ideas how this can be accomplished have changed vastly in recent times. Before psychoanalysis, people were convinced that morality could be taught, by word of mouth, by lecturing, almost as if the difference between "good" and "bad" were a school subject. By now we know that this is not the case; that where morality is concerned, children take their cue from their love objects, and that they acquire a conscience indirectly, by identification with them. What the parents teach in this respect weighs very little in comparison with what they do themselves.

With id and superego thus removed from directly aimed-at influence, what remains as the main recipient of education is the child's ego. Psychoanalysis teaches that it is the ego on which the responsibility rests for the maintenance of mental equilibrium and mental health. To mediate between the demands of the environment, the demands of the superego, and the pressing requirements for instinctual satisfaction is a formidable task for it. While the mature ego of an adult may feel equipped for it, the child, throughout his formative years, lacks the capacity to carry it out.

An application of this insight leads to the realization that the mother's role for the infant goes far beyond providing comfort, satisfying his needs, and offering herself as the first object for his emotional strivings. Her task lies equally with the developing ego. It is the mother who has to act as a protective shield against undue stimulation until the child's own stimulus barrier becomes established. It is the mother's management of the infant's wishes and the balance struck by her between fulfillment, frustration, and postponement which has to serve as a prototype for the childish ego's own later dealings with his drives. Her introduction of familiar routines and regularities stimulates the infant's time sense and facilitates such ego functions as memory and orientation. Her sense of reality is leaned on heavily by the child until his own testing of reality and distinguishing it from fantasy begins to function.

To apply these insights to the practical task of child rearing is no easy matter. What is needed, above all, may be to steer mothers away from the lessons of the previous phases during which they were made to feel that it was their prime duty to make the child "happy," disregarding the fact that the developmental processes to which the child is subjected contain in themselves innumerable factors which cause unpleasure, unhappiness, frustration, etc.

What is necessary, further, may be some mother guidance. Doubtless there are mothers whose natural affection, protectiveness, and possessiveness toward their infants equips them emotionally for taking over the role of being the child's "auxiliary ego." Others may find themselves unable or unprepared to do so and need help. Where the mother's own personality difficulties or her needs are not too overwhelming, this help can take the form of giving her insight into the developing ego's very specialized requirements.

17

The Child Guidance Clinic
as a Center of Prophylaxis
and Enlightenment
(1960 [1957])

As opening speaker of this convention I have the privilege
of offering some general considerations concerning the role
of the child guidance clinic in the community as well as
discussing the interrelations between child analysis and
the allied field of child guidance work.

Presented at the Symposium on Child Guidance and Psycho-
analysis at the 35th anniversary of the Youth Guidance Center of
Worcester, Mass., on September 19, 1957.
First published in *Recent Developments in Psychoanalytic Child
Therapy*, ed. Joseph Weinreb. New York: International Universities
Press, 1960, pp. 25-38.

CHILD ANALYSIS BEFORE THE
CHILD GUIDANCE ERA

I begin with my personal recollections about the development of these relationships, recollections which make me feel that analysts and child analysts owe the child guidance clinics a debt of gratitude. Before such clinics existed, we analysts felt that we were in possession of much solid analytic knowledge potentially useful for the upbringing of children, their teaching, and the treatment of their problems. But there were no recognized channels of communication, neither with parents nor with the professional workers within the children's services. All that the analysts could rely on in this respect were chance contacts: parents while or after undergoing a therapeutic analysis themselves could not help but apply some of their newly acquired insights to the handling of their children; teachers who, for personal reasons, underwent analysis were expected to carry back to the teaching profession some analytic findings concerning child development.

It was a thrilling occasion when in Vienna (approximately in 1930) an inspector of nursery schools invited us to conduct a seminar for a small group of nursery school teachers to discuss their problem children; or when an inspector of municipal play centers invited me to give a series of introductory lectures to his workers. Actually, one of the first schools to make systematic use of analytic child psychology was the Walden School in New York, a fact which Ferenczi learned on one of his early visits to the States and reported on most enthusiastically after his return. But these hopeful signs of possible cooperation between analysis and work with children remained few and far between.

There was another side to the same picture which was no less frustrating. We knew that there was a large amount of child material near at hand from which we, as child analysts, could have profited greatly. There were all the initial states of mental disturbance, as they show up in childhood, the many transitional stages between health and illness, the common developmental difficulties of all young children, their relationships to the more circumscribed syndromes of the infantile neuroses—all this was potentially available in our environment and, still, we were denied access to it. The children brought to us in private practice or within the hospital services were those in whom mental illness had passed the initial phase of behavior disorder or symptom formation and had become ingrained in the personality in a massive way, causing severe breakdowns or permanent deviations of character. Again, there was little or nothing that we could do to alter this condition.

But it is precisely this situation which has changed with the advent of the child guidance clinics. Since they have come into being, they have opened up a two-way traffic between parents and professional workers with children on the one hand and child analysis or child psychiatry on the other. It is the child guidance clinics which at present act as mediators between the two fields and serve as clearing houses between them: they receive material from the public to pass on to the child analysts and child psychiatrists; and conversely, they receive information from child psychiatry (or analysis) to hand out to the public. This is an important and formidable assignment, and it seems worthwhile to me to investigate how far the child guidance clinics of our knowledge have been able and equipped to fulfill this double task.

THE CHILD GUIDANCE CLINIC
AS A CLEARING HOUSE

Collection of Material

As regards the first side of the assignment, the collection of available case material, there is no doubt that the existing clinics are eminently successful. Probably on the basis of their status as public institutions, they have done what the private child analyst had been unable to achieve: namely, to gain the confidence of the public.[1] As director of a child guidance clinic, or when talking to one of the directors, you will find that collecting the material presents no difficulty. If anything, trouble arises in the opposite direction: there is too much material. Clinics are swamped with the cases sent in to them by the parents themselves, by teachers, youth workers, general practitioners and pediatricians, almoners of hospitals, probation officers from the courts, child welfare organizers, etc. There is everything from the most common difficulties of management, with which parents used to deal on their own (such as the early sleeping, feeding, and toileting troubles), to the severe retardations, borderline and autistic and atypical states.

---

[1] It was August Aichhorn who remarked first on this difference between private and public work with parents. When he was praised for the hold he had on parents and the amount of information he gathered from them, he would answer: "Don't forget what I represent for the parents. As official advisor, appointed by the authorities, I am backed up by the whole Municipality."

There is, indeed, more than the diagnostic skill of the child psychiatrist or child analyst can cope with at present. The bewildering variety of pathological, or seemingly pathological, manifestations seems to call for new diagnostic categories based not on symptomatology but on developmental considerations. But, however this may be, the case material is there to be looked at by the analyst, studied, sorted out for therapy, understood, and, perhaps in the future, to be newly classified.[2]

There is, as said before, no lack of confidence in the clinic on the part of the public; again, if anything, there is too much. For many people, the concept of treatment in a clinic has acquired a magical connotation. Little distinction is made between children who suffer from environmental neglect, unsuitable parents, tragic bereavements, and those cases in which something has gone wrong in the development and personality structure for internal reasons. In both instances, to know that a child is in treatment seems to spell safety to parents, welfare agencies or public authorities, as if every nonorganic disturbance were automatically suitable for psychological treatment, and as if treatment guaranteed a cure in all cases. Paradoxically enough, it will soon be necessary on the part of the clinics to disabuse the public, i.e., to induce people to lower their expectations of therapy to a level more justified by the conditions and limitations imposed by reality.

[2] In our Hampstead Child-Therapy Clinic, our Psychiatrist-in-Charge, Liselotte Frankl, is conducting a diagnostic study of this kind.

[See also the Diagnostic Profile in Volume VI as well as the other papers on the Profile listed in the Appendix at the end of Part I of this volume.]

The Application of Analytic Knowledge

I find that the clinics have been less successful where the receiving and application of analytic knowledge are concerned. There is, at least in this respect, a wide gap between the "analytic" clinics as they exist in some of the big European and American centers, usually in close collaboration with a local psychoanalytic society and training institute, and the ordinary, although frequently "analytically oriented" child guidance clinics as they exist in larger or smaller numbers all over the countries. The analytic clinic usually has a fully trained analyst as psychiatrist-in-charge with several younger staff members in analytic training. The analytically oriented clinic may base its whole connection with psychoanalysis on some contact with analysis which a senior staff member has had at one period of his career. What he brings back from such contacts often consists of no more than single pieces of analytic findings which bear the hallmark of a certain phase of analytic thinking.

In the preceding chapter I have described these phases in detail. Here I shall simply name them: emphasis on the pathogenic role of repression of infantile sexuality (resulting in therapeutic emphasis on sex enlightenment, dealing with guilt arising from oedipal fantasies, masturbation conflicts, etc.); emphasis on the pathogenic repression of aggression (with therapeutic emphasis laid on the discharge of the child's aggressive and destructive tendencies); emphasis on the mother-infant unity in the earliest years (treatment being directed toward the aftereffects of traumatic separations); emphasis on the pathogenic role of the mother's abnormal personality, emotional withdrawnness, severely neurotic or psychotic traits (with consequent inclusion of the mother in the child's treatment). Not that these findings do not represent all-important parts of the analytic knowledge of child development as it stands at present, but they have to be pieced together and fitted into the framework of analytic child psychology before their clinical application can be wholly useful. When they are used in isolation, the diagnostic as well as the therapeutic issues become distorted, a frequent occurrence for which psychoanalysis has had to take much blame.

Perhaps in the future our distinction between analytic child guidance clinics and others should be based less on the therapeutic time available for each patient (once weekly versus daily treatment) than on whether the whole analytic knowledge of children is available for application or merely selected portions of it.

We are left with the question where to place the responsibility for this, to the analyst, unsatisfactory state of affairs and where to look for remedies. The fault may lie mainly with us analysts, who are notoriously bad at public relations and known to publicize findings all too often in unsuitable language or with exaggerated emphasis on the most recent discoveries. On the other hand, the fault may lie with the clinics, where people fail to sift, weigh, and integrate data before applying them to therapy and guidance work. The necessity for such discrimination in this field is not so different, after all, from the corresponding one in the medical field, where knowledge of new findings, new methods, and new drugs has to be pursued constantly and integrated with former knowledge before its application.

The Distribution of Analytic Knowledge

For discussing the distribution of knowledge I turn once more to the experience of those clinics where a considerable fund of reliable and comprehensive analytic data is available for use. The points of contact with the public open to them are of various kinds.

DIAGNOSTIC ASSESSMENT

There are, for one, the constant demands for the assessment of children, as they are made in all child guidance clinics for purposes of the juvenile courts, or placement for adoption, with foster parents, in residential institutions, for selection of school, etc. Where the assessment is made not in terms of symptomatology but from the wider point of view of personality structure and development (as mentioned above), and where the language is nontechnical, more than the immediate practical purpose can be served. Here is a legitimate channel of communication which can be used to acquaint the referring agencies with the clinical (and theoretical) aspects on which the clinic's understanding of the child is based. In time these case histories will illustrate many of the main issues of analytic child psychology, such as the interdependence of environmental and internal factors, of body and mind, of emotional and intellectual capacities; the overriding importance of drive activity and its position in the personality structure; the role of anxiety and of defense activity leading to inhibition of function or to symptom formation; the developmental aspects of social or dissocial development, etc.[3]

[3] In the East London Child-Guidance Clinic Augusta Bonnard has carried out valuable work of this kind for a number of years.

INSTRUCTION OF PROFESSIONAL WORKERS

A second and more direct channel of communication is opened up by the constant demands for instruction which arrive from the professional workers in the field, such as pediatricians, nurses, or teachers. It is true that many of us feel that the teaching role of the clinic is a very temporary one with regard to these. By rights, instruction in child development should be an integral part of the medical or nursing courses as well as of the teachers' training colleges. But while developments in these institutions have to be waited for, there is a gap to fill, and it may be worthwhile to discuss how to do this constructively, avoiding past mistakes.[4]

So long as the general knowledge of child development has to be introduced as an afterthought to the majority of the members of the medical, nursing, and teaching professions, the success or failure of such ventures will depend on three factors: (1) the selection of the right teaching method; (2) the selection of the right facts; (3) some overall considerations which provide a framework.

To take the last point first: in work with doctors, nurses, or teachers, it is essential to remember that not all the psy-

---

She has done an effective teaching job with the school and welfare authorities in her area through answering their requests for diagnostic assessment by means of elaborate and enlightening developmental pictures of the children referred to her.

[4] The next speaker in the Symposium, Grete Bibring (1960), reports on the manner in which the analytic theory of child development is taught today to pediatricians and other residents in the Beth Israel Hospital, Boston, Mass. And Anny Katan (1960) describes the way in which such knowledge is integrated with the medical course from the first year onward in Western Reserve University, Cleveland, Ohio.

chological data which we can offer are suitable for immediate application, since the conditions under which they work are different from ours. It is only a short time ago that teachers learned that the child's intellect does not function divorced from his feelings and that, therefore, some connection with their pupils' emotional life is indispensable for teaching. For the medical world it is a similarly recent discovery that the child's body is not divorced from his mind and that, therefore, physical and mental matters are sufficiently interrelated to influence and interfere with each other. But schools and hospitals as institutions have antedated all these new findings. The application of the latter, therefore, implies a whole host of changes which range from the free entry of parents to schools and hospitals to the rota of changing nursing personnel and the very arrangements of schoolroom or ward, changes which especially for nurses and doctors may mean a more or less complete upheaval in the established conditions of their work.

As regards teaching methods, many of us agree that formal courses in child development remain ineffective before links have been established between the data offered in these courses and those contained in formal professional training on physical matters. On the other hand, openings are provided by those patients or pupils who remain "problems" in medical practice or schoolroom, i.e., where the physical or intellectual data fail to explain the picture. For these reasons, teaching "on the case" has been found satisfactory by many analysts.[5]

[5] Our Hampstead Clinic is lending an experienced child therapist, Bianca Gordon, to the Paediatric Department of the Woolwich Memorial Hospital for weekly consultations—an experiment which has proved successful.

As for the selection of facts for teaching, I emphasize, as before, that few analytic data are beneficial if applied out of context. Schools, for example, may profit greatly from applying the analytic concept of *sublimation* to the teachers' work. By deflecting libidinal energy from its original sources and harnessing it to school subjects much drudgery in school can be changed into activities almost as pleasurable as play. On the other hand, progressive schools will come to grief if they base their schedules too consistently on this single piece of analytic knowledge. Psychoanalytic theory also has much to say about the essential differences between *play* and *work*, the first being governed by the pleasure principle, the latter by the reality principle. It is one of the main tasks of education to lead each individual child from the earlier to the later mode of functioning. Only the integration of the knowledge of sublimation with the more intricate knowledge of mental functioning on the various stages of development will be of real benefit to the psychological orientation of the modern schools.

Pediatricians might be similarly misled if they meet the present psychoanalytic campaign against hospitalization of small children unconnected with other facts. It is true that a first early separation from home for purposes of medical or surgical intervention may prove traumatic to the individual child and that the psychological damage done by it may go as far as outweighing the physical benefit in health. On the other hand, doctors should not be impressed exclusively with the fact, or the effect, of separation. It is equally necessary for them to learn what part physical illness as such, even when undergone at home, plays in the mental development of children. Again, it is only the combination and integration of both these lines of inquiry which will lead to beneficial application.[6]

WORK WITH PARENTS

This leads us to the third and last channel of communication with the public, the work with parents, which will remain the clinic's domain, whatever the developments.

There is at present the widespread belief, held by all clinic personnel, that work with parents (or, in the case of young children, with their mothers) is effective only if directed toward changes in their personalities. Consensus on this point has been reached, I believe, on the rebound from earlier and outmoded attitudes toward the parents, attitudes which included much teaching of facts on a purely intellectual basis, advising in an authoritative manner or, at worst, preaching and exhorting. Our analytic discoveries have laid bare the intricate emotional relationships between child and parent; the role of internalization of the parents' personality traits and attitudes, and identification with their qualities; the consequences of love and hate; the subtle or crude forms of seduction; the overriding importance of any one of the developmental phases, whether libidinal or aggressive, being acceptable or repulsive to the parent. Once the parent-child relationship is seen in this light, work with a parent ceases to imply a teacher-pupil attitude and takes on the aspect of a therapeutic relationship.

Most analysts subscribe to these arguments, which are, after all, derived from their work, although with the proviso

[6] For the effect on children of severe physical illness and immobilization, see Thesi Bergmann (1960), Bergmann and Anna Freud (1965). For an enlightened discussion of hospitalization as a beneficial psychological influence in some cases, see Solnit (1960).

that experience in analytic practice also teaches one to be modest in the expectation of personality changes through any but the most intensive therapy.

For my own person, I remain a heretic in some of these respects. I am far from denying the effect on a child from a beneficial change in the parents' attitudes. Still, I cannot help believing that this therapeutic approach to the parents is no more than one among a whole series of possible approaches, all of them serving the same ultimate purposes of beneficial change, prevention, and enlightenment. In what follows I shall try to justify this rather unpopular view of mine by outlining a number of these possibilities as I have learned to see them.

Therapy with Parents. I begin with those instances where I have no hesitation and no reservation in joining the popular demand for therapy for the parents. There are the cases, by now known to most clinics, in which the mother's and the child's pathology are completely intertwined. We believe that very young children have some primitive pathway of communication with their mothers' unconscious which render them sensitive and vulnerable to the latter's unconscious libidinal or aggressive impulses and fantasies. A young child may merely act out the mother's fantasy in play,[7] or may defend himself against it in some complicated way, or may build a complex pathological structure of his own on the basis of the mother's secret or manifest disturbance. In the most extreme instances, the mental disorders of mother and child will be fitted together as if they were pieces in a jigsaw puzzle or— to compare it with adult disorders—as in a *folie-à-deux*.

[7] As described by Dorothy Burlingham (1935).

In our Hampstead Clinic we have studied a number of such mother-child couples over the years by analyzing both partners simultaneously under different therapists and analysts and coordinating the results. Our aim is to determine the limits of dependence and independence in their disturbances and to assess the therapeutic chances for those other cases in which only the child, i.e., the more passive factor in the partnership, is taken into treatment. On the basis of several of these investigations we have concluded that there is some hope in altering the condition by the child's analysis alone so long as the pathogenic agents from the mother's side remain in the realm of thought and fantasy; but that nothing except simultaneous treatment will alter the situation when these mental influences are reinforced by actions of the mother which tie the child to her as a result of pleasurable or painful actual excitations.[8]

The therapeutic approach to the mother is equally vital in those cases in which young children show the various signs of deprivation of mothering, though in the mother's presence. This may be caused by a depression of the mother, or a period of actual mourning which causes withdrawal of feeling from the object world, including the child. The mother's incapacity to fulfill the task of mothering may also be caused by the consequences of a pathogenic masculinity complex, as well as many other factors. Again, nothing except therapy will have a chance of altering the condition. But, since, the therapeutic results are slow to come, we have seen repeatedly that the change in the mother comes too late for the child in whose handling the deficiency be-

[8] See ch. 30 in this volume. See also Burlingham et al. (1955), Hellman et al. (1960), Levy (1960), Sprince (1962).

came apparent and that it is the next-born infant who benefits from the preventive measure.[9]

*Guiding the Parents through the Child's
Analysis.* The close interdependence of mother and child at
the beginning of life, and the exaggeration of this factor in
some abnormal cases, should not make us ignore the fact
that children are growing personalities in their own right
with a wide range of possible disturbances and conflicts
within their structure. But while they need treatment in
their own right, their mothers will be severely affected by
this procedure and will need to be helped and guided
through this period.[10] To safeguard the child's future in
the family after the conclusion of treatment, the parents,
and especially the mother, should be allowed or even urged
to accompany the analytic process to some degree. This
implies facing their own adult resistances to the repressed
remnants of infantile sexuality and the cruder forms of
infantile aggression, all the more so since the child's impulses are directed against their persons and, as a rule, become increased temporarily during treatment. The child's
treatment acts as a threat to the defenses of the mother,
quite apart from the violent feelings of jealousy and competition with the child analyst which are aroused by the
young patient's positive attachment to the latter's person.
Much human tact plus therapeutic skill on the part of the
clinic's representative (whether therapist, psychiatrist, or

[9] Kata Levy is responsible for drawing our Clinic's attention to
the difference between the mother's disturbance being (a) a direct
agent in the child's pathology through identification and excitation;
(b) an indirect agent through incapacitating the mother for her
task of mothering.

[10] See in this respect Dorothy Burlingham (1932).

psychiatric social worker) will be needed to handle these difficulties of the parents and to safeguard treatments.

Mothers of Handicapped Children. The approach is different again where the mothers of abnormal children are concerned, i.e., those who either are born physically or mentally defective (blind, deaf, spastic, deformed, mongoloid, etc.) or have acquired such abnormalities in early life, or undergo some unusual experience or fate (traumatic separations, deprivations, adoption, fostering, motor or dietary restrictions). There is no reason to expect that mothers are automatically equipped for the specialized task of bringing up such a child in a manner calculated to minimize the handicap. On the contrary, the mother's natural hurt and despair concerning her child's defect, the injury to her pride and pleasure in the child, will all work toward estranging her from the task of mothering, thereby increasing the initial damage. There is here a specially difficult therapeutic task with the mothers which has been tackled in few places. But there is, besides it, also the need for expert advice, based on knowledge of the abnormalities concerned, such as the following: how to ensure with the blind infant that contact with the object world by sight is substituted for through other channels; how to provide motor outlets for the blind toddler, thereby preventing many of the abnormalities following motor restriction; how to prevent necessary dietary restrictions from being understood by the child as punishments and experienced as intolerable deprivations; how to minimize the effect of inevitable separations from the mother; how to prepare for operations and meet their equally inevitable aftereffects, etc. There are a whole host of emergency situations of this kind in which the normal mother will feel helpless without guidance.

Treatment of the Young Child by the Mother. A number of analytic clinics, besides ours, have recently devised a procedure in which an intuitive and willing mother, free from severe pathology herself, is helped to guide her own child through the phases of an average developmental disturbance or infantile neurosis.[11] Such work implies close contact with the mother, usually through weekly sessions, in which the child's difficulties, his tantrums, his behavior, his play, or whatever other material has been elicited are discussed, assessed, and elucidated for the mother, who then bases her handling of the child on her understanding. Inevitably this also implies much reassurance of the mother, so far as the severity of the pathology, the comparison with other children, the confidence in her own ability as a mother are concerned.

I have had personal experience with two cases of this kind, one a case of soiling in a two-and-a-half-year-old boy (see Volume IV, ch. 16); the other, an incipient but violent school phobia in a six-year-old girl (see this volume, ch. 8, example ii). In both instances, satisfactory results were achieved, in spite of the therapeutic aspects of the work being concentrated on the child alone. That the mother's attitudes during the cooperation have to be met with understanding, patience, and sympathy goes without saying. Also, the mothers suitable for this type of cooperation have to be selected carefully; but there are more than a few who

[11] See in this respect Erna Furman's report (1957) and that of Robert A. Furman and Anny Katan (1969) on work done at Western Reserve University, Department of Psychiatry. See also ch. 35 in this volume.

will be able to respond positively to the appeal to their reason, common sense, and goodwill, who will cope with their own resistances and succeed in the task, helped by the satisfaction that their child need not be handed over to a stranger for therapy.

The Indirect Approach by Way of Public Opinion. It is not only on the basis of the foregoing considerations that I refuse to believe that mothers need to change their personalities before they can change the handling of their children. Assertions of this kind, I find, are not based on facts, above all not on historical facts. Even in the last thirty to forty years, during which I have been able to observe the methods of upbringing, changes have been remarkably great. *Breast feeding,* for example, has been adopted, given up, is being adopted again, and may be on the way out once more. *Feeding schedules* have been extremely strictly observed for two or three decades (with some disastrous results as the later severe feeding disturbances show), have given way to feeding on demand (with other disturbing results), and show some indication at present of returning with more moderation. *Toilet training* before the war in England began with official hospital approval soon after birth, was delayed in the postwar period until the end of the first year, and is postponed now by many mothers until the second or even third year. To widen the picture we need think only of the question of *sexual enlightenment,* now accepted as a must by almost all parents; of the immensely increased freedom given to the child's *aggression,* even if directly expressed toward the parents; of the altered attitude to *corporal punishment* as a recognized tool of education, etc.

Far-reaching developments of this kind are due not directly to personality changes in the individual mothers but indirectly to alterations in the social atmosphere to which the mothers cannot help but respond. My contention is, therefore, that in rearing their children, mothers are not only guided by instinct and misled by distorting personal influences, but they are to an even larger degree dependent on tradition and public opinion, both of which are open to change.

For the child guidance clinic this opens up the possibility of playing a part in the setting up of new traditions. As described above, they have already gained the confidence of the public where the treatment of problem children is concerned. It should not be difficult for them to establish a similar position of trust with regard to the handling of normal children during the all-important first four or five years of life, very much in the manner in which the well-baby clinics have established their traditions with regard to the healthy infants' physical needs. This will be slow work, supplanting gradually what is left of religious, national, and class traditions, but it will be no less effective so far as influence on the mothers is concerned.

CONCLUSION

I foresee even a further role for the child guidance clinics. At present all the workers in the children's services, whether in schools, hospitals, courts, clinics, suffer from the effects of specialized training and lack of coordination and integration in the field. It is as rare for a teacher to deal with a sick child as it is for a hospital nurse to handle a healthy one, or a pediatrician to come in contact with the juvenile courts. This limits each specialist's outlook on childhood, of which the various tasks show no more than a single aspect. I can envisage a future when a basic training in understanding all the developmental manifestations of childhood will become the rule for any worker in the field. Whenever this happens, the child guidance clinics as places of demonstration and instruction may be called upon to play a central part in the new scheme.

18

The Assessment of
Borderline Cases
(1956)

GENERAL REMARKS ON ASSESSMENT

Infantile Neurosis

The assessment of borderline cases in childhood is only a subdivision of the assessment of early infantile disturbances as such. There is a general framework, which can be left aside after a while, and which concerns the infantile neurosis as such. This is relevant not only from the aspect of diagnosis, but also from the aspect of technique. It hardly needs to be repeated here that the technique of child analysis was derived from the technique for adults to be

---

Based on a lecture presented at the Hanna Pavilion, Cleveland, on September 22, 1956. It is here published for the first time.

used with children who had developed an infantile neurosis in the strict sense of the term. When psychoanalytic clinics for children were set up initially, it was done with the idea that it would be most profitable to treat the infantile neuroses, since these were known to be the forerunners of the adult disturbances. Even though, as is well known, spontaneous cures of infantile neuroses do occur, it was thought safer not to wait for such spontaneous cures but to treat an infantile neurosis whenever it appeared in a significant form.

The concept of infantile neurosis may need a definition. We assume that an infantile neurosis develops in the period of the oedipal conflicts; that the child, unable to solve either the oedipus complex or the castration complex, or a combination of both, regresses to earlier fixation points. At these earlier fixation points, the child's ego is confronted with primitive modes of satisfaction which it cannot tolerate; as a consequence, an inner conflict arises and the resulting compromise solutions appear on the surface in the form of symptoms. If prototypes of such infantile neuroses are looked for, they are found best in cases such as the Wolf Man, Little Hans, Jenny Waelder Hall's case of pavor nocturnus (1946), my case of an obsessional child (see Volume II, pp. 40-41; see also pp. 74-79, 86-91), etc.

To return to the opening of clinics. We were uncertain at that time whether we would be able to convince parents that such children should undergo treatment for an infantile neurosis and that parents should not wait for the child to "grow out" of it. In actuality, this proved easier than expected. Clinics for children were opened, and they were swamped with demands for treatment, an experience that can be met with anywhere.

The Nonneurotic Disturbances

What came as a surprise were the types of cases with which clinics were confronted. The majority of children who were referred did not fit the picture of the infantile neuroses. Many children were seen whose difficulties or conflicts were far removed from the oedipal scene, who had in fact never reached the oedipal level and consequently could not be described as having regressed from it. It was far from easy to bring order into the chaos of clinical pictures.

There are, for one, children who suffer from disturbances of their vital functions, such as eating, sleeping, later on learning; or who show unusual delays in acquiring vital capacities such as movement, cleanliness, speech. There are many whose development has been arrested, especially at the points of transition between one developmental phase and the next. Cases of this kind crowd out those with phobias and incipient obsessional neuroses, even though the latter two are not completely absent.[1]

There is an important problem of assessment here which is not easy to solve. We doubt whether all these arrests of functions and capacities represent prestages of neurotic development, which would imply that such children would develop an infantile neurosis later on if they went untreated. Such disturbances may also represent attempts at neurotic formations which have miscarried and could be called abortive neuroses.

There is no doubt that this enormously varied material

[1] We know that the absence or the mitigation of the masturbation conflict has done a great deal to change the picture of the infantile neurosis. On the other hand, this does not explain why we see the disturbances so much earlier now.

cannot be contained within the old diagnostic categories that distinguish between neurosis, psychosis, dissociality, intellectual deficiency, etc. Whether we call some of them psychotic, i.e., schizophrenic, depends largely on the diagnostician's viewpoint. However this may be, these child patients' symptomatic manifestations and forms of behavior show a close resemblance to the adult patients who come under these classifications.

It is an added difficulty that during the last decades our former clear-cut distinction between emotional and intellectual difficulties has been shaken. We lost this distinction when we learned that emotional deprivations in the first year of life can act as a severe check on intellectual development. A child under investigation may to all intents and purposes appear to be mentally deficient, but this will leave us quite uncertain whether he was born with a defective mental apparatus, or whether his ego apparatus was not sufficiently stimulated and motivated at the beginning of life. Infants who are emotionally deprived fail to cathect the environment with interest and consequently fail to develop their intellectual functions.

Metapsychological Assessment

If, on the basis of the foregoing, we decide to abandon the usual diagnostic distinctions, we are left in a void which we need to fill. Leaving labels of any kind aside, we may find it profitable to turn to metapsychological assessments and in this way try to approach the whole problem of diagnosis from a variety of angles. It may take some time until these disparate aspects can be collected again and turned into a unified whole.

ASSESSMENT FROM THE ASPECT OF DEVELOPMENT

Since children of all ages are unfinished human beings, whose future normality will be decided by the fact whether or not maturity is reached, the state or rate of their development should be of greatest concern for the diagnostician. There are some more or less highly disturbed children who nevertheless are still progressing from one developmental level to the next. There are others whose development has been arrested either in some areas or altogether. There is a third group where development has progressed satisfactorily to a certain height, from which regression to certain fixation points then has taken place. Only where the regressive moves concern primarily the libidinal side will the outcome be an infantile neurosis; where libido and ego regress simultaneously, conflict does not arise and the child's whole personality is reduced to a lower level—we might say, an infantilism.

It would not be out of the way for an analyst to use these three points—progression, arrest in development, and regression—as a basis for diagnostic grouping. Such a grouping could still be improved if we examine the various parts of the child's personality from the developmental levels that have been reached. There are children who are fairly normally developed so far as their instinctual drives, including their emotional relations, are concerned, but who simultaneously lag behind in ego functioning, in the building up of their defense organization, or in their moral functions. Our former judgments on a child as "precocious," "backward," etc., would thus be refined, each part of the mental apparatus being assessed in its own right and the developmental levels reached compared with each other.

ASSESSMENT BY TYPE OF CONFLICT

There is another angle, so striking in its usefulness that it is difficult to understand why it has not been exploited more for diagnostic purposes. What I have in mind is the ascending severity of conflicts with which we are presented in the individual and which are highly significant in determining the pathological result. Psychoanalytic study has made us familiar with three types of conflict: first, the external conflict, i.e., the conflict between child and environment; secondly, the intersystemic conflict between the various agencies within the personality, i.e., id vs. ego, ego vs. superego, superego vs. id; thirdly, the intrasystemic conflict within the id between opposing drives such as activity-passivity, masculinity-femininity, love-hate. The assessment of disturbances according to type of conflict also provides clues to the type of therapy which need be used. Guidance or educational methods will help in external conflicts; analysis is ideally suited for intersystemic conflicts, for which essentially it was designed; whatever intensive method is used, the task will be a difficult one when a child is treated whose conflict is between the drives.

ASSESSMENT AT THE DIAGNOSTIC STAGE

It is to be expected that the suggestions mentioned so far will meet with major objections in the psychoanalytic world. As analysts we are used to make no assessment of the patient's state except on the basis of material gained from his analysis. But if we adhere to such a cautious approach to the diagnostic problem, we are left at the beginning confrontations with the patient with no more than an enumeration of his symptoms and a descriptive qualification.

What I suggest here is a more courageous approach which can take us further.

Once we decide to disregard the diagnostic categories derived from descriptive psychiatry for adult psychopathology and to play down the importance of symptomatology as such, we can hope to be alerted more vigorously to these other aspects of the patient's personality. Where children are concerned, these will be mostly developmental ones. Also, where children are concerned, we do not commonly restrict ourselves to what the child has to say about himself, but we are offered a great deal of circumstantial evidence, i.e., descriptions given by the parents, school, the social history, etc. Not all items of this collection will be relevant, but there are many behavioral and surface manifestations which can be turned into diagnostic clues and pointers by the knowledgeable child analyst.

THE ASSESSMENT OF BORDERLINE CASES

To return to our question of the borderline cases. There exist many definitions of this concept, the most common one being a clinical picture on the border between neurosis and psychosis. It is perhaps an unwarranted licence to use the term—as we do in the Hampstead Child-Therapy Clinic —for a whole series of disorders which do not fit into our notion of an infantile neurosis, but, deviating from such a structure, lead over to other, usually more severe pathologies.

If we understand the concept in this way, we arrive at cases not only on the border between neurosis and psychosis, but also on the border of mental deficiency, of delinquency, of the perversions, etc.

It is easy to understand that the distinguishing lines between these disorders are not always drawn sharply. We know that all children of certain young ages have their delinquent features, or, to say it more clearly, that there are ages when antisocial or asocial behavior is still to be expected. It goes without saying that the same is true of the perversions. There even is, to our mind, a "border" between the neurotic and the autistic child insofar as the autistic features (withdrawal) can manifest themselves within the picture of an infantile neurosis.

The Problem of Quantity vs. Quality

Before we label a child borderline, i.e., beyond the framework of the infantile neurosis, we ought to ask ourselves whether this distinction is made on the basis of the quantity vs. the quality of the observed manifestations. Massive, quantitatively increased symptomatology is seldom distinguished from qualitative differences between the manifestations.

A useful example, in this respect, are the anxiety attacks of phobic children. These can reach such a height of frantic intensity that they are frequently confused with the temper tantrums of near-psychotic children. Another example of this kind are the seduced children, e.g., Erna Furman's case (1956). Their behavior following the trauma may be so abnormal, so erratic, so out-of-the-ordinary that there is every temptation to classify them under the heading of schizophrenia. The same is true of boys with heightened castration anxiety. Even though their disturbance is based on the castration anxiety of the phallic phase and represents an infantile neurosis, their behavior is undoubtedly "crazy," i.e., apparently psychotic.

To separate off quantitative increase from qualitative difference seems to be an important first step in the assessment of borderline phenomena.

The Problem of Qualitative Difference from Neurosis

This leads us to the cases that are qualitatively different from the neuroses. Such differences can be located in the *id content,* so far as the depth of regression or the massiveness of developmental arrest is concerned. In either instance, these children do not function on the oedipal level. But while the regressions of the neurotic child are halted at the anal-sadistic or the later oral fixation points, the borderline ones return to much earlier levels if they have not been arrested in them altogether. There is of course also the possibility that neurotic manifestations, i.e., regressions to later fixation points, manifest themselves simultaneously with very early fixations and produce a mixed clinical picture.

Another important qualitative difference concerns the child's libidinal attachments. We feel that a child is nearing the "border" if his libido is on the point of being withdrawn from the object world and attached either to his body or to the self. It is a frequent occurrence with such children that they do what no normal child would dream of doing. Instead of fighting for the right to stay up and not to break their contact with their environment, they withdraw voluntarily into bed and into sleep, preferring their own company to that of their objects.

It has often been stressed that the inability of a child to receive comfort from his objects is an early sign of severe pathology. The border we are considering here is that between autoerotism and object relations, with preference given to the former.

Differential diagnoses of this kind are not always easy. I remember the assessment of a thirteen-month-old baby who showed severe disturbances in her relationship to the mother at whose approach she invariably screamed. She would accept no comfort from her mother and would go into withdrawal states that sounded ominous. Her best times were in bed when she was left alone, free to indulge in thumb sucking.

Surprisingly enough, this child, suspected of mental deficiency, reacted perfectly normally to an observer—a fact from which we had to conclude not that the capacity for object relations had been lost or had remained undeveloped, but that some traumatic event had shifted the sources of comfort from the figures in her environment to her own body.

Our diagnosis was confirmed by the information that for a while the child had been in the care of a nurse who developed schizophrenia and had ungovernable outbursts of jealousy and quarreling with the mother in the infant's presence.

To return once more to the differential diagnosis: I have no doubt that this particular infant, if not helped, would at a later date have appeared not as a traumatized child frightened of the object world, but as a severely mentally deficient child who also lacked the capacity to form meaningful object relationships.

There are further qualitative differences for which we look within *the sphere of the ego.*

The first that comes to mind is the security of the so-called ego boundaries (Federn). We expect children from the second year onward to have a clear delimitation in their minds between their own body and self and those of the people in their environment. We consider it natural and normal for an infant to treat parts of the mother's body as if they were his own, or to treat his own body as being merged with hers.

This state of affairs is manifested frequently by children of that age sucking the mother's finger instead of theirs or, for example, at a slightly later date, leading the spoon interchangeably to their own mouth and that of the mother. It is true that in certain respects the mother will for several years to follow consider the body of the child as part of herself (or at least her concern) and that so far as health and hygiene are concerned, children almost up to the age of adolescence feel that it is the mother's, not their own, function to look after the safety of their bodies.

But even if remnants of such merging with the mother are counted among the normal manifestations up to the end of childhood, the normal or neurotic child will have a clear body image in his mind from early on and it will need severe upheavals in his life to make him lose his sense of personal integrity and separateness.

It is particularly in this respect that the differences between the neurotic, psychotic, autistic or mentally defective children are outstanding. We are treating a number of borderline children who are constantly confused in this respect.

I mention here an eight-year-old boy, Peter, a highly intelligent child who frequently does not know whether he is in fact himself or whether he is his therapist. At home the same confusion exists in his mind between himself and his mother. For example, after destroying one of his own toys, he will scream accusations against his mother for having done this.

An atypical girl, for instance, has the compelling need to carry a teddy bear or doll thrown over her shoulder. On the other hand, this can be replaced by her mother or the therapist carrying a doll or teddy bear or even herself in the same way. The doll, therapist, mother, and her own person are used interchangeably, with no distinction made between them. Such confusions between self and others can be regarded as valuable pointers for the diagnostician.

It goes without saying that qualitative distinctions between the various types of cases are found within the *ego functions*. The important function of reality testing can be used as an example. This of course is complicated by the fact that the perfection of this particular function is a question of age, that the very young are apt to confuse reality and fantasy and that we do not know with absolute accuracy at what age reality testing should be firmly and unmistakably established. Normal children may play, for instance, that their dolls are alive, need to be fed, clothed, kept warm, put to bed, etc. There are few clues in their behavior whether this is "play acting" or whether in fact they believe in their own fantasies.

What we still condone at the age of three or four may begin to alarm us by the time the child is five and will give rise to serious concern once the latency stage should normally have been reached. I quote in this respect another highly intelligent schoolboy treated at our Clinic who at times seemed completely oblivious of reality. There was an incident one summer when he rushed into the Clinic carrying an enormous sunflower in his hand. Analytic interpretation would say that he treated this flower as an obvious penis symbol and that this, in itself, is not unusual. But then he described to everybody how he scared his therapist to death with that sunflower, how she nearly fell down in a faint when he took it into the room, how he waved it before her, how people right and left were amazed at what he had brought, and so on. What for another child would have been a daydream was convincing truth for him. I think we can agree that such absence of reality testing indicates that the borders of neurosis have been overstepped.

The conspicuous absence of the synthetic function, once early childhood is passed, points in the same direction.

So far as we believe in a chronological sequence of defense mechanisms from the most primitive to the sophisticated, we view a retrograde development with suspicion. We are equally suspicious of the presence of a nonneurotic disturbance when children never develop beyond the primary mechanisms of denial, projection, introjection, with repression, reaction formation, sublimation playing no part. Likewise, the retrograde steps from secondary to primary process thinking or arrest on primary process level is an ominous diagnostic sign.

So far as differential diagnosis between neurosis and psychosis is concerned, the concretization of thought processes and the use of body language are important items. We differ very little from this in our assessment of children's cases. Some borderline children lose speech altogether and become preverbal; others retain speech but use words concretely. I name here a four-year-old withdrawn child who was fascinated by the London station called King's Cross. For him this was not a name but the image of a king, cross with his subjects, who chops off their heads.

A borderline schoolboy, referred to the Clinic because of

a dangerous compulsion to walk on the Underground lines (which meant to him the intestines in his body), had an uncanny ability to memorize names of stations. Likewise he memorized not only the names of the forty children in his classroom, but the addresses, each name of a street constituting a vivid image in his mind: Hobden Lane, e.g., was a man who hobbles. According to his borderline withdrawal, he had no normal social relations with his peers, the place of these being taken by their names.[2]

I should like to mention as a last distinguishing item the barriers between the agencies of the personality, especially the barrier between id and ego. In the very young child we do not expect these barriers to be very stable: we are prepared for id content to burst through occasionally and to lead to what we know as emotional outbursts or temper tantrums. But as the child grows older, and especially in neurotic children, we expect these barriers to become relatively stable structures.

SUMMARY

In concluding, I would like to emphasize that none of these points taken by itself is diagnostically significant. They become significant only when they appear in combination. The more of them are present in a given child, the more certain one can be that we are dealing with a nonneurotic, i.e., a borderline case.

[2] For a detailed discussion of this case, see Singer (1960).

19

Entrance into Nursery School:

The Psychological
Prerequisites
(1960)

May I add to the introduction made by our Chairman,
Mr. R. W. Ferguson, that I am not really a newcomer to
the Nursery School Association. About twenty years ago
I was an active member of the Executive, and repeatedly
a speaker at the Summer Schools of the Association. I
think back to those times with pleasure but also with some

Presented as a lecture entitled "Why Children Go Wrong" to
the Nursery School Association of Great Britain, National Conference, July 1, 1960.

First published in *The Enrichment of Childhood*. London: The
Nursery School Association of Great Britain and Northern Ireland,
1960, pp. 23-34.

misgivings. They left me with the feeling that, although I tried my best to fulfill the needs of the Association as I saw them, I did not really succeed in fulfilling their wishes.

As a psychoanalyst I was occupied then, as I am now, with the disturbances of children, whereas the Association thought of their teachers as dealing with healthy, normal children. When I talked about the hidden motivation of behavior, they would have preferred me to deal with its manifest and visible aspects; when I laid stress on the emotional life of the child with all the ensuing complications, this appeared to them rather as neglect of the child's skills, intellectual needs, and interests; my emphasis on the past events and their impact on the building up of personalities appeared to distract attention from the conditions actually present, etc. Anyway, our direction of thinking did not coincide in those times and that was the reason why, after a few years of cooperation, we began to drift apart.

At the time I am referring to, the nursery school went through what may well be called a heroic period. The needs of thousands of young children were made urgent by wartime conditions. Many day nurseries and nursery schools had to acquire residential status and take over full-time care of their charges. Teachers had to be equipped hurriedly to deal with homeless, derelict, bombed-out children whose family life had been broken up. These were urgent practical problems which left little time for other considerations. It is very much to the credit of the Nursery School Association that its members played a significant part in fulfilling these tasks, thereby safeguarding the mental and physical health of large numbers of young children.

Since I did not know where the next developments lay, I was surprised to receive the title of my present assignment.

An interest in the reasons why the development of certain children takes a turn to the wrong betrays a definite acceptance of the idea that the normality of development in childhood is a precarious matter and the acknowledgment that it may be necessary for every teacher of the young to be aware of disturbances and abnormalities. It gives no hint, though, of the influences which may have been at work to bring about this change.

Looking for such influences, one is immediately reminded of the fact that the London County Council has given very important leads in recognizing the existence of the problem child, and in making provision for problem children of many types. There are the so-called "special classes" in the London County Council elementary schools for children who fail to adjust to the ordinary course of learning; there are the schools and hostels for maladjusted children who do not fit into the lives of their own families; there are the child guidance clinics of the London County Council and the cooperation of the school authorities with clinics set up by other agencies; there is provision for organically handicapped children with their resulting mental difficulties, etc. All this has had a far-reaching influence on all workers with children. The knowledge that there are difficult children has become acceptable and respectable, and has spread to wider circles. So far as the Nursery School Association is concerned, members of the audience merely need to look over the library table filled with recent publications to find booklets dealing with the disturbances of the child's sleeping and eating habits, the difficulties of their toilet training, their jealousies, etc.

The question with which we are faced in this new situation is the following: what is the best line of approach for

introducing all teachers, either during their period of training (i.e., within the training colleges) or during their work
in the nursery schools, to the differences between normality and abnormality in childhood? There are, of course,
places where the problematic behavior of children is reported, collected, sifted, diagnosed, and treated, namely,
the child guidance clinics. But I do not consider it a satisfactory solution to recommend that teachers, either during
their training or during their career as teachers, merely pay
visits to such clinics, even though they would see much
there to create an impression. They would realize how many
workers in the field are puzzled and mystified by the behavior of young children. Parents, doctors, teachers, hospital almoners, the police, the courts, the local authorities,
etc., all play their part in referring children to the clinics.
It can be a most upsetting experience to read the reports
which accompany the children. There are the urgent complaints from young mothers that their infants will not sleep
properly, or not feed, or refuse to be toilet-trained; or that,
after being successfully trained, they have reverted again to
wetting and soiling; some will even starve themselves or interfere with their own bodies to the extent of causing
serious damage. Some are described as being hesitant and
inhibited in play and missing most of the legitimate pleasures of childhood; others are inhibited in learning and remain far behind their contemporaries in spite of good
potential intelligence. Many are frightened without apparent reason, cannot approach certain harmless animals,
or go out into the streets, or go to school. Many are difficult to control; many are overaggressive; many lie, play
truant, show signs of dishonesty, etc.

The picture is such a bewildering one that to me it does

not seem right to expose all teachers of nursery schools to this comprehensive psychopathology of childhood. Many of these details are far beyond the teachers' scope of experience, others arise only later in a child's life, so that nursery school life does not show evidence of more than the faintest trace of beginning disturbance. Introducing teachers to too many of these complexities—and cursorily at that—may well have the effect of confusing the whole issue, instead of clarifying the pictures of normal and abnormal development.

I suggest, therefore, that a different approach to the problem might be chosen. Nursery school teachers can be taught about abnormality and normality on the basis of the child population they see in their own classrooms, and I am convinced that the average group in every nursery school contains sufficient material to illustrate the links between the two states. Before embarking on this task it is useful to sift the teachers' ideas about children who seem to them to have developed on the right lines (i.e., to be normal) or on the wrong ones (i.e., to have become abnormal).

I begin, therefore, with the average teacher's expectations of the normal child at the date of entry into nursery school. There may be a general consensus of opinion among teachers that not much is expected of the child and that the rules laid down for normal behavior are rather tolerant ones. I doubt whether there is any truth in this belief.

More than twenty years ago I was connected with an experimental nursery where children between the ages of one and two were received and where it would have been true to say that our expectations concerning the entrants were low indeed. What qualified for entry was one achievement only, namely, the beginning of independent movement, whether crawling or walking. But that is not so with the nursery school proper where the child usually enters at the age of three and a half and where the list of necessary qualifications is a long one. This list includes independent movement; speech; toilet training with some ability to use the lavatory independently; the ability to eat without much help; orientation in new surroundings; the ability to separate from the mother for a number of hours without undue distress and to accept the teacher as a substitute; the ability to accept and enjoy playmates; the ability to use toys either with skill or with imagination, or both.

It is true that teachers do not really object if the individual child fails to come up to standard in one or two of these respects or if occasional lapses occur in all of them. But if such lapses are too frequent or if substandard behavior occurs in too many areas, the teacher will be alarmed and consider the child as one who "has gone wrong" in his development. I believe, therefore, that successful teaching about abnormality can be effected by examining such lines of development in detail and by bringing it home to the teachers which complexities in the external life experiences and the inner mental processes of the child determine success or failure in living up to the demands of the nursery school. Such examination could be carried out on all the demands made on the child entering nursery school as mentioned above. Since we lack the time for such a lengthy procedure, I select from them merely three important ones, namely, (1) the tolerance for temporary separation from the mother; (2) adequate behavior in the nursery school; (3) tolerance for group life and enjoyment of it.

TEMPORARY SEPARATION FROM THE
MOTHER FOR NURSERY SCHOOL PURPOSES

There is perhaps no other nursery school routine in which more changes have occurred in recent years. In the not so very distant past it was assumed that a child who had reached the age of three and a half would be able to separate from his mother on the first day of entry at the outer door of the school building, and would further make himself acquainted with the new physical surroundings, the new teacher, and the new playmates, all in one morning. A blind eye was turned toward the distress of the new entrants; their crying for their mothers and their initial lack of participation and cooperation were considered inevitable and of little significance.

What happened under those conditions was that most children went through an initial stage of extreme unhappiness, after which they settled down to the nursery school routine. Some others reversed the sequence of events. Surprisingly enough, they began with a period of acquiescence and apparent enjoyment, which then, again surprisingly, was followed a week later by intense unhappiness and a breakdown in participation. These children, too, adapted themselves to the new conditions after the first weeks. What seems important now is the fact that in those times no one gave much thought to what happened inside the individual children in their periods of desolation and how these affected their later attitudes and performances in school.

We all know that this procedure has changed in our times and that at least all progressive nursery schools base their entry routine on the recognition that the first separation from home life is a significant event in the child's development, i.e., one which has to be handled with care. Nowadays the young entrants are often shown the playrocm before their first school day; they usually meet the teacher for the first time with their mother, no other children being present at the time; above all, their mothers are permitted to take them to the school room on the first day and, in many nursery schools, to remain as spectators in the background for a day, several days, or even more, until the child has become adjusted to their absence. These are far-reaching changes in attitude, and it is worthwhile to draw the teachers' attention to the new insights to which we owe these innovations.

What is now known under the name of "separation anxiety" (i.e., the protest of the infant and young child against prolonged absence of the mother) has been observed and described above all in three settings: in the residential war nurseries of our evacuated children; in hospitals where young children are admitted without their mothers for stays of varying lengths; and in residential institutions of peacetime such as orphanages, foundling homes, etc. Studies of such children who grow up in separation from their mothers, or whose contacts with their mothers are interrupted, have been correlated with knowledge gained from the analytic treatment of disturbed individuals and have led to a new attitude toward the significance of the young child's tie to the mother, a tie which cannot be broken or interfered with without serious consequences for the whole of the young child's emotional development.

It will be useful, then, for every teacher to learn that normally the child's ability to separate from the mother is the end product in a line of development in which a series of consecutive steps can be distinguished from each other.

There is a first stage, beginning with birth, when an infant can hardly be considered as a person in his own right. Just as in intrauterine life he has been part of his mother's body, he remains part of his mother's living presence during the first months of his extrauterine existence. No infant can survive without his mother's or a motherly person's constant nearness and attention. No one doubts that at this time of life nothing is gained by separating the two partners of the mother-child couple and that much distress is caused whenever such separations become necessary owing to illness, death, or other circumstances which are beyond control. We may call this stage the period of biological unity between mother and child.

But even the next stage, approximately the time of the second year of life, remains one in which close and unbroken contact with the mother is demanded. Here the infant is still dependent on the mother for the fulfillment of all his needs which arise either from his body or from his awakening mind, and usually no unfamiliar substitute for the mother will be in a position to gratify his wishes and bring comfort, a fact well known to all sick-nurses and even baby-sitters. The greater the individual need, the louder is the infant's clamor for the presence of the mother, who is released from duty only when the child is asleep or, for a short while, satisfied.

The demandingness of the infant develops further in imperceptible steps into the clinging of the toddler, who loves his mother with an attachment of the most possessive, dominating, savage kind. Adults who have no personal experience of the upbringing of a toddler are usually convinced that this relationship is an abnormal one and is the mother's product, that it is she who has "spoiled" the child, who will not separate from him, or who teaches him to cling. Actually, nothing could be farther from the truth.

Careful observation shows that at this stage it is still normal for mother and child to live in close contact; that the child protests violently about separations on this level because they are unnatural and not helpful to him; that mothers suffer a good deal during this period, which, luckily, does not need to last longer than the toddler stage itself; and that the mother is not yet "loved" by her infant on this level, at least not in the true sense of the word: she is needed.

Finally, there comes a third stage when the child finds himself ready to separate from his mother for short periods. He does not need her all the time any more. He is ready to reach out to new people, to widen his circle of intimate acquaintances, to accept new ventures and adventures, of course in the beginning only if the periods of independence are not too long and if return to the mother is open to his choice. Several inner factors have to work together before this development is achieved. The most important one among them is a change in the quality of the mother-child relationship, which has ceased to be determined wholly by the child's needs. By now the mother is appreciated not only as the giver of satisfaction and comfort, but also as a person in her own right. The child can retain a loving relationship to her even in her absence, and even in situations when she does not serve the fulfillment of his wishes. He has acquired what we call an inner image of the mother which does not change easily any more and which sustains his relationship to her during the periods of her physical absence, always provided that this absence does not last longer than adequate for his level of development. Within this limit he can now let the mother go, remember her with positive feelings, accept her absence without distress, and receive her happily when she returns.

To return to our requirements for nursery school entrance so far as the separation from the mother and acceptance of the teacher are concerned: it seems clear from the foregoing descriptions that entry into the nursery group will be profitable only for those children who have been successful enough in their development to reach the last of the described stages. But even then it will be necessary for the teacher to know the preliminary ones which had to be gone through first, since they seldom disappear without leaving visible traces of the past. Furthermore, no young child remains on the height of his developmental achievements for long periods. Often it needs no more than a little tiredness, some disappointment, a small accident, some anxiety, a slight bodily indisposition to change the whole aspect of the child and to make the infant or the toddler reappear in the apparently well-adapted nursery school child. What the teacher is then confronted with are tearful scenes at parting in the morning; or angry ones when the child is fetched by the mother; signs of distress which would seem appropriate only for the two-year-old; noncooperation with the teacher, etc. The teacher who can assess these outbreaks as throwbacks to former stages of development will be less puzzled, less inclined to criticize the mothers, and better able to intervene helpfully. She will understand "abnormality" in this respect as the return to former levels of behavior and development.

ADEQUATE BEHAVIOR IN THE NURSERY SCHOOL

There are many teachers for whom the intimate and violent emotions of the child are a strange and uncertain matter and who will prefer to assess the normality or abnormality of his development on the basis of the general ease or difficulty with which he is able to adjust his behavior to the life in the nursery group and to follow the existent rules. Somewhere in her mind even the most tolerant nursery school teacher carries the image of the "ideal" nursery school child. Such a child exhibits no outward signs of impatience and restlessness; he asks for things instead of grabbing them; he can wait for his turn, whether in the playroom or on the swings; he expects no more than his fair share. He can stand disappointments; for example, he does not throw a temper tantrum if another child's favorite record is played rather than his. If his building topples over, he does not kick and scream but begins to erect a new and steadier one, etc. Of course, the teacher knows that no single child will have acquired all these desirable forms of behavior, but on the whole they will be found in the group, in one or the other child, with regard to one or the other daily event. Couched in psychological terms, this means that at this age the children are on the point of learning one of the most difficult tasks in life: to master their feelings and impulses instead of finding themselves at the mercy of them.

Teachers will be able to grasp the magnitude of this achievement only if they are able to compare this state of affairs with the stages which have gone before. No baby or infant can wait for his food, or for the attention of the mother, or for being taken out of his cot, or for the removal of any discomfort without showing the extreme urgency of his need and discomfort by kicking, screaming, and clamoring. An infant who remains quiet and accepting under such conditions is not considered normal; he lacks drive and impetus, and his very peacefulness gives rise to apprehension with regard to his development.

It is thus the extreme urgency of impulses and wishes which has to be mastered to a certain degree before the child can enter nursery school life. Something has to develop within the child himself, a kernel of a new personality, a reasonable center, by means of which the child can take charge and master the unruly and demanding inner world of drives and impulses. As shown with regard to the mother relationship, the growth of this reasonable center is a gradual process which takes time, is not completed all at once, and the influence of which extends slowly from one set of impulses to another.

For the understanding of the teachers it will be useful if they train themselves to observe their charges from this particular point of view of behavior. Describing their individual children, they could show how far each one has mastered his needs and wishes and the extent to which he is still overwhelmed by them; and which of the needs have come under the child's control and which others still swamp the child. There are the child's greed with regard to food, his possessiveness for toys, his desire to show off in front of all others, to be singled out for preferential treatment; there are his aggressiveness and destructiveness, his curiosity, his attraction to dirt, etc. Such observations will convince the teacher that what she calls "normal" behavior is no more than the child's partial or complete success in mastering these impulses and impulsive attitudes; what she calls "abnormal" means failure in this particular respect.

As shown above, no young child maintains a high level of performance for long periods. Whenever a child is tired, anxious, or for physical reasons below par, he will revert to earlier, easier, i.e., more childish forms of behavior. At the end of a long nursery school day, for example, temper tantrums will occur, good manners will disappear, impatience and urgency of wishes will be more obvious, even in the most adapted child. This is "normal." No development goes forward in a straight, progressive line. It is usual for every human individual during his period of growth constantly to take temporary steps backward, without on the whole giving up or harming his forward development. An understanding of these developmental necessities will go far in helping teachers to be less puzzled about the changing behavior of their children, and, perhaps, to be less worried and more skillful in dealing with their periods of "abnormality."

ENJOYMENT OF GROUP LIFE

The situation becomes more complex and the lines of development need even closer watching where not only the behavior of the individual children but their interactions with each other come into the picture. As my example I take here a happening which is familiar and welcome to every teacher: a small group of four- to five-year-olds who cooperate in setting up a railway system. Some of them are busy laying the tracks and running the train, two are building bridges and setting up stations; if the play takes place in the garden, some enterprising ones may even add rivers or some lakes. There is very little talk to accompany the work. In spite of this, there may be perfect understanding and cooperation in carrying out a common, preconceived plan. Every teacher in whose group such play is taking place is justifiably proud. The skills, the speed with which the work is carried out, and the peaceful atmosphere in which it proceeds are proof to her that these children are well adapted, happy, and successful—in short, that they are "normal."

I wonder whether teachers also realize all the difficult stages through which the individual child has to pass successfully before he can participate in such play. Apart from the two important developments mentioned before, it seems to me that at least three further lines of growth have to be completed, and almost brought to perfection, to equip the young individual for such a group task: he has to be able to play constructively with toys; his play has to be brought to a level not far removed from what will later be called "work"; and he has to accept other children as his partners. All three achievements (play, work, partnership) have a long history which it is useful for the teacher to scrutinize.

Development toward Constructive Play

Although toys of all descriptions are often given to infants from birth onward, the ability to play with them is a gradual acquisition. Actually, the child's first play takes place on his own body, and on his mother's body. His fingers, his hands, his feet, the surface of his skin, his sexual organs, as well as the mother's face, her hands, her breasts are the baby's first toys, which are used and explored for all the possible ways and means to obtain satisfaction from them. Remnants of this normal stage of development can be observed in a category of highly abnormal children, the so-called "autistic" ones, who ignore all possibilities of pleasure to be gained in play with objects offered by the world outside and continue (or revert to) constant play with their fingers, their hands, etc.

Normal children soon grow beyond the satisfactions which can be obtained from their own bodies or the mother's body, and become attached to toys, the first ones usually being the cuddly toys which serve as the transition between the body and the constructive toys. Cuddly toys are loved, used for comfort, as an outlet for loving as well as angry feelings. It is only after the cuddly toy that the constructive toys begin to play a role: the building blocks, railway tracks, etc. These latter are not just loved by the child; they are used for an ulterior purpose, and they are cherished for that purpose. Naturally, it is this stage of play with the constructive toy which has to be attained before a child can join in group play of the kind described above.

Development from Play to Work

Again, the ability to use constructive toys does not in itself qualify the child for carrying out a preconceived plan. Other abilities have to be added to it. In the beginning, building blocks may be used merely for throwing; sand and water, for messing; train engines, for being taken apart to satisfy the child's curiosity; the building of a high tower may lead merely to pleasure in the noise when it is destroyed again.

All these impulses—to mess, to take apart, to use things destructively and for aggression—have to be brought under control and placed in the service of a higher purpose. Sand and water are then used for building; curiosity for understanding engines; building for constructing something which will be pleasing to the eye and satisfying to the child's imagination. Furthermore, no plan will ever be brought to completion before the child has acquired the ability to persevere, to overcome difficulties instead of being overcome by them—in short, before some of the attitudes which will later characterize the adult's work have been added to the child's ability to play.

Developments toward Partnership

Teachers have a right to be proud of their children's growing ability to accept partnership, since development toward this goal is one of the most important items in the whole list of achievements necessary for normality. Infants and toddlers, as we know, are self-centered; they are asocial rather than dissocial; they have little use for other infants or other toddlers, and a children's party at these early ages usually ends up with each individual child playing in an individual corner of the room after successfully appropriating some toy or plaything which is individually pleasing. In residential or day centers where toddlers must live together, we can observe that the other child, if not merely a disturbance, is at best treated by them as a lifeless thing, a toy that can be used, pushed away, treated in all sorts of ways, and maltreated.

Normally this stage is outgrown at the end of the second year when new attitudes toward the contemporaries appear on the surface. Other children are now accepted as helpmates for short periods of time on the basis of a common wish. They are considered useful to build something together, or destroy it together, the interest in these instances still being centered on the occupation or the goal, to which the other child is merely incidental.

It needs a further advance until the other child becomes a partner, that is, a person in his own right, whose wishes are considered, whose feelings are taken into account, whose friendship is valued, and who is either admired or at other times criticized for his personal qualities. Only from then onward will the associations between children proceed on a basis of equality and comradeship. It is this final step which has to be taken before group cooperation of the type described above can be achieved.

Falling Apart of the Group; Regressive Behavior

It seems to me that all teachers should be taught to view their children's behavior as the outcome of consecutive developmental steps.[1] They would then understand more readily why children differ so greatly in their adjustments to nursery school.

There are, as we know from other areas of life, no two individuals whose rates of development proceed at the same pace. There are those who develop fast and are "forward" for their age; there are others who are slow developers and show up to their disadvantage when compared with their

[1] [For a more detailed discussion of this point, see ch. 27 in Volume IV.]

contemporaries. But this, in itself, means little for the final results of growth. The fast developers may slow up later, the slow ones take sudden moves forward, as is well known from the acquisition of speech, of independent movement, of the pleasure in learning, etc.

It is of equal importance for teachers to realize that in the three lines of growth which lead to group play, steps backward to former behavior are as common as the forward steps. No group play among four-year-olds lasts longer than, perhaps, half an hour. After that, the participants tire of their high level of group performance and the play falls apart. One of the children may retreat once more along the line from the toy to the body, i.e., he will withdraw to a corner and begin to suck his thumb; another will cease to construct, tear things apart or throw utensils which a short while ago had served a building purpose; a third child will begin to act aggressively toward his companions, grab what they are working with, or turn his back on them. These are temporary lapses, in themselves normal. Observation of them will be useful to the teacher, not only for understanding the length of the way these children have already come in their development, but also for being tolerant of their short span of attention and achievement.

CONCLUSIONS

To sum up: it seems to me that teachers of young children should be taught to understand the variations which exist within normal childhood development before they approach the difficult subject of the pathology, i.e., the abnormalities of childhood. Some of the abnormal children they see in their classrooms are merely backward ones, i.e., those who have remained on lower levels of development and are not yet able to come up to the standard set for their ages. Their difficulties can be understood if we compare their everyday behavior with the regressive moods and attitudes of normal pupils. Other "difficult" children who puzzle the teacher may be those whose development is uneven, high levels being achieved in some respects (for example, speech, or ability to separate, or play), while development in other, no less important areas (for example, toilet training; adapted, social behavior) has lagged behind. Other children again may not fit into the nursery school scheme because their periods of good performance are too short, i.e., their lapses in behavior being more conspicuous than their good achievements.

I hope that it will not be too disappointing to my audience if I say that there is no simple answer to the question why children go either "right" or "wrong." On the contrary, I should like to warn teachers not to trust the simple solutions, wherever they are offered. It is not true that children become abnormal for any one reason, whether this is found in not being loved enough by the parents; or rejected; or not being given a feeling of security; or being overprotected; or separated; or clung to, etc. The truth is that the growth and development of the human individual (body and mind) are a complex matter. Human individuals are born with varying endowments into environments of infinite variety. Their development will in each case depend on the interaction between the inner and the outer forces which come into play. A favorable environment will help those whose endowment is poor; on the other hand, children with a good endowment will show more resilience under the pressure of adverse outside influences. Every child is born different, has a different rate of growth, and experiences different growing pains and conflicts. But I certainly do not think that it is beyond the teachers' reach to gain insight into these complicated and fascinating processes.

20

The Emotional and Social Development of Young Children
(1962)

I should first like to give an explanation of why I am here at all today. When Miss Pickard came to visit me about a year ago in order to invite me to speak at this assembly she made it quite clear what her motive was: namely, that she felt that the right person to speak to you about the child's emotional and social development would be a psycho-analyst, since psychoanalysis is the discipline most concerned with fact finding about these areas of the child's life. This seemed to me a very great compliment to psycho-

First published in Report of the 9th World Assembly, London, July 16-21, 1962 (World Organisation for Early Childhood Education, Organisation Mondiale pour L'Éducation Préscholaire).

analysis, and was something I could not let go by without answering. However, I still had many misgivings about appearing here. I thought I would probably need to give a lengthy introduction to my talk to make it helpful to you, and in this mood of concern I decided to listen to the opening session of this convention. I therefore came along yesterday, and found, to my enormous relief, that all the necessary introduction was already done for me by yesterday's speakers.

I believe I could have found no better words to introduce what I have to say than Miss Pickard's yesterday, when she said that dealing with the older child as compared with the younger child meant a turning away from logic and reason to the illogical and the irrational. I also echo your president's words, that the step from preschool education to school education was a step over the most extreme and last frontier of education. This is exactly what I had in mind. I felt that my talk today would take you very much across this borderline, and that what we all have to do in training teachers for the young is to make them feel at home in this other country where reason and logic do not count, and where one must proceed according to different mental principles altogether.

Now for the detailed characteristics of the country of the small child and of the language that is spoken there. I have always been interested, when working with parents or with teachers, in the many misunderstandings that arise between them and their children. The parents and the teachers make arrangements for the child with the best intentions, based on external circumstances, based on an insight into the conditions, based upon reason and logic. But these are looked upon by the child in a very different spirit: namely, they are understood in terms of the child's wishes, fantasies, fears, and thereby are completely altered. The child may be sent to nursery school by the mother for excellent reasons, perhaps to avoid boredom at home. The mother may feel that the company of others would be good for the child at this particular stage of his development, because she herself is very busy with other matters. The child understands this as banishment from home. The mother, with the best intentions, makes plans for a term of hospitalization—for a tonsillectomy, for example, or for some other necessary repair to the child's body. The child understands this as an attack on his body. Or the child has to be subjected to a diet. This means to him punishment and deprivation.

Struck by examples of this kind I have tried to look to our knowledge of children, in the hope that it would be possible to pinpoint the areas in which these grave misunderstandings between adults and children arise. I have found quite a number of them, and of these I want to present to you roughly four—four important points in which the child differs from us adults so that we have to relearn to understand the world of his emotions. But in this difficult task for the parent or teacher there is one saving grace; namely, that this way, characteristic of the child, is still alive somewhere in the adult, only unknown, repressed, and continues to exist in a dark area. But this confronts us with the task of understanding such areas in ourselves; when this is done, we shall find it easy to understand the child.

1. Let me give you four illustrations. We adults dream, and we also daydream. There is one important fact about our dreams and daydreams. Have you ever noticed that we are always the center of that dream world? We may appear

to dream about other people, but when we look into it more closely, it is always ourselves. We may daydream, but has anybody daydreamed about a neighbor having a wonderful experience in his life? Saving somebody, being acclaimed as a hero, amassing riches, and so on—it is always ourselves. What is left over in the adult in these rather isolated and dark areas is the functioning of the child, because this egocentric way is the way in which the child sees the world around him.

There are no objective facts in the early years, only subjective ones. When the mother has a headache or when the teacher has a cold, the child does not feel that the mother has a headache, the teacher a cold. He probably feels, "They are cross with me, I must have done something wrong." When the mother is ill in bed, the child feels, "She does not want to play with me today." When she expects a new baby, the child feels, "Why doesn't she lift me up any more? Evidently she does not like me." And I remember one patient who in later years could talk of the mother's death only in terms of: "When she deserted me. . . ." It is this egocentric way, that nothing happens in the world which is not immediately connected with the child's own feelings, wishes, experience, which makes it so difficult for us to understand the child. The feelings of other people do not count. When it rains, it probably rains to spoil the child's outing. When it thunders, it is probably because the child has done something wrong. The child never thinks, "It also rains for the people who have done everything right." When we find such beliefs in adults, we say they are superstitious. I am thinking of a specific adult who is quite convinced that when he goes on holiday it rains. I am quite convinced that this is left over from his childhood.

To give you an example of not understanding other people's feelings: the children of my own little nursery school were on an outing with their teacher the other day, and when they got near to the school the teacher said they could run to the door of the nursery. But one little girl, who is new to the community, pulled the teacher's hand after they had started and said, "Tell that boy not to run so fast. I want to be first." What about the little boy who wanted to be first? That played no part in it.

This is what we may call, without any criticism, the child's egocentric view of the world: it is natural to the child; it is natural for us to understand it; and it only ceases to be natural when the child does not outgrow it gradually in the years of nursery-school age. So much for the first point.

2. Another point has more to do with the contrast between reason and unreason, logic and illogic. To start again with the adult, we all know that under the provocation of very strong feelings the adult can do anything, can commit crimes, *crimes passionnels*, for which a judge or jury will sometimes even make allowances, feeling that the emotion, the urge of that moment in that particular adult person was too great to be held in check by the forces of reason, morality, convention.

But again this is exactly the state in which we continually find the child. Here it is mostly the parents who misunderstand, who feel that the child has let them down. The child has understood so well that one should not do this or that; that cars on the road are dangerous; that strangers should not be accosted; that desirable toys should not be taken, or even touched, in a shop. The child has understood, but the understanding has not governed his actions.

I think the great difference between ourselves and the children of nursery-school age, or younger ones, is not that they are so much less clever than we are, because they are quite reasonable. I think the difference lies in the fact that our reason is supposed to govern our behavior; whereas in the young child reason may be present, but behavior is governed by fears, wishes, impulses, and fantasies. You in this room listened to me so patiently; perhaps I have something interesting to say, but imagine that my talk became very dull indeed. You would still sit there to the end of the hour, because this is what is done. But if you were members of a nursery school and I failed to interest you in the continuation of a story, you would drift away, some out of this door, some out of that; some would collect in a corner and do something else. No convention and understanding of the difficulties of the teacher or speaker would keep you in your places. It would be the cessation of the wish to listen which would govern your behavior.

When I still had the Hampstead War Nurseries, we had children from the baby stage—from ten days—until eight years, very much the age of the children in whom you are interested here. Our young nursery teachers and helpers used to take the children out for walks in London, and, as there were so many children, I said, "Take them on reins." But the teachers said, "Not our children, They know all about the traffic. They are only two or three, but they would be offended if you put them on reins." The child knows that one does not run into the road. But what if a visiting mother appears on the sidewalk on the other side of the road? I will guarantee that these clever children will run through the traffic to the mother, because at that moment the wish is stronger than reason and understanding. Or let us say that a mother takes her child to the doctor or dentist. The child promises beforehand to be very good and very sensible, and has every intention to be so. Yet he will let the mother down, as she says. He screams when the dentist approaches his mouth, because by that time reason has gone and behavior is governed by fear.

There is another area in which adults find it difficult to understand the level of the child's functioning. Adults have long-term views, while children have short-term views. This means that we can tolerate the postponement of our wishes, and it is only in states of high emotional tension and impatience that we have to act immediately and under the pressure of impulse. But the child always has to act immediately: there is no postponement; there is no waiting period for the child, and the frustration that sets in when a wish is not fulfilled is enormous. This means that urgency of feelings and wishes is so much greater in the child than in the adult, and it makes nonsense of promises such as "We will learn that next year," or "In six months we shall take a trip to this or that place," or "Just wait until you are grown up." These are phrases that are absolutely meaningless to the child, as meaningless as if one were promised something in adult life a hundred or a thousand years ahead.

3. This leads me to the third point. I think we as teachers, parents, and teachers of teachers do not make enough of the fact that all young children have a time sense very different from our own. As adults we measure time objectively and by the clock, which means that we know the length of an hour. Again it needs a state of extreme anxiety —waiting for somebody to arrive, sitting it out during a

near relative's operation—that makes time stretch endlessly, so that one hour, three hours, four hours could just as well be one hundred hours.

It is only in states like these that we can understand the child's experiences with regard to time. Parents say, "We only go away for the weekend, two and a half days—that is nothing." Two and a half days' separation in the life of a child of two or three is an eternity. It could just as well be two and a half months or two and a half years. One may say to the child who is crying in the nursery, "Never mind, your mother will come in an hour." But an hour has sixty minutes, and every minute has sixty seconds. To a child it is an eternity. On the other hand, we say to the child, "You can still play for five minutes." But the five minutes seem to the child only one, because he wants it to be longer. We treat the child on the basis of our time sense, when we should treat him on the basis of his own time sense.

Again I shall give you an example from the Hampstead War Nurseries, where we learned so much because we had the opportunity of applying the knowledge gained in the complicated process of psychoanalysis to the apparently simple process of the upbringing of children. We had eighty children in these nurseries, fifty in one house and thirty in the other, broken up into groups and families as well as we could in wartime. We realized very soon the enormous distress that one induces in a toddler if you put him down at the table and then go and get his food. The toddler cannot wait. So we thought, "We will do it the other way round. We will put the food on the table and then we will bring the toddler to the food." You have no idea what a revolution that meant in our nurseries.

When you try to dress thirty little children in the morning and then take them to breakfast, what do you do with those who are dressed first? I have seen other residential nurseries where games are played with them until everybody is dressed, or where they even sing. Well, who wants to sing before breakfast? We made a breakfast room, with one young teacher in charge, and the children trickled in as they were washed, dressed, combed, and so on, and they received their breakfast as one does in a cafeteria. Again we saved enormous distress.

It struck me at that time how much distress one could save children if one understood no more than their different sense of time. We had one little girl in our nursery who wanted to be big the whole time, because she had a bigger brother. It was a sign of her healthy personality. She asked over and over again, "When will I be big? Is it soon? Is it in half an hour?" We had a little boy who wanted to stay and not be fetched by his mother, and who said to the teacher, "When will my mummy come?" The teacher said, "Do you want her to come soon, or do you not want her to come for a long time?" He replied, "I want to play. Is half an hour long?" He had no idea.

4. If you want a very impressive example of how different is the language of the child from the language of the adult in all these respects, I can give you no better example than the children's understanding of sex life—that means of the difference between boy and girl, of what father and mother do together to produce a baby, and of the way in which babies are born. We have learned a good deal from observing children's reactions in this respect, and, as you probably know, the first exhortations to parents not to feed children stories about the stork or gooseberry bushes but to tell them the facts of life came from the psychoanalyst. What should

also come from the psychoanalyst is the explanation of what the children do with these facts.

At present we have several children in our nursery school who in the last six months have had younger brothers or sisters and who are therefore very much concerned with the birth of babies. Their parents, young and enlightened, and not too repressed, tell them exactly how it comes about. The children give lip service to it; they understand that the baby is in the mother and understand how boys and girls are made. But when you watch their play you realize that they do not understand it at all. For example, they blow on a brick and pretend that this "makes a baby." Or they play "family" and, as mummy and daddy, pretend to go to bed at night. What emerges then are usually scenes of "messing each other up," fighting, shooting, almost killing each other: love and violence seem to be inextricably mixed up with each other. They also betray in play that according to their feeling, all children should be boys by right, and that the girl's body is really a broken one from which something is missing or has been taken off as punishment.

In short, the child translates the real facts of sex life into the terms which are appropriate to his immature mind and body, and these terms are very crude, primitive, and brutal ones, resembling most nearly the content of certain fairy tales. Therefore, whenever you want to convince yourself of the great difference between the child's emotional language and the adult's factual language, you find no better area than this particular one.

Let us assume now that we have helped the teachers to understand some of the child's peculiarities, such as his egocentricity, his irrationality, his different time sense, the difference in his sexuality. But what then? After all, this is only the prerequisite for entering into an understanding of the processes of development that go on in the child as he grows toward maturity so far as his feelings and social sense are concerned.

We have to find our way further, and for the purpose of doing so I offer you an example from another sphere of life. When I was still a teacher of schoolchildren—that is how I started—I was very impressed by something I heard a grammar school boy say. He said, "School could be so pleasant if one were not always dragged along. Hardly have you learned how to add when you have to learn how to subtract; and hardly have you found it easy to subtract when you have to do long divisions; or you learn enough Latin to read a very simple author—but are you left at that? Oh, no. You are dragged along to read the most difficult and complicated works." But at the same time I listened to a clever little girl, who said she could really enjoy school "if it were not so boring. You are always expected to do the same thing over and over again, to wait until everybody has understood. Why can't one go on to the next thing?" That made me think that it is not easy to fulfill children's wishes: there are those who want to go ahead; and there are those who want to enjoy their achievements and be left in peace.

Since this happened teachers of schoolchildren all over the world have learned that intellectual development proceeds in stages: that a particular child should neither be hurried beyond nor be held back below the stage of his development; that you should let everybody grow intellectually at his own pace. I think that this is a valuable piece of insight which you, as teachers of the very young, should take over from the realm of intellectual development to the realm of the emotions and of social growth. Here, too, there are stages the child has to master, through which he has to pass, and it is no good either hurrying him on where he cannot follow, or holding him back where he feels like a prisoner held down in an atmosphere which he has already outgrown.

In our analytic studies of children we have tried to establish such stages in various respects: stages in development of the relationship to the mother—which really means the bulk of the child's earliest emotional development; stages in development toward companionship in school; stages in development from play with various kinds of toys, up to work; or the stages a child goes through in managing his own body, his feeding processes, his evacuation processes, looking after his own health, hygiene, etc.

Watching step by step the development of young children in detail, I have become very impatient with the one-sided views of people, some of whom say, "Mother and child should be kept together just as long as possible. Do not separate them"; or those others who say, "Children need companionship. Try to get them out of the home as soon as possible. Have them in groups." Either opinion is right if it is based on the child's stage of development. Either opinion is wrong if it is based on no more than a sentimental attitude of the adults. Nowhere else would we dare to base the handling on sentimental attitudes. We could ask pediatricians, for example, whether it would be right to choose the child's diet on the basis of the feeling that mother's milk is best until the child is six. "No," the doctors would say, "We can give you many proofs that this would not do justice to the requirements of the growing body." Or it is as if somebody else said, "Cut out the mother's milk and start the child on minced beef." This may sound ridiculous, but it is exactly what we do regarding the emotional development of our children today.

In recent years you have probably heard a great deal about the gradual development of the mother-child relationship. For this reason I shall not go into that today and instead present to you something that is of more immediate concern to the teacher: namely, the fact that here are similar stages in the child's life which take him from the comparative isolation of the family relationships into community life.

We all know what we want of children in the nursery school: that they enjoy their surroundings and make good use of them. But do we always ask ourselves, "What has to happen before they can do so?" In my Clinic we have the very good fortune that we can look after a small number of children from birth. We collect the mothers of the babies at the Clinic during the first sixteen months to see the children on certain play afternoons—strictly with the mother. Then they enter our nursery school, so far as we can accommodate them, when they are three or three and a half. This makes it possible to observe their growth toward companionship—not companionship with brothers and sisters, but companionship with children outside the family.

We have established roughly four stages. At the first stage, mother and child are together and are a unit, and whoever comes between them is a disturbance. For instance, if another child tries to climb on the lap of such a mother, he is pushed out of the way. These other children are not wanted. You can say that the child behaves asocially, egoistically. After all, that is his way: he is asocial and should be at that age. That is stage one, where, as I have said, the other child is a disturbance.

Then comes stage two, where the other child becomes rather interesting. For instance, somebody in the room has very crinkly hair and all the children pass and just touch that hair a bit. But it is not the child; it is the hair that is attracting them. Or a child pushing a doll's pram walks through the room and another child is in the way: the child pushes along as if the other child were a piece of furniture. If the child falls over, well, to the child it is a piece of furniture that has fallen over and somebody will come and lift it up again. This means that the other child at this stage is not treated as a human being. It is treated like something inanimate—almost like a toy.

Teddy bears are such very good playmates because you can do anything to them and they do not respond. The child throws his teddy bear in the corner because he is angry. The teddy bear suffers it, the child reclaims the teddy bear, cuddles it, and it is all right with the teddy bear. That makes toys such valuable playthings. But at this stage children are treated in exactly the same way, and if a response comes from them, it is unexpected. With our little ones, aged sixteen months to two years, you see on such occasions the surprise spreading on their faces as if a "teddy-bear child" had given a squeak or hit out.

Then comes the next stage, where two children begin to be interested in the same toy, sometimes in a very conflicting way. I remember seeing two children of two and a half playing in our nursery school kitchen. One little boy was extremely intent on taking out all the cups and saucers from the children's dresser and putting them on the table, and the other little boy was equally intent upon putting them back again. They played on for a good while, not noticing that their purposes were cross-purposes, until in the end some distress was caused and they stopped.

But this initiates a further stage where children become playmates: namely, they ask, invite, use each other to carry out play projects as we have them in all nursery schools. The project may be to build a garage for a car; and one little boy may come running up to another saying, "Who will help me build a garage for this car?" and they may play for half an hour or an hour and build something beautiful; or they may have some big project involving sand, water, trains, tunnels, etc., and cooperate beautifully—not on the basis of personal friendship, but on the basis of a common aim. That is an extremely important stage in the child's life. When the aim is achieved, the group falls apart; the children again go their own ways.

This in its turn initiates the fourth stage, when the other child is valued, not only as a playmate but as a person in his own right: somebody to be loved, hated, admired, competed with, chosen for friendship. I do not know what your own observations are, but we in our nursery school have observed several couples of this kind, sometimes boy and girl, sometimes two boys, sometimes two girls, with real personal feeling and liking for each other. We see distress when they are separated.

What is interesting to me is that you can no more make a child in stage two, where other children are treated as toys, behave like the children in stage three or four than you can do the opposite. These are processes of growth and adaptation which are achieved gradually; just as it is not possible for the parents to get from the toddler the mutuality in relationship which can come about only when the child has already reached the phase of constancy in his loving relations with people. It seems to me that the understanding of such phases of emotional and social growth gives us the lead to a grading of our children which compares with the lead the teachers of schoolchildren get from the psychological tests in their intellectual grading of the school population.

21

Clinical Problems of Young Children

(1962)

In spite of my close association with the Hampstead Child-Therapy Clinic, I am not, strictly speaking, a member of a Clinic team; neither psychiatrist, nor psychologist, nor psychiatric social worker, nor even a child therapist. I decided therefore that I was invited to speak here, at the Inter-Clinic Conference, as a representative of the field to which I belong—psychoanalysis—just as John Apley,

This paper was presented under the title "Assessments of Normality and Pathology" at the 18th Child Guidance Inter-Clinic Conference for the Staffs of Child Guidance Clinics, chaired by A. D. B. Clarke, on April 14, 1962. It was first published in *Clinical Problems of Young Children: The Proceedings of the 18th Child Guidance Inter-Clinic Conference*. London: National Association for Mental Health, 1962, pp. 22-29.

who follows me as a speaker, has been invited to represent the field of pediatrics (1962). What the audience expects of both of us, I imagine, is a description of the contributions which we in our fields have made to the specific work of the child guidance clinics. Such an interest of the child guidance workers in allied disciplines seems to me an interesting and important step toward more intimate relations and a closer integration of their work with ours.

INTERRELATIONS BETWEEN THE SERVICES FOR CHILDREN

In my own working life, moving around freely from one of the services for children to another has played a decisive part. While training and working professionally as a psychoanalyst, I also taught normal children; acted as a consultant for teachers of problem children; treated neurotic children; cooperated theoretically in work with delinquent adolescents; organized a day nursery for toddlers, residential nurseries for evacuated war children, a nursery group and advisory service for the blind, etc. This brought me into closest working contact with the mentally normal and abnormal; the bodily ill and healthy; the socially, financially, and emotionally deprived; the adapted and maladjusted; the traumatized and handicapped of all childhood stages.

The variety of experience which I was able to collect in this way left me with the feeling that there might be something lacking in the training and the working opportunities which we offer to our next generation of workers. By this I do not mean to underestimate the advantages and the importance of specialization, only to stress the point that all those who deal with children might profit from what one might call a "basic training in childhood" before they qualify for their specific tasks in schools, nurseries, clinics, hospitals, courts for children. It is not that I wish other people the hardships of my own career; rather that I should like them to share the intense pleasure in possessing a background of wide and varied experiences together with the opportunity of applying them to a wide range of practical work.

To be confined to one small circumscribed field of work or even to one age group is a restriction from which teachers, nurses, probation officers suffer even more than guidance workers; psychiatric social workers perhaps least of all. On the other hand, it is easy to prove that it is impossible to understand adolescence without understanding toddlers; to deal with ill children in bed unless one is familiar with the motor restlessness and bodily impatience of the healthy child; to understand what happens to young children when they are separated unless one has had intimate contact with them in their homes, and the reverse.

A basic training in childhood, shared by all workers in the children's field before specializing begins, might also allow for some freedom after qualification to change from one type of professional work with children to another. To continue to teach normal young children the rudiments of knowledge for one's entire professional lifetime can be a devastating and crippling experience. The same is true for work with the backward, the autistic, the handicapped, the institutionalized, who have a depressing and disheartening effect on the adult if the work with them continues unrelieved. That a child is ocmposed of body, mind, intellect, emotions, drives is a refreshing experience which ought to be explored separately in the various fields, with some possibility given not only for interchange and contact but for actual exchanges.[1]

THE CHILD GUIDANCE CLINICS
AS CENTERS OF COORDINATION

If ever such a training scheme became a reality, the child guidance clinics would play a central part in it since, so far, they are the only places where coordination of the services can be effected in a serious way. This is demonstrated most clearly if we compare the present position in this respect with the conditions as they were before the majority of child guidance clinics came into existence.

From my own memory I can assure you that psychological work with children at that time was a frustrating and unhappy experience. I worked, then, with a small group of child analysts, engaged like myself in the treatment of neurotic children. We could not help feeling that due to our work we had collected data which were potentially useful to parents and teachers and all others engaged in the upbringing of the young. The difficulty was that we

[1] [In a paper entitled "Childhood Neurosis" (1957), not included in this volume, the author discusses not only what should be taught but also who should receive instruction in psychoanalysis, and especially in child analysis. She discusses the coexistence of the two prevalent points of view in our time: one that would restrict training in psychoanalysis to physicians only, the other that would give training to all who seek it. She proposes that the solution to this controversy could be based on our knowledge of the nature of personality development, both normal and abnormal. In brief, if personality development is viewed not exclusively as either a "medical" or a "social" problem but in terms of the complementary series, it becomes obvious that the teaching of psychoanalysis can under no conditions be limited to any one professional group.— *Editor's note*.]

had no means of reaching that public and that the parents, although in need of help, felt ashamed of their children's problems and did their best to hide them. Contact was confined to chance occurrences and depended on a parent, a teacher, a pediatrician coming into analysis himself for personal reasons and in the course of time carrying some knowledge back for application in his work.

On the other hand, the parents and schools were in possession of the case material for which we longed for our studies. In those days a child had to be in a severely disturbed state before the parents decided to look for psychological help. This meant that we were deprived of the clinical pictures of all the initial stages of the infantile neuroses, psychoses, delinquencies, deviant development in general. We had no entry to the homes, the schools, the hospitals, the orphanages, and the material remained unavailable to us.

ADVENT OF THE CLINICS

All this changed dramatically with the advent of the clinics. The clinics became the intermediaries between the public needing information and the disciplines engaged in fact finding. They emerged as clearing houses where knowledge was received and handed out, and this view of the child guidance clinics really determined my own personal attitude to them and finally prompted me to have a child guidance clinic of my own.

It may be of interest here to examine more closely how the child guidance clinics managed to fulfill the double task which was assigned to them by circumstances.

First, the relationship between the clinics and the parents: we all know that it became excellent quite soon—almost too good for our purposes. It is a universal wish among all clinic personnel that parents should not have more, but rather a little less, trust in the clinic's work; that they should not bring all children, from the most common difficulties of management (which they ought to be able to solve on their own) to the most seriously ill, who defy help and often even diagnosis. It is of concern to us that parents often presume that all will be well the moment they have handed over the child and "treatment has begun." As I know from our own experience in the Hampstead Child-Therapy Clinic, all is not well, and not everything is treatable.

Children are often referred quite regardless of the reason and the type of their disturbance and of the therapeutic possibilities, as, for example, for the aftereffects of homelessness, neglect, wanderings from one foster place to another, i.e., for understandable reactions to adverse external circumstances which—though they can be explained and sometimes ameliorated—are not "treatable" in the same sense as the genuine mental disturbances. Still, it remains a fact that trust between the parents and the clinics was established quickly. Probably after the first task of establishing confidence is over, the clinics will have to embark on the second task—to teach parents a more realistic evaluation of their potentialities.

PARENT GUIDANCE

It was the same confidence, and even overconfidence, of the parents which opened up for the clinics possibilities of guiding the public which were previously undreamed of in private practice. Parent guidance in its various aspects seems to me an essential part of clinic work since it constitutes the main agent of prevention. As such it deserves a treatise, which cannot be given here. It includes the spreading of information concerning child development; the gradual changing of public opinion with regard to educational methods, punishments and rewards, the timing of interference, the balance between satisfaction and frustration, discipline and freedom; the supplanting of traditional or religious support on which the mothers used to rely in child rearing by support based on the child's psychology; the understanding of the parents' own personal difficulties and their relevance for the child, an aspect which leads in many cases to the demand for treatment of the parents.

As matters stand today, few child guidance clinics are equipped for all these tasks. Considerations of staffing, finances, time, the slants governing training and, above all, public demand weigh the scales in favor of treatment and against preventive work even though many people (I among them) would prefer to see the bulk of the clinics' efforts distributed in the reverse way.

I turn in what follows to the other side of the picture, namely, from the handing out of information to the receiving of it. Naturally, the child guidance clinics depend for the success of their work with parents, teachers, and allied workers on the knowledge which is an integral part of that particular clinic's staff. Where does that knowledge come from? It is taken from disciplines where, as I said before, fact finding about childhood is proceeding—it comes from psychology, child psychiatry, and child analysis.

I feel I am authorized to talk only about the side that

concerns analysis and child analysis. Here, I would say from personal experience that the relations between the clinics and the psychoanalysts have not been happy ones; and if you ask me who is to blame for it, I would accept the blame for my side, the psychoanalysts. Fact finding in psychoanalysis was not undertaken primarily with a view to its clinical application to children but was a by-product of the treatment of neurotic adults. Its progress was linked to the advances in treatment technique and even though a psychoanalytic child psychology was built up gradually, the nature of the facts and the interests of those who did the explorations were centered above all around the problem of prevention of neurotic illness.

SUM TOTAL OF THE FACTS

Perhaps we, as psychoanalysts, were not active enough in warning the practical workers with children that the prevention of neurosis in itself does not safeguard mental health and that it should not be given preference over the prevention of delinquency or any other of the many possible disturbances of childhood. From our side it should have been emphasized more that there is a long way from the bulk of analytic data to their orderly application to the understanding of children, and that data used out of their context are as misleading as one-sided information about one part of the personality which is not balanced against knowledge about other parts.

There are many examples of the latter kind which can be used here for illustration. Facts about the child's need for sexual enlightenment—one of the early analytic discoveries

—led to disappointment in their application because they were given out without the warning that sex knowledge is never received by young children as it is given because whatever the child learns about the activities of the adults in this respect is translated by him into the terms of his own infantile sexual level, i.e., that all sexual knowledge in the early ages has to take the form of the so-called infantile sexual theories.

Facts about the pathogenic role of anxiety led in their application to abortive attempts to eliminate anxiety from the child's life since they were not accompanied by an explanation that anxiety in its various manifestations is an inevitable by-product of personality and character development: where fear of parental authority is reduced, guilt, i.e., fear of the child's own conscience, may take its place; where this is avoided in turn, a deep anxiety about being overwhelmed by the drives will show in the child's ego.

There was another mistake made by the analysts in their relations with the public. They did not guard sufficiently against their most recent work at any period being given undue emphasis in application. In their own activity of fact finding, one element of the human mind after the other moved into the center of attention and naturally received prominence in publications: infantile sexuality and the sequence of libidinal stages; repression and the unconscious mind; the division of the personality into various agencies and the conflicts between them; the oedipus and castration complexes; the role of anxiety; aggression as an independent drive; the relationship between mother and infant and the consequences of early interruptions of the mother-child relationship. Yet, no single one of these factors was ever meant to be considered the only or even

the foremost pathogenic agent, as happens all too frequently in clinical evaluations and publications.

In short, no application of single facts can be useful in
the work of the clinics, whether this work is in therapy, in
guidance, or in prevention. It is the sum total of the facts
—the all-round picture of the child which analytic knowledge might help to establish, which should be aimed at,
and which would be well received.

AN ASSESSMENT OF THE CHILD IN
PSYCHOANALYTIC TERMS

It is my ambition as a clinical child analyst to replace this
piecemeal and frustrating application of psychoanalytic data
by an assessment of children which includes all the areas
of the child's mind and avoids the fallacy of explaining the
child's development or his pathology predominantly in
terms of either his drives, his emotions, his relations to
his love objects, his reasonable functions, his conscience,
his conflicts and complexes, or in terms of his upsets, traumatic events, separations, hospitalizations, operations, object losses. It is true that it is not easy to put weight fairly
and appropriately on each of these factors and on their
interaction with each other. On the other hand, this is
precisely what is done successfully in every comprehensive
medical assessment of a child's physical state, where the
child is weighed, measured, one organ system examined
after the other, defects excluded or explored, etc.

There seems to be no reason why the sound psychoanalytic assessment of a child's state of mind should not come
up to and compare favorably with a medical diagnosis. Nor
is there a good reason why the child guidance clinics' rela-

tions with psychoanalysis should remain worse than they are with experimental and educational psychology. It is true that the psychologists had something to offer to the clinics in a finished and entirely useful form, namely, the intelligence and personality tests, ready for application. But this should be an added incentive to the psychoanalysts' efforts to work out equally usable schemes on the basis of their own theoretical assumptions.

Stimulated by the example of the psychologists and the medical practitioners, we began to experiment in our own Clinic with something which—for want of a better term—we called a "Diagnostic Profile," a scheme meant to prevent us from seeing the child one-sidedly, the direction being determined by preconceived inclinations within our own theoretical framework. Without disregarding any historical, environmental, or internal factor which we can elicit, the Profile is intended to help the diagnostician place the factors in a certain order and highlight their relations to each other. Incidentally, this eliminates some of the dangerous shortcuts which are only too frequent in diagnostic work, namely, the direct inferences drawn from known, potentially traumatic events in the child's past for the causation of his present state. Separations, operations, hospitalizations, as the parents record them, are historical facts, i.e., external events. It is not legitimate to accept them as traumatic, i.e., to attribute to them internal significance, without a further thorough investigation of the child. What seems important to the parents may be a negligible experience in the child's mind; on the other hand, small happenings, hardly noticed by the adult world, may have had major traumatic significance in his development.

SCOPE OF THE PROFILE

Now for the Profile itself. It is meant to convey a picture of the child under examination irrespective of the question of mental health or illness and equally suited to the assessment of either. What the diagnostician should carry in the background of his mind for the purpose of apperception of the clinical facts is a fairly comprehensive knowledge of the various aspects and stages of normal childhood growth—a body of knowledge which is not always sufficiently stressed in the training and mental equipment of child psychiatrists and other clinic workers.

The Profile makes use of all the material elicited in the psychiatric examination, the social history taking, the tests, home or school visits, etc., by summarizing the results in a given order. It resembles the case histories taken in all clinics in a *first part*, which contains *the reason for referral, the description of the child, his family background* (including the personalities of the parents and their potential abnormalities), and the enumeration of obvious *environmental influences* which are of possible significance (with the *proviso* given above that no direct conclusions regarding the causation of pathology should be established on this evidence).

The *second part* of the Profile, based on the analytic assumptions of normal childhood growth, is developmentally oriented; i.e., an attempt is made to establish the child's position on the scales of drive (sexual and aggressive) development, of ego development, and of the interactions between the two which manifest themselves in the various steps toward social adaptation.

With regard to *drive development* we inquire as to the

level of libidinal sequence which has been reached, or from which the child has returned to earlier ones. Has the oral, anal, phallic phase been passed through in an age-adequate manner? Has the oedipus complex, i.e., the triangular relationship to the parents with its jealousies and rivalries been established, or (with the older child) solved and overcome? Is the child's attitude to himself sufficiently positive to create a healthy self-esteem, pleasure in his own body and his achievements, or is he self-derogatory and dissatisfied in this respect? Can he love other people besides himself, and, after passing through the infantile stages of egocentricity, demandingness, clinging, has he reached age-adequate forms of give-and-take, constancy, and loyalty in relation to his love objects? Can he use his aggressive drive, not only for destructive purposes but for positive construction and activity? Is there enough of it, or too much? Is it inhibited and is it mainly directed toward the child's own person, or body, or against the outer world?

Ego and Superego Growth

There is an equal number of questions to be asked about the child's rational, social, and moral development, i.e., about his ego and superego growth. What has to be established here is the intactness or defectiveness of the apparatus which serves perception, memory, motility, etc.; further, the age-adequateness of the most important ego functions: whether the child can make use of experience, can distinguish between sensations and perceptions, can integrate what happens to him; how far he is advanced in speech, in logical thinking, etc.; whether he has acquired any moral values, and if so which, and whether his behavior is governed by them irrespective of the presence or absence of the parents.

When inquiring into the relations between the ego and the drives, we try to see whether the child is a prey to his impulses or has established control over them, too much perhaps or too little for his age; we ask by what methods such control is achieved: by repression (exclusion from consciousness), reaction formations (substituting welcome for unwelcome qualities), sublimation (deflection of drive activity from primitive aims), projection (ascribing to objects in the outer world what belongs to the inner world), etc.[2]

To help our assessment of details further, we ask the parents to describe the child's functioning as a total personality with regard to a particular event such as the birth of a sibling, absence of the mother, illness and surgical intervention, entry into nursery school or school, reaction to a community of children, etc.

Aspects of the Child's Personality

So much for the developmental part of the Profile. Further parts of it consist of inquiries into aspects of the child's personality at the time of examination.

1. Behavior, fantasy activity, and symptomatology are scrutinized to single out those items where the relations between the surface manifestations of the personality and the repressed depth are well known to the analyst, not open to variation, and therefore betray genetic material, i.e., specific difficulties encountered by the child in any of his developmental stages, trends which have been warded off

[2] For a brief description of the various mechanisms of defense, see Anna Freud (1961).

and modified but where the repressed impulses have left their unmistakable imprint.

Familiar examples of such revealing behavior are the personality characteristics of the obsessional children (slowing up, excessive cleanliness, excessive conscientiousness, compulsive questioning), which are derived from the events of the anal-sadistic phase; fears for the parents' health, which betray repressed death wishes; food fads, which point back to difficulties of the oral phase. In contrast, symptoms such as lying, stealing, bed wetting have a multiple and varying causation and, at the diagnostic stage, supply no information regarding the causes of a child's disturbance.

2. The conflicts around which a child's life revolves, i.e., his battles for wish fulfillment, seem to us to offer a convenient shortcut toward assessing the complexity and maturity reached by the structure of his personality. We distinguish three types of conflict: with external authority (the earliest and most primitive form); between the child's wishes and his own conscience (after identification with the parents); between contrasting drives and impulses (such as love and hate, femininity and masculinity, passivity and activity). From the type of conflict which governs a child's disturbance, we can also draw conclusions with regard to the type of therapy to which he will respond.

External conflicts are affected and can be dealt with by external measures (such as removal from home or foster place, change of school, or educational handling); conflicts within the personality or between the drives are amenable only to therapies which alter the balance of internal forces.

3. Finally, we find that there are certain general characteristics in each child which are worth describing since their presence or absence, strength or weakness have a

definite bearing on that individual's chance to remain healthy or not, to respond favorably to treatment or not. Such characteristics are, for example, the children's differing ability to stand disappointment, pain, frustration, anxiety.

Since all these various forms of unpleasure are potential starting points for mental trouble, a high degree of toleration for them acts as a safeguard for the child's stability; a low tolerance for frustration and anxiety can transform minor unpleasant events into traumatic happenings which initiate pathology.

4. Children also differ widely with regard to the health and strength of their progressive developmental forces in comparison with their regressive tendencies, both of which are normally present in the immature personality. To illustrate this with a simple example: one child, in his jealousy over the birth of a sibling, will stress that he is "big" and in rivalry with the newborn will make a forward move to assert his rights; another, in the same situation, will give up his own greater achievements, compete with the smallness and helplessness of the baby, and through jealousy regress once more to the baby stage. There is no doubt that the chances for maintaining mental health are better where progression outweighs regression.

CONCLUSIONS

The diagnostic scheme outlined above may, to the majority of clinic workers, seem unduly complex. For this eventuality I should like to stress the point that not all the questions asked or aspects enumerated in the given sample are essential for building a Profile of a given case. What the scheme is meant to do is to point out directions, outline possibilities, and, above all, to remind the diagnostician that the picture of the child should not be seen from one angle but be an all-rounded one. For the ambition of the child analysts it will be satisfying that cases can be seen and described in dynamic, structural, genetic, economic, and adaptational terms even at the diagnostic stage.

22

Interactions between Nursery School and Child Guidance Clinic
(1966 [1965])

Links between the therapy of children and their education are few and far between in our times. For the student of the subject this makes it all the more important to look for information to the small number of organizations in the United States and in England where the two types of work are found side by side. The benefit which they derive from each other under such conditions is not difficult to demonstrate. Nevertheless, before entering into an account of these practical advantages, it seems appropriate to go

Presented at a symposium held on the 35th anniversary of the Leyden Child Guidance Clinic, July, 1965. First published in *Journal of Child Psychotherapy*, 1:40-44, 1966.

further afield and to give evidence of the thinking which underlies such ventures.

THE DISADVANTAGES OF SPECIALIZATION IN THE CHILDREN'S SERVICES

Adding educational to clinical work represents the attempt to right a wrong which is being done to the children's services by specialization, i.e., by a method which has been taken over from the adult field and applied to them unchanged. In the case of adults, we find no fault with the idea that their needs are split into medical, psychological, spiritual, legal ones, etc., and that there are specialized professions offering specialized aid. Even here the fields may overlap, as they do where psychological or mental health problems enter into and complicate the legal ones, or in psychosomatic medicine where organic and mental etiology is intermingled, or in cases where medical specialization has gone too far and the independent function or dysfunction of an organ is overemphasized at the expense of its interaction with other organ systems. Nevertheless, on the whole, the structuralization and differentiation of the adult's personality are in tune with the differentiation of the services which are available to him.

Our practical experience with children as well as our psychoanalytic knowledge of their mental processes leave us in no doubt that none of these assumptions are valid if transferred to their case. Whereas the mature individual is differentiated and structured, the immature personality is undifferentiated and unstructured. In infants, there are no sharp demarcations between the physiological and psychological processes, which implies that life at this time is truly

"psychosomatic." Nor is this blurring of the borders between *body and mind* the only one of its kind in childhood.
There is a similar lack of discrimination between *self and
object* until the child learns to distinguish his own body
ego from the person of the mother. There is, until a much
later date, an unshakable unity between *intellect and emotion,* which causes attention cathexis to go where the events
are charged with libido, and to be withheld where the
child's feelings are not involved. In the early years it is
equally difficult to draw the dividing line between *perversity
and normal sexual development,* or between *delinquency
and progressive social adjustment,* since by definition normal infantile sexuality is perverse, and normal infantile
behavior is asocial or dissocial. Altogether, normality and
pathology are less divided from each other in childhood
than they will be later: many quasi-pathological formations
are common accompaniments of normal phase development; and, vice versa, in the mental disturbances of childhood, apart from the most severe forms, there are almost
invariably areas of growth and development which have
remained intact.

Insights such as these, if taken for granted, make nonsense of the specialized services which we offer to children
and of the specialized training which is all that is available
to their personnel. Under present conditions, the medical
and nursing staff of a well-baby clinic or a pediatrics ward
find themselves badly equipped for disentangling the neurological, physiological, and emotional factors which play a
part, for example, in the infants' feeding and sleeping upsets, since the staff members are at best trained for two, and
hardly ever in equal measure for all three, sides of the
child's nature. Teachers feel helpless when confronted with

learning failures in their pupils as soon as these are due to influences outside the intellectual processes with which they are familiar. Trained nurses, who know everything about the ill child's needs, are rendered incompetent when expected to look after and satisfy healthy children, as they were supposed to do in the residential nurseries for evacuated children in the Second World War. Juvenile courts and probation officers possess no developmental yardstick to help them determine from which precise moment onward lying, stealing, destructive acts, etc., cease to be normal and age-adequate expressions of impulse, anxiety, or defense and begin to signify failures on the road to moral development and social adaptation. All workers in education, and quite especially teachers, suffer from the fact that their training applies only to specific age groups —toddlers, under-fives, schoolchildren, adolescents—and that they are deprived of the opportunity to see human growth in progress in an unbroken line, with the events of each successive phase being understood as influenced by previous experience and as predetermining the later stages.

In short, all workers in the field suffer from the fact that schools date back to a period when thinking was believed to be capable of development independent of feeling, and hospitals to a time when the needs of the body were considered to be independent of those of the mind; to a period, that is, when both types of institution dealt with children as if they were separate entities and ignored their utter dependence on the parents with whom they form a unit. It is only in the most recent decades that belated attempts are being made to remedy such errors. I list under these the parent-teacher associations which forge links between home and school; the new visiting rules in children's hospitals which take account of the child's distress when separated from his parents; the turn against residential institutions and toward fostering of orphans in recognition of the young child's psychological need for individual mothering; the interest shown by some pediatricians in the emotional side of the child's life; the introduction of courses on child psychology into the program of teachers' training colleges and into training for child nursing; finally, the introduction of some nursery schools into the fabric of some child guidance clinics.

AN EXAMPLE OF COMBINED SERVICE: THERAPY AND EDUCATION

I owe the invitation to participate in this Symposium to the fact that in the Hampstead Child-Therapy Course and Clinic of which I am the Director, a large outpatients' clinic coexists with a well-baby clinic, two prenursery groups, and two nursery schools, one for blind, one for sighted children.

So far as the Nursery School for Blind Children is concerned, this is the prototype of a therapeutic nursery school, which implies that here the aims of education and treatment are intermixed, to the degree of being almost indistinguishable from each other. Since the absence of vision in itself acts as a hindrance to normal progression, the children's development depends on the measures taken to minimize the effects of their handicap, or to compensate for them by the systematic stimulation of the remaining senses, by their use for intimate libidinal contact, by pleasure derived from the musculature, etc. Whether these dealings with the child are therapeutic or educational in nature then becomes a matter of terminology rather than of fact. Whatever they are called, it is the therapeutic intervention which renders the children educable. The combined procedure, devised to serve this purpose, is based on the analytic understanding of the unsatisfied developmental needs of these children's personalities, and it is carried out by group activities alternating with intimate individual contact.

The interactions between the other service departments and the clinic itself lie in a different field, benefiting on the one hand our students, on the other hand our patients.

Our child therapy students are taught from the outset that mental pathology in childhood cannot be understood per se, but has to be viewed against the background of normal child development, including all the variations and distortions of the latter; also, that instinctual phase development with its vicissitudes, in spite of being an invisible internal process, reveals itself by significant alterations in the child's behavior. The well-baby clinic where the mothers of infants receive physical-psychological guidance, the prenursery groups where toddlers attend with their mothers, and the nursery school for sighted children are rich sources of material for observation, demonstration, and study of these facts. This assures that students do not begin with the therapy of problem children before they have become familiar with the main characteristics of normal child development.

Constant confrontation in discussion of normal with pathological phenomena leads, further, to the constant weighing of the claims of education against the claims of therapy. Our child analysts may be apt to feel that every educational restriction imposed on a child will create neurotic inhibitions, while our teachers are eager to prove that without such educational restraint no normal outcome can be envisaged for the individual. We agree, finally, on the definition that educators work with the healthy part of the child's personality, help build up ego defenses, develop ego interests and functions, promote sublimations, and facilitate adaptation; that they use as a vehicle for progressive change the child's relationship to the teacher as a superego representative as well as the child's increasing pleasure in the social interaction with contemporaries. In contrast, the therapist deals with the ill part of the child, and it is legitimate for him to be concerned not with growth in the first place but with regression in the analytic setting, which enables him to explore the past, to give interpretations, and to undo crippling defenses and archaic superego formations. By doing this, therapy clears the field for the forces toward progressive development which take over after its completion.

There is no doubt in our mind that both teachers and therapists benefit equally from this interchange.

So far as the needs of our clinic patients are concerned, these are served in a variety of ways by the availability of the nursery school with a basic population of normal children.

In the diagnostic assessment of cases we may find that what is required for the disturbance is not therapy but a *therapeutic environment*, or not analytic but *educational help*. If this happens, and if vacancies are available, referral to the nursery school is resorted to as the method of choice.

In other instances, closer acquaintance with the child's

behavior may be thought necessary before a diagnostic assessment can be made at all. For these cases, nursery school becomes the place where prolonged *direct observation* of the child in question can be carried out.

Some of our young patients need attendance at the nursery school concurrent with analytic treatment to provide them with a *protected environment* where the regressive moves engendered by the license of the analytic process can be contained and development be promoted. In these instances, close contact between teacher and therapist becomes not only imperative but also most profitable and most informative.

The nursery school is, further, the logical place where young patients *after treatment* are helped systematically to employ their freed energies, i.e., where new opportunities for ego interests and sublimations are opened up for them.

A VISION OF FUTURE TRAINING FOR THE CHILDREN'S SERVICES

Combinations of educational with therapeutic work, as they are described above, are constructive efforts for the organizations which provide for them and satisfying experiences for the workers by whom they are carried out. Nevertheless, their main value lies not in this but in their significance as forerunners of bigger and more sweeping developments in the children's field.

Once we have convinced ourselves of the insufficiency of present provisions, it becomes a natural ambition to create for the future an altered state of affairs in which the child's life will no longer be split up into parts which are catered to by different professions and even administered by different authorities. On the other hand, so long as the training schemes for the various categories of workers remain as compartmentalized as they are today, teachers, nurses, health visitors, children's officers, probation officers, house parents, pediatricians, etc., will remain strictly within their own functions and will regard their charges in the light appropriate to these, namely, as pupils (in school), patients (in the hospital), dependents (of the family), wards (of the court), inmates (of residential institutions), etc., forgetting that these temporary roles may at times be no more than the dissociated aspects of one and the same human individual. Obviously, drastic changes in this respect can originate only from the side of training.

On the strength of our present state of knowledge it is not too difficult to envisage future training schemes by means of which a revolution in the field can be brought about.

What is needed, above all, is a basic training in child development which is common to all professions in whatever role and is concerned with children of all ages and in all conditions. This would have to include the principal facts of neurological, physiological, instinctual, emotional, intellectual, and moral growth with their age-adequate and phase-adequate interactions; the child's gradual mastery of his external and internal world and the means by which this is brought about; the child's gradual advance from emotional and moral dependency to independent status; the environment's tasks with regard to the immature individual's needs for body care, affection, stimulation, and stability.

Where specialized professional training will make its departure from a common basic course of this nature, the professions, instead of being closed off hermetically against each other, will retain the possibility of lively interchange. Given a common grounding, there is no reason why a children's nurse should not try her hand at nursery school work or why a nursery school teacher, or other teachers, should not leave their classrooms periodically to serve as aides in hospitals, to function in residential institutions, to act as helpers, observers, or even as consultants in juvenile courts. High school teachers will return with increased understanding to their preadolescent or adolescent pupils after spending some time with toddlers or in nursery schools. Pediatricians will derive profit from seeing healthy children develop. Juvenile court personnel will develop a new outlook on juvenile delinquency if given the chance to observe the first stages of social adjustment and law-abidingness as they are on show in any nursery school.

To work with one single aspect of the child's life only, as it is done today, can become as frustrating and limiting in outlook as automation is for the workers in a factory. What is essential in our particular field is every single worker's involvement with the total growth and development of the child, even though his own efforts may represent only one single contribution to its future fate.

Seen in this wider context, our present successes in counteracting specialization are no more than very small steps taken toward an ambitious goal.

23

Answering Pediatricians'
Questions
(1961 [1959])

When I came here this afternoon I came quite unprepared
—or you might say, prepared for the worst—namely, ready
to answer questions that will be difficult to answer as such.
Each question which will be asked here would probably
be quite easy to answer in a wider context. Therefore, I
thought that it might be useful for me to have an idea in
my own mind how to deal with your inquiries.

Presented at the Study Group of the Society for Psychosomatic
Research at the Royal College of Physicians, May, 1959. The
meeting was chaired by Dermond MacCarthy. Among the partici-
pants were Drs. Percy Bray, D. Gairdner, C. B. Hindley, W. S.
Inman, C. Koupernik, A. Victor Neale, T. E. Oppé, Ben S. Wood.
First published in *Psychosomatic Aspects of Paediatrics*, ed. Ronald
MacKeith & Joseph Sandler. New York & London: Pergamon
Press, 1961, pp. 27-41.

There will, I hope, be a time in the future when all medicine will have a double orientation—namely, an orientation directed simultaneously toward the body and the mind. This will then presuppose that all people who practice medicine will also receive a double training: that they will learn approximately the same amount about the body and the mind. In this future, distant and improbable as it now seems to us, people will handle questions of this kind in a specific way. They will call on their own double knowledge, and they will weigh the claims of the body and the mind against each other; knowing all sides of the human personality well enough, they will be able to do so.

Until then one has to use one's imagination, and I shall therefore try to give my answers as this perfect medical practitioner or consultant of the future might do; in his thoughts, he would weigh whatever he does to the child's body against its repercussions on the mind; and whenever he interferes with the child's mind, he would think of the body at the same time.

Do you feel that the use of suppositories is justifiable as a medical procedure, e.g., suppositories of aminophylline at the very beginning of an asthmatic attack; or the giving of medicines by rectum, as is frequently done in France? Is there a difference in the cultural pattern in France which enables this to be tolerated, and does it do any harm or not?

I would like to apply the point of view outlined above to this particular question. What about suppositories, and why is the question asked at all? Suppositories and enemas have been given and temperatures taken in the child's anus for countless years without any such question being asked.

Then came the discoveries of the people who worked

with the child's mind and who found that this particular body opening has a number of functions. One is a purely bodily function, namely, that of elimination. But there is also a secondary function, which is to provide excitation for the child and, especially at certain ages and stages of development (approximately between two and four years), excitations of a very strong and pleasurable kind. Thus, whenever doctor, nurse or mother, for purely medical reasons, interferes with that part of the child's body, a secondary effect is set in train. The child feels excited; this is pleasurable until he learns that this is not a very nice kind of pleasure. After that he feels violently upset by such interference with his body. This reaction has in time become rather widely known and has made people wary of interfering with that body opening.

Then an additional piece of information was added. These actions not only provide bodily excitation at the moment, but the accumulated bodily excitation in the anal region may set up certain trends of development which will be unwelcome later on. They strengthen the importance of these anal sensations and keep them going at a time when the child should have outgrown them and substituted other, for example, genital, excitations for them. This is, I would say, how knowledge stands at the moment.

I return now to the physician who keeps body and mind in his thoughts simultaneously. He will have to ask himself in each case: Is it imperative that I carry out this particular action? If it is imperative, then I have to risk whatever side effects may develop. Can I instead use a medical procedure of some kind which has no such side effects? If so, I would prefer to do that.

Thus, the question will have to be answered in a different manner on different occasions. If temperatures can be taken under the arm, there is no need to excite the child anally. If suppositories have to be given for some important reason, then it has to be, and one has to risk the side effects.

In our present imperfect state of knowledge and training does the greatest safeguard lie in the parents or the doctors not fussing too much when they recognize that they may be doing some damage? An overscrupulous attitude which embodies so much concealed anxiety but does not express it as concern can do every bit as much harm. It seems to me very important not to get caught up in a kind of obsessional attitude in which the harm is known and one dare not apply the remedy but would still like to, and is not sure what to do. This is perhaps an attitude that one sees more in parents than in doctors. Nevertheless, one can sometimes reassure parents and allow them to do the wrong thing firmly and happily if that is what they feel they must do.

I can see what the questioner means, but I also think that what has been described here as overanxiousness is a consequence of the newness of our psychological knowledge. If you imagine people who for years and generations have performed certain actions without realizing their effect on the mind of the child, then it is not so difficult to imagine that, when their eyes are opened to some of the possible consequences, they may become overanxious. If this is harmful, perhaps the opposite attitude is equally harmful. So much has been done for so many years unthinkingly that in the preliminary stages of knowledge about the mind some overanxiety may be a healthy sign of new knowledge coming in. Once the new knowledge is firmly established, there should be no room for overanxiety. Nowadays we can very often choose, in the attitudes of the parents, only between lack of thinking on their part, their not caring at all about what happens, or caring too much.

Supposing one is faced with a child with asthma, do you think it is less harmful to insert a suppository against resistance than to inject a vein against resistance? Is it more harmful to give a suppository without resistance than to give an injection into a vein without resistance? I will give you one particular example of a small girl cyanosed with asthma. In the next room was her mother with a day-old baby; this girl was absolutely livid about this situation. I popped a suppository into her bottom and went away and told the general practitioner to let me know if she was not better, and I heard no more. Would it have been better under those circumstances if I had struggled with her— and it would have been a struggle—to give her an injection of aminophylline into a vein?

I am here to ask questions as well as to answer them, and there is room here for an intermediate question, asking what kind of side effect we see after injections. When that has been answered, all we have to do is to weigh the effects of injections against the effects of suppositories. We find children who will take an injection without much upset and fight violently against the insertion of a suppository, but we also find children who will take a suppository without fighting and scream violently when given injections. We know that there are big guardsmen who will faint when they are given an injection.

    Let us compare the two events. We know now that suppositories have an unexpected effect on the child's mind, representing to the child, not to the adult who is carrying out the action, interference with a body opening, therefore an attack of a certain kind. To other people injections also represent an attack, but of a different kind—not on a body opening, but an attack with a sharp, long, pointed instrument. Both happenings have a symbolic meaning: the one represents an anal attack, the other represents a sexual attack of another kind, namely, a phallic one. As I said before, there are individuals impervious to the one and highly susceptible to the other, and the other way round. Still, we know injections have to be given; but I think doctors who know the possible meaning of injections for the child will know better how to prepare, how to quiet the child, and how to diminish the possible shock.

By the way, it is an interesting experiment, for anybody who wants to make it, to observe how different children of the same age react to routine injections, their behavior ranging from complete panic to heroic indifference. These reactions, when we learn to compare them, give us valuable information about the personality of the particular child.

My answer to the above question is thus as follows: in some moments of stress, when action is immediately necessary, it may not be possible to weigh the side effects against each other; afterward the pediatrician will have the opportunity to see whether the child is upset or not, to think again, and to come either to the same or a different conclusion with regard to the next patient.

The point has been stressed in France that the use of suppositories would be more harmful in boys than in girls be-

cause it would favor some latent trends toward homosexuality. I would like to have your opinion about it.

This is perfectly true. The aftereffects are more dangerous for boys than for girls.

Is rectal manipulation inadvisable particularly between the ages of two and four or earlier in infancy or later, or is it a general relative prohibition?

The possibility of side effects is there at all ages. Between the ages of two to four the rectal manipulation falls in most readily with the child's own inclinations; if you look for children who manipulate their own rectums, you will probably find them at this particular age. Therefore, at that time you may get compliance from the child for the manipulation; at later stages you may get violent revolt against it, which means that the child has outgrown this place of excitation and fights against being tempted to regress to it.

When I first qualified I had the idea that a good doctor was an applied physiologist, and then I thought a little more, and thought that a good doctor was an applied physiologist who was also kind and a bit understanding. Then I changed round and thought that a good doctor was a kind and understanding person who knew a little physiology. Well now, a lot of us are trying, rather late in life perhaps, to apply this also to the physiology of the emotions, but we do not know very much about it as we are amateurs. There must be certain situations in which an amateur dealing with the problem makes a worse problem, or uncovers a worse problem, and kindness, understanding, and an elementary knowledge of the physiology of the emotions cannot be

*enough to deal with it. Can you give us any hints on how
to avoid this or is that too naïve and simple a question?*

I do not think that the question is either simple or naïve;
I think it is justified. I remember that in a small discussion
group with a few pediatricians, which we kept going in recent years, this same question was put very often without
our arriving at an answer to it.

I also remember being asked by the members of this discussion group in what way a pediatrician, who is, as you
say, probably a good physiologist and a kind and understanding person, can equip himself in what you call the
physiology of the emotions, what we would call psychology.
They asked, for instance, whether an intensive summer
course in psychology would be a great help to doctors. My
answer was that it would help the doctors approximately
as much as it would help me as a nonmedical person to
take an intensive summer course in medicine. It would
leave me very much an amateur, and I think it will leave
the medical man in very much the same state.

I do not think that, as medical training stands now, this
situation can really be avoided. It can be avoided in the
future in a manner which is already in practice in some of
the big American universities, namely, by giving medical
students psychological training from the first or second year
of medical studies onward, with the intention of bringing
in the psychological side not as an afterthought, to be
added to their medical knowledge, but to be integrated
with it from the beginning. It is hoped that the products of
these medical schools will differ in important respects from
the present products of medical training.

But until that happens, and until it happens in many

places, I think only a close symbiosis between people with a full medical training and those with a full psychological training will bring about similar results. Both are amateurs in the other's field, but both can quite happily contribute to the solution of the individual problems. It would be, I think, as wrong for the medical people to overstep certain limits as it would be for the nonmedical ones to give medical treatment.

I have very rarely heard cuddling discussed, and it seems to me to play a big part in human relations between parents and children in the first few years of life. One notices that when one asks mothers or fathers whether their children are cuddly, what a tremendous variability there is. One notices this with one's own children. Some children like to be cuddled in a very nice babyish way, at least for some time in the day, up to about five, six or seven years; others, often perhaps little boys, never like it. Mother will say he is a nice little boy, she has never had any trouble with him, but no, he has never, even as a baby, liked cuddling. It obviously gives immense satisfaction to many parents to have a child who likes being cuddled. Would you care to discuss the question of cuddling?

In psychological discussions that have gone on in recent years, cuddling has come into its own again—I would say with a vengeance. There was a period in the upbringing of children here in England, the Truby King period, in which cuddling was discouraged, in which it was not thought necessary to give the young child extra satisfactions and bodily attention apart from those actions which were necessary for bodily health and growth.

Recent developments in psychology and in psychoanalysis have shown a very different picture, namely, that as the infants grow and develop, the needs for contact with the people in their environment become as imperative as the needs for food, sleep, and warmth (i.e., the basic bodily needs), and that children whose basic physical needs are fulfilled do not thrive well if the corresponding emotional needs are not fulfilled at the same time. It is perfectly true that the need for cuddling, that is, for pleasurable close contact with the parents, especially the mother in the earliest years, is not expressed to the same degree by all children.

I think it makes the mother so happy to have a cuddly child because she can feel quite certain that this child is in very good contact with her. With the child who refuses cuddling, the mother feels that this is not only a refusal of a certain form of skin contact, bodily warmth, and nearness, but that it may be a failure to have good emotional contact with her altogether. If it were that, then it would mean a serious lack in the personality development of that particular child. Actually, if you follow the early histories of highly abnormal children, the so-called atypical or autistic ones, you will invariably hear that they have never been cuddly, that they have not achieved the normal nearness to the mother in their first and second years of life, and this points to a deeper defect.

This does not mean that all children who are not very cuddly are abnormal. When the mother complains, for instance, that her child is not very cuddly, I think I would ask further questions. I would inquire whether that child looks for contact with the mother in other ways, always wants to see the mother and follow her with his eyes, or always wants to listen to the mother and is frightened if the mother is not heard at least walking around in the next room. It means the child may express his desire for nearness to the mother in various forms. Cuddling is one way, a normal way certainly in the first two years of life. And I think it would not harm pediatricians to inquire, at least with every difficult child, how matters stand in this particular respect.

I would like to raise the ever-present problem of the crying infant. Most of us are faced with this from time to time; we find various causes—feeding, colic, overanxious parents, and so on—but many of us are finally reduced to the regular administration of barbiturates. I recently had a patient who has, I think, moved about ten times because the neighbors complain. One need not emphasize the importance of that effect upon the child. How can we as pediatricians investigate this problem at our level? Or should this problem be referred for a more careful psychoanalytic study, and at what stage?

The crying infant is a problem equally to you and to us, and the referral for investigation at a psychoanalytic level is less promising because it is not so easy to investigate infants psychoanalytically. You will find, therefore, that our reasoning when such a mother and child come to us is very much like yours. Namely, our first thought is of a physical reason. Is there any physical disturbance which the mother has not found, which the pediatrician has not found, which makes it impossible for the child to be comforted? Let us see then that all these possibilities are excluded by experimenting with the feeding, by instructing the mother, and so on.

Then there is a further question which we ask ourselves: is this mother unable to give the child the comfort that other mothers are able to give? We all know that it is not unusual for children to have times of crying and discomfort, but the normal situation is that if there is no physical reason, the mother will be able to bring comfort and quiet to the child. Here, I believe, we arrive at the stage when we look for the reason either in the mother or in the child, and the less serious case would be if it is in the mother.

I have very recently had occasion to go through the files of our pediatrician at the Clinic concerning contacts with infants in the first year. When I sorted out the crying infants who were finally in need of sleeping pills, I thought in one or two cases that the child was in need of this physical method because of a failure in the mother; another mother might have been able to supply what the drug has to supply here—a quieting, soporific effect—but something in the mother, a restlessness, an anxiety, an inability to relate to the child, may have prevented her from doing so.

I think it would be interesting to pool resources here. I am very much against the easy solution that wherever there is something wrong with the infant, there is something wrong with the mother—I do not think that is true at all. Infants have a right to their own disturbances—they are people. But with the crying infant, I believe, we have one of the many instances where one has to go into the situation very carefully, and compare the methods of comforting of one mother with those of other mothers.

I saw an instance of a crying infant, really a wildly shrieking one, the other day in a shop. This was a perfect baby of about eleven months. The mother had taken him in a pram into a big store where she was about to buy him a beautiful pale blue spring coat—a big day for the baby. But she put the pram with the baby at one end of the store and went to the counter at the other end, where she had to wait for her turn. The baby felt deserted and began to shriek. One would not have known that she was the mother of the shrieking baby. She never turned her head. In the end, the people in the shop got so disturbed that she went and picked the baby up and he was quiet. Then the whole thing started all over again, about trying on the spring coat; every time the mother did the right thing, the baby was quiet; every time she failed to do it, the baby shrieked. It was evidently a battle between the two, the mother thinking, "I'll see who wins," and the baby thinking, "*I'll* see who wins."

This is a crude illustration and does not fit our case completely, except that I believe that the inability of a mother to stop a crying baby may have causes of which she is not aware at all, and then the two enter into a battle with each other which can increase many times over. This diagnosis would be the less serious one; besides, I think there are infants who cannot be comforted for psychological reasons, just as others cannot be comforted because of an organic disturbance, because there is something wrong in them. There is something wrong in their development, they are oversensitive, they get more anxious, more excited, more frightened, more upset by events than a normal child. Therefore, this kind of early screaming can really point to serious abnormalities. Again, in the history of the very abnormal children, we often hear about unmanageable crying in the first year. That is as far as we have gone in our explanations. I know it is not very far.

When should one have a sort of showdown with a child? I am thinking particularly of sleep disturbances: of the child who will not lie down unless the mother goes to bed with

the child, lies down with the child; or the child who wakes
up at night, who screams, is quiet when the mother goes
in, and then starts screaming again. This goes on week after
week, perhaps with very poor response to heavy sedation
for a short period. When should one leave the child to cry
and for how long a period should one leave him? One is
often asked if one should advise this sort of treatment.

That is one of these difficult questions to answer because
there is not one type of sleeping disturbance: there are
many types. It might be good to let a child "cry it out" in
one case, and it might be very harmful in another. I never
like the word "showdown" because it signifies that mother
and child are already involved in a big battle; and once that
has happened, whatever action is taken is usually wrong. In
most of these "showdowns," it is the child who wins, usually because the situation is already spoiled.

Perhaps I might use an illustration from my own experience here. During the war we ran a residential nursery
with fifty very young children aged from ten days to five
years, and as the children had to have a communal sleeping
place in our shelter, we were, of course, confronted with
innumerable sleeping difficulties, especially difficulties in
falling asleep. The handling of these difficulties was the
basis of much discussion among us, as we trained a number
of young nurses at that time. I remember feeling quite
proud of our training once when I overheard one of these
young nurses, while handing over night duty to another,
say to her successor: "If this child cries, don't go to him.
He always cries himself to sleep. You will only disturb him.
Let him cry for twenty minutes and he'll sleep. But if *that*
child cries, go immediately, because he will cry himself into

a panic, and if you don't qiuet him, there will be no sleep for anybody this night."

It meant that she recognized differences, on the basis of her training in observing the children: in the first child, crying was only a sign that he found it rather difficult to withdraw from the activities of the day and the people to whom he was attached, and that there was a short period of unhappiness before sleep took over; whereas the second child evidently had real anxieties which, if you did not quiet them, led to shrieks and a panic. Thus, I would suggest that mothers on such occasions find out what the crying means to the child—and then arrange the handling accordingly.

As we are talking about sleep disturbances, I should just like to mention a finding that we have come across in research at the Child Study Centre, where we found that many babies (in a normal sample of the population) who had already started to sleep well through the night at the usual age, which might be at two or three or four months, a little later began again to wake up during the night and to cry for their parents. Sometimes there was a clear reason for this, but very often there was not a clear reason that the mother could give us. Is there an inherent factor in the development of children between five and eight or nine months to account for this? Secondly, the treatment of disturbances of this kind is, of course, a problem for parents. We have just had a salutary reminder that what suits one baby will not suit another, and of course it is very easy for parents to feel that the disturbance is becoming a habit, as indeed it does if it is not effectively treated. Thus, what is the best way of handling this? Is it a question of trial and error with the baby you have? Or is there one method which in general is better than others?

This question really belongs in the wider context of the study of sleeping disturbances and that is not an easy subject at all. Sleep disturbances certainly have something to do with age and development. There is a simple form of infant sleep that we know and that we and many other people have studied. The infant sleeps when all his needs are fulfilled, and wakes when he is disturbed by any inner bodily demand. The very young infant then goes to sleep again when the excitation is removed. This is the simplest physiological pattern.

The whole problem of sleep becomes complicated with personality development. When the child's person, what we call his ego, develops, knowledge of the environment and attachment to the environment develop as well, and these interfere with the ease of falling asleep. Usually at that time the mother's struggle to put the child to sleep increases.

You probably know all the old methods of putting a child to sleep, methods which remove all outside stimulation, as if we were saying to the infant: there is no environment; look, it is dark, there is no noise, there is no one around, you don't miss anything, you might as well fall asleep. When people did that very consistently, I suppose the infant believed them and fell asleep.

But in reality the infant is alert to the signs of life that are going on around him and wants to take part, and the difficulty at that age is to achieve detachment from the environment. That is why the dummy was such a useful aid in putting the child to sleep because it substituted for all the pleasures and satisfactions offered by the environment, something which the child could take with him into the cot. Children who have no dummy use, as we know, their own thumb for sucking, or some other part of their body for satisfaction, or, as Winnicott (1953) has explained, they use some toy, a so-called transitional object, something which is neither the body nor the outer world, to help in this transition from waking life to sleep. I think that many of the developmental sleeping disturbances can be explained by some such reasoning. Can the child detach himself sufficiently to blot out all inner life, which is, after all, what sleep means?

There are also other influences at work. Children not only have difficulty in falling asleep, but often wake in the night and then cannot fall asleep again. If it is not a physical disturbance that disturbs sleep, then it may be some excitation left over from the day, an excitation with which they cannot deal.

Again, I take as an illustration our war children between one and two years old, who lived a much too exciting life, in a group in which there was too much battle, too much attacking of one another. They would wake in the night and fight their battles, they would cry out "No, no," defend themselves against an attacker, protect some possession, and so on. What I want to say is that it was the difficulty of detachment from the environment and the remnants of waking life that acted as disturbers of sleep.

With each child it is a matter of trial and error to find what will help. I think parents are greatly reassured by the idea that it is not just *their* child who has these difficulties, that these are developmental phases. I believe there is hardly any child who escapes sleeping difficulties, although mothers differ very much in their skill in dealing with them and therefore the problem does not always arrive at their pediatrician's door; most of it is fought out in the family.

I would appreciate some guidance on the child who refuses to eat. We tend to work on a rule of thumb, trying to induce indifference in the parents, trying to get them to give up the struggle or to send the child to live with his grandmother. But we do meet those who persistently go wrong. We meet those who get into states of severe malnutrition. I have seen a child in a state of anorexia nervosa that was indistinguishable from that found in older children; and I do not think we deal with this situation very well. I am sure we would all be very grateful for a word or two of guidance.

I wish a word or two of guidance would do away with the feeding disturbances. It is indeed a big chapter, at least it is a big chapter in *our* books, and I think it should be a big chapter in *your* books too.

It is a comparatively straightforward matter if one is able to organize the feeding of the child from the beginning, and to guide the mother through the various phases of breast or bottle feeding, drinking from a cup or spoon, introduction of solids, variety of foods, and following the child's preferences or avoidances. If the pediatrician or psychologist guides a mother through these phases, he will probably nip many feeding disturbances in the bud. The situations that come to him when a child absolutely refuses food for no organic reason are already end results, usually of years of battle between mother and child. There are many people who have written about feeding disturbances and I am one of them (see Volume IV, chs. 2 and 21). It is not an easy subject, and also not easy to summarize.

But perhaps it helps to keep in mind that, again, for the child, food is not only a material matter. In the first year of life, food and mother are more or less one and the same. The child cannot feed himself without the mother, and hunger, the sight of the mother, and the experience of satisfaction become for the child one whole. The mother herself feels this. She feels that when the child refuses food he refuses her, and takes it as a personal offense, very often quite rightly, since this close unity between mother and food endows the feeding process with all the difficulties of the mother relationship. It is the mother who gives the food, who refuses the food, and who is refused by the child. Very many children know that control of the mother is possible for them by eating or not eating.

I think, therefore, that one type of feeding disturbance is to be viewed from the aspect of the child's relationship to the mother. In modern feeding methods one tries to combat this unity between food and the mother by urging the child, as early as possible, to feed himself. At least we establish for the child a direct way to the food, bypassing the mother, in the second year, but still it will be the mother who gives the food or refuses it. I was greatly impressed when I read in the Platt report, in the discussion of the feeding of children in hospitals, that while many children will refuse to eat in hospitals when they are separated from their mothers, there will be an equal number of children who will eat in the hospital even though they do not eat well with their own mothers. This is perfectly true; there are many children who will eat in the absence of their mothers but not in their presence. This, I think, is the diagnostic sign which you can use if you want to deter-

mine whether the type of feeding disturbance you are dealing with is the one closely connected with the mother.

There are of course other types. There is a feeding disturbance that comes roughly between two and four years,
at the time when the child first becomes overinterested in
anal products and then turns against the whole subject;
much of the child's disgust of feces is apt to go over to food
and to exclude certain forms, consistencies, and colors in
food. These are the children who suddenly refuse to eat
spinach or chocolate sauce or sauces of any kind, who are
very suspicious of brown things and of certain shapes. I remember a little three- or four-year-old boy coming to the
table in the nursery and finding on his plate some small
sausages and mustard. He looked at the plate with horror
and gently picked up the small sausage, and with an expression of disgust put it on the ground, where he thought
it belonged. He felt this was not edible and should hardly
be touched. The disturbances in this group are not serious
since children outgrow the phase of disgust, usually when
their toilet training is fully established.

At a somewhat later stage we may encounter another
type of eating disturbance which is connected with the
child's ideas of impregnation, pregnancy, and birth. On a
certain level of sexual development children believe that
babies grow in the stomach as the result of the mother
having eaten something specific (as in some well-known
fairy tales), and such fantasies, when warded off, may lead
to an avoidance of food and a fear of getting fat. Other
children again may feel that eating is an aggressive act
which destroys the food, and they may restrict their diet
to a vegetarian one for fear of being "murderers." With
other children, the aggressive and destructive tendencies

are turned against their own bodies. In the well-known anorexia nervosa, the refusal of food is placed in the service of self-destructive suicidal impulses which often enough succeed in reaching their aim. There is a long path from the early, common feeding troubles based on the relationship to the mother to these later, very complex pathological structures.

As you see, it is as impossible to give general prescriptions for the handling of feeding disturbances as it would be to prescribe in general for stomach upsets or fever; their treatment depends not on their surface appearances but on the underlying meaning which is expressed by them.

As pediatricians we are, of course, increasingly getting involved with obstetricians, in an advisory capacity as well as that of clinic responsibility. I refer, of course, to the generally bad arrangements of obstetric departments, of the housing of the newborn. What would you give us as reasonably good advice to help us put up a stronger case to obstetricians so that they will gradually arrive at an ideal situation in the hospital that would better the mother-baby relationship? And to what extent do you really think, in the light of psychology, that the infant in the first weeks calls for any particular or special consideration in regard to general care, not only feeding? And I think you might include in your remarks a little note on the relationship between mothers, midwives, and doctors and the baby.

I do not want to pretend to know more than I do, and therefore I can only say in answer what I have recently heard in discussions of this question. You probably know that in the United States there has been a strong movement in the direction of returning to a more natural condition in the beginnings of life shared between mother and baby in the hospital. This is the so-called "rooming-in" project, carried out at Yale under the direction of Dr. Edith Jackson, who is one of our colleagues in the United States. She found in her work that the situation between young mother and young infant is very often spoiled by the time the two are brought together and arrive at home, the father also being excluded from the situation until then. She succeeded at Yale in opening a hospital section which returned to natural family conditions by keeping mother and infant together from the first day of life, with help given to the mother by the nursing staff, and with the father having free access to mother and baby. This project has been in action for approximately ten to fifteen years, and the results have been observed and published. It was very interesting to see that requests for admission to that special section have been very numerous.

In contrast, I can quote the story of the mother of a child patient who still remembers with strong feelings of guilt that one night in the hospital she got out of bed, unnoticed by the night nurse, crept to the room where the babies were kept, again was not noticed by the baby nurse, and tried to feed her baby, because she had heard the baby cry across the corridors. She thought she had committed a most dreadful act, but she could not help herself. Well, I think any hospital rule that places a wedge between mother and infant at that time is not a good arrangement. After all, the further care of the infant depends on the mother's empathic attitudes toward the child; to cut them off for a week or ten days and then to expect them to be there as if nothing had happened is not very reasonable. That would be my answer.

I am bothered these days by a great many mothers who seem to suffer from psychological misinformation. There is the mother who is so anxious to breast-feed, because she is told it is the right thing psychologically, that she fails. She then feels guilty for ever after that she has destroyed a very important relationship with her baby. Then there is the mother who fails to pick up the early cues of toilet training in her child, because she has read somewhere that early and coercive toilet training is a bad thing. Or the mother who has a child in the hospital and can never treat that child naturally afterward, because she is terrified that "separation" has occurred. Now the poor pediatrician, in trying to reassure this mother, is immediately told, "Well I have heard it on the television," or "I read it in a certain paper or book," and that printed word carries much more value than anything he could tell her anyway. I wonder, do you recognize this danger, and what can we do to protect mothers from it?

We certainly recognize this danger. I often feel that the mothers of young children are the most maltreated individuals in our community, because they are made responsible for whatever happens to the child, whatever is found in the child, without being given the possibility to do something positive about it or even to defend themselves. Young mothers are usually insecure. They are always insecure if they are not backed up by a strong social tradition that tells them what to do without questioning. Our young mothers nowadays have no such social tradition to back them up. Instead, they have conflicting psychological opinions, which they hear, as you say, on television or over the radio.

What they want, above all, is a reassuring authority to

tell them what to do, and they have found one, as you probably know. Perhaps not your own patients who have invested you with the necessary authority, but many other mothers look to Dr. Spock for guidance. He, quite intentionally, accepts this role. He tries to set himself up as a benevolent, and at the same time firm, authoritarian figure, in order to return to mothers the self-confidence which they have lost. I had a discussion with Dr. Spock about it once in which I took another point of view. I said I think all this advice to mothers is not really what is needed; the spreading of knowledge is what is necessary. He answered, and I suppose quite rightly, that spreading of knowledge would be quite all right if it were not so conflicting. How is the mother to know what is right and what is wrong? She wants somebody to decide for her.

Would it perhaps be right to say that mothers find themselves in such a harassed position because they have taken their lead from such public sources as radio, television, and popular books, and because pediatricians have not been active enough in taking over the role left empty by religion and social tradition? Here then is the place for the pediatrician to establish a new authority, to show the mothers what is right and wrong, in the medical and psychological sense. The mothers would be only too glad to follow any lead. But unless such a strong lead is given by people in authority, the mothers will be in a most unhappy position, and their position will be made worse by the fact that in the social services a transitional phase has existed, and to some extent still exists, where all the blame which in the more distant past had been put on the bad children is now put on the bad mothers. I believe it is high time that we got past that period.

I would like to ask whether in respect to what you have just said, you know of a comparative study of childhood behavior disorders in the United States and this country. It is all very well to say that the pediatrician should do this and that, to provide continuity of service, but he sees a very, very small minority of babies and infants. In this country, they are in the medical care of, and are the property of, the general practitioner. I do not know whether mothers register their children antenatally in the United States, but certainly within a few hours of birth they have a pediatrician who gives continuity of service, and he, together with Dr. Spock, will provide a continuity of service. I was wondering, therefore, whether your thesis is one which bears analysis. In the United States there is more continuity and consistency of approach all the time, as distinct from the haphazard approach in this country, where the practitioner may give some advice, the doctor at the Welfare Centre may adivse something very different, and then the patient comes to the hospital to receive yet a third lot of advice.

I can only say to that that if I were a pediatrician, I would fight for the pediatricians' influence from the start. The case which comes to the consulting pediatrician is often in such an advanced state of disturbance that measures that would have helped in the beginning are no longer applicable.

I have noticed you have once or twice used the term "abnormal" children. We accept the fact that some children are born with low or high IQ's, with red or black hair, and who may develop big or small physiques. Do we accept the fact that some children are born with easy temperaments and some with difficult temperaments? When faced with some of the problems we have been discussing today, can we accept the idea that some of these disturbed children are just born difficult? One sometimes sees striking examples coming in the midst of a family of easy children, where the mother had no difficulty in bringing up most of the children, and then one, from the moment he is born, rejects the breast, is difficult in every way, and is, as one mother very aptly expressed it, "bloody-minded" from the beginning. Do you accept the fact that there are some children who are born bloody-minded, and that it is realistic to accept that fact and not try and adduce environmental factors to explain what is really a congenital disorder?

I have no doubt about the existence of congenital differences, quite apart from the big congenital disorders. But in discussions of this kind, to point to the congenital differences is not very helpful. We can be quite certain to find them at the bottom of all the situations we study, when we have gone as far as we can in the understanding of what has happened during the child's lifetime. On the other hand, recent studies have revealed that much happens in the first six months of a child's life that determines the child's later behavior, for instance, his inclination to turn toward the outer world or to withdraw into himself, to show free aggression or to turn aggression against himself, to be a good or a bad feeder, and so on. Before we looked at the beginning of life more closely, we were always apt to say that these tendencies are inherited. I think that it does no harm to explore these early influences on the child as far as we can. The fact will remain that people are born different.

I now have a question to ask the pediatricians here, and it is probably not a question that you will find easy to answer. When we went through the program for this particular study group, I was very struck by your growing interest in the psychosomatic disorders; this means that you are becoming very interested in the reaction of the body to the mind. Not all the disturbances that manifest themselves as physical, you now say, have physical causes; some of them seem to have their origins in the mind. Certain things going on in the mind have certain repercussions in the body, and you would like to know more about that.

I always wonder why you are not equally interested in the other side of the picture, namely, what repercussions the truly organic disturbances which you treat have on the mind of the child. I often regret that pediatricians care more for the psychosomatic side and are less interested in the psychological aftereffects of physical illness.

There are questions such as the following: take, for example, a digestive disturbance in the first year of life, with a great deal of pain and discomfort, one that cuts out the pleasure in nourishment which belongs to that age. Will this have a lasting effect on the child's personality? There has been pain at a time when there should have been pleasure; there has been an overemphasis on the digestive tract; there have been times of revulsion against food or unsatisfied hunger.

I think whenever you handle a physical disturbance of this kind, you should ask at the same time what it means in psychological terms, just as you have asked today what rectal manipulation means in psychological terms. Whenever you interfere with the body of a child in some massive way, you should ask yourself: what will the child make of this? Perhaps some day there will be another study group dealing exclusively with the other side of the subject, namely, with the question of what illness and medical interference mean in terms of the child's psychological development.[1]

---

[1] [For a further discussion of this issue and related ones, see Volume IV, ch. 11, and this volume, ch. 25. See also Bergmann and A. Freud (1965).]

24

The Role of Regression in Mental Development

(1963)

Psychoanalysis as a clinical and theoretical field offers its own workers possibilities which range from developmental to normal and abnormal psychology. But psychoanalysts have always had the reputation of straying in their work beyond their own confines and, with the aim of "applying" their theories, to make contact with other disciplines. Psychiatry, education, the social sciences, mythology, religion, literature, art, etc., are among the earlier realms of applica-

First published in *Modern Perspectives in Child Development,* ed. A. J. Solnit and S. A. Provence. New York: International Universities Press, 1963, pp. 97-106.
[The same topic addressed to analysts, rather than specifically to pediatricians, was dealt with by Anna Freud in a paper (1963b) not included in this volume. See Volume VI, pp. 93-107.—*Editor's note.*]

tion. General medicine (under the term of psychosomatics) and pediatrics are among the later ones. On every one of these occasions, the gradual approach between the two fields depended on a few pioneering figures, rooted either on one side or on the other. In pediatrics the name of Milton Senn will remain connected with the groundwork for such linkage with analysis.

It has been felt for a long time that the pediatrician and the child analyst share much common ground. Both have as the object of their observation the immature individual who is in a fluid state of incomplete development, characterized by rapid changes, where the interaction between inborn and environmental influences is more open to view than it will be in maturity. Both, therefore, have to reckon not only with the child himself but with his management. For both, the experiences gained from the sick lead automatically to application to the healthy and to methods of prevention.[1] In therapy, both suffer from the uncooperativeness of their patients, since young children seldom, if ever, seek help actively or are ready to describe their symptoms. Where symptomatology is concerned, in both instances, the similarity between child and adult is frequently a superficial one, the same pathological manifestation carrying different weight and outlook in the growing individual. Both pediatrician and psychoanalyst are in a situation where the maturational forces work simultaneously with their own therapeutic efforts, and where in the final result of recovery it is not easy to distinguish how far the patient has responded to treatment and how far his ills have been "outgrown." Above all, it can be said with justification that

[1] As in the Well-Baby Clinics.

both, the pediatrician as well as the child analyst, assist the curative factors which are normally active in the young organism. Therapy is directed toward freeing the child from "obstacles to his growth so that he can move with reasonable security through succeeding developmental stages."[2]

While these identities in themselves might have led to an earlier, and profitable, link-up between the two professions, there are other and theoretically more essential differences which were effective in keeping them apart. The pediatrician who has been trained in the conditions governing organic growth does not take readily to the different principles which are governing the mental side. Brought up in chemistry, biochemistry, biology, anatomy, physiology, genetics, he has acquired a high valuation of laboratory methods and experiments which are not valid in the other realm. Trained as an exact scientist, he feels a natural bias against a field in which—to his mind—assumptions, conclusions, hypotheses, and subjective interpretations reign supreme. In the long run, it was only the "illogical" behavior of the child patients themselves which impressed the pediatricians: their conversion symptoms such as headaches, pains, constipation, digestive upsets without visible organic cause; asthma and eczema with their fluctuations in intensity and their unknown origin; the sleeping and feeding troubles of the young; anorexia of the adolescent; enuresis and incontinence where they are purely functional. In spite of his readiness to diagnose and treat, exactly and scientifically, these psychosomatic (as they are now called) troubles of the child left the pediatrician helpless, and gradually more pre-

[2] See for this and some earlier formulations, Report No. 38, *The Diagnostic Process in Child Psychiatry*, of the Group for the Advancement of Psychiatry, 1957, p. 316.

pared than before to contemplate an approach which, itself inexact and to all appearances erratic, proves capable of following the child patients into their psychological intricacies.

It is the object of the present paper to describe in detail the process of *regression*, this being one of the specific principles which is operative only on the mental side and as such is strange to the physician. To acknowledge and learn to diagnose the results of the regressive process may contribute toward familiarizing the pediatrician with mental manifestations in the child, both normal and abnormal, which otherwise remain inexplicable.

The physician is familiar with the processes of growth on the organic side. Bones, once formed and developed, do not reassume their former infantile appearance; physiological or neurological processes, once risen to a certain level, maintain it; glandular action matures, sheds infantile forms, and substitutes others. The more mature levels of development replace the earlier ones. In short, growth proceeds in a straight progressive line until maturity is reached, invalidated only by intervening severe illness or injuries, and at the end, by the destructive, involutionary processes of old age.

The pediatrician may assume automatically that the same is true of the child's mental and emotional equipment, i.e., that here, too, a developmental line is selected by the individual and pursued to its conclusion.[3] But expectations of this kind are not borne out by facts, and therapeutic actions based on them will miscarry. That does not imply that orderly maturation fails to play its part in drive development, or in the gradual perfection of the rational part of the

[3] [For a detailed discussion of the concept of developmental lines, see Anna Freud (1963a) and Volume VI, pp. 62-92.]

child's personality, the ego. It means to say merely that progression is not only the force in operation and that equal attention needs to be paid to the regressive moves which are its inevitable accompaniment and counterpart.

REGRESSION IN DRIVE AND LIBIDO DEVELOPMENT

Where sex development is concerned, for example, we observe in children the now well-known sequence of libidinal stages, each named after the body zone which plays the leading part in providing autoerotic, i.e., sexual, stimulation: oral, anal, phallic stage. On each libidinal level of development we find, also maturationally coordinated with it, the corresponding manifestations of the aggressive drive: biting during orality; sadism, destructiveness during anality; competitive masterfulness in the phallic stage. This line corresponds further with a distinct sequence of emotional attitudes toward mother, father, siblings, etc.: dependence, helplessness, demandingness, greed in the oral stage give way to clinging and possessiveness in the anal child; these again to the jealousies, rivalries, demonstrativeness on the phallic level, the latter being the bodily equivalent of the emotional experiences which belong to the oedipus and castration complexes. So far, these are lines of progress, comparable in their forward direction to any similar developmental line on the organic side.

Now for the other aspect of the picture. We conceive of this development in the sense that the consecutive positions (and the persons which serve as satisfying objects at each stage) are invested with drive energy, and that this energy (libido, aggression) moves forward from one position to the next. But in spite of forward movement taking place, no station on the way is ever fully outgrown, as it is on the organic side. While one part of the drive energy is on its forward course, another part—of varying quantity—remains behind. For example, the thumb-sucking infant will not give up his interest in sucking automatically when the bulk of his drive energies already centers around anality; some of the former pleasure in oral erotism will remain intact and will survive. Similarly, some of the anal interests will survive the child's transition to the phallic stage. In short, no drive position once held, however obsolete it may appear, will really be abandoned.

It is not essential here whether the survivals of the former stages remain in consciousness or are relegated to the repressed unconscious. In either state they are capable of binding and retaining drive energy. Whenever difficulties, disappointments, frustrations occur, then, at a later date, these stations of the past, or "fixation points" as they are called, come into their own again by exerting a retrograde attraction on later energies. Libido will flow back to them, to the impoverishment of the later levels. This creates the puzzling pictures where older children, or adolescents, or adults, lose interest in the libidinal or aggressive outlets which are appropriate to their ages and hark back to childish wishes and concerns.

Such regression may be temporary, the drives—after a pathological interval—may pursue their forward course again. More often it is permanent, meaning lasting complications, repercussions, and damage to the individual's sexual normality or the age-adequate, constructive employment of his aggressive powers.

Surely, there is nothing on the organic side of human

development which prepares the physician for the appreciation of the importance of such fixation points and nothing which matches the regressive pull exerted on the organism through this formation.[4]

REGRESSION IN EGO DEVELOPMENT

Regression appears different where it occurs on the side of the child's ego, although the same principles are active in the process: return to earlier mental structures and, with it, return to more primitive modes of functioning, representation, and expression.

Temporary Regressions in Normal Development

There is, first, regression as a normal, never-failing accompaniment to all newly acquired achievements of the child, as is well known to all mothers, nurses, or teachers of the young. It is taken for granted by them as a characteristic of childish behavior and as such rarely mentioned. In their mental growth, children do not take a straightforward path, but, as it is popularly expressed, take "two steps forward and one back." This refers to all their functioning, from control of motility, speech, bladder and bowel control, manners, to such ethical virtues as impulse control, ability to wait, social adaptation, honesty, fairness, etc. The capacity to function

---

[4] It may be useful for the pediatrician to know that, apart from the usual hazards which a child meets in his development, any deliberate interference with the legitimate quantity of gratification at any stage can set up fixation points. Examples are deprivation as well as overindulgence in the management of the child by the mother in general, or on the medical side: dieting as deprivation in the oral phase; enemas, suppositories as overstimulation in the anal phase, etc.

on a high level of achievement is in itself no guarantee that the performance will be stable; on the contrary, it is more normal for the child, and a better guarantee for later mental health if, during the state of growth, he reverts occasionally to more infantile modes of behavior before these are abandoned: from being toilet trained to messing, from sensible speech to nonsense talk, from play with toys to body play, from constructiveness to destructiveness, and from social adaptation to pure egoism. What mothers describe as surprising in diagnostic interviews are not these relapses but, on the contrary, those other instances where their children have taken a single step forward which, for once, was not reversed. This may have been a sudden transition from the breast to the bottle, or bottle to cup; in toilet training one single incident, after which there were "no more soiled nappies"; an incident at bedtime after which there was "no more calling out"; in habits a sudden weaning from the dummy, or the thumb, or from sleeping with a favorite toy, etc. These happenings are recognized as exceptions, and we know that they are in general not to be welcomed. To use the method of trial and error, progression, and temporary reversal is more appropriate to healthy mental growth.

Temporary Ego Regression Under Stress

It is another fact, well known to educators, that ego achievements are not maintained at their height when children are under the influence of fatigue, anxiety, pain, or any other strain. Every mother knows that the tired child at bedtime behaves like a much younger child; although well adapted in daytime, he may begin to fret, to whine, to babble nonsense, to be unreasonable, clinging, and demand the physical attentions of the toddler stage. Every nursery school teacher knows that her pupils at the end of the morning will be less concentrated than in the beginning, that construction toys will be thrown about, that tempers are shorter, manners lapse, and partnership with playmates ends more easily in quarrels. Mothers and nurses are aware that pain, fever, bodily discomfort, and fear of medical examination bring out the infant in the child. Not all child patients who are unruly in the pediatrician's waiting room, or who kick and scream during examinations are really backward in upbringing or behavior. The examining pediatrician, although able to record an accurate account of the child's organic growth, will rarely be in a position to see his patients at their mental best. As regards their food and sleeping habits, their cleanliness, their occupations and behavior, ill children are usually regressed children, with many of their age-adequate functions in abeyance.

Regression has also been studied in young children who are separated from their parents, in wartime institutions or in hospitals. There the state of distress, caused in them by the experience, reveals itself in various forms, of which the loss of such functions as speech or toilet training is an important one. That in such regressions they return step by step along the line taken previously in forward development, is borne out by the fact that it is invariably the latest achievements which are lost first.

Such regressive lapses receive little attention if they are temporary. The healthy child at home or in nursery school will next morning be once more in full possession of his faculties. The ill child will resume his former status when recovered. The hospitalized children or those separated for other reasons may take longer to overcome infantilisms in behavior, especially their clinging and demanding, if separation has been of longer duration and has been traumatic.

But, taken as a whole, regression under stress is a normal mechanism and is based on the immature individual's flexibility. It is useful as an answer to the strain of the moment and an attempt to adapt to it; it is always available to the child as a response to frustration which otherwise might be too difficult to bear. As such a response, it is short-lived and reversible.

Perhaps a device comparable to it on the physical side is the ability of some children to lower all their reactions during illness and "sleep through it."

EGO REGRESSION RELATED TO DRIVE REGRESSIONS

Regressions in the ego lose their beneficial aspect and turn into a threat to development and mental health as soon as they become permanent, i.e., irreversible. In the immature individuals, this happens predominantly following a regression in their drives.

When, as described above, drive energy flows backward after frustrations in the phallic phase to fixation points in anality or orality, the ego, i.e., the side of the child which represents adaptation, morals, and intelligence, has to choose between alternative reactions. He may acquiesce in the occurrence, accept once more the infantile, primitive desires and fantasies as they return from the unconscious, and, with it, lower all his demands on himself and his standards of performance. The result will be what both child analyst and pediatrician regard as an "infantilism." Children of this kind seem younger than their years and, although no "obvious" reason can be found for it, they lag behind their contemporaries in behavior, habits, play, school performance, or general adaptation to the environment. They may soil or wet with indifference; or attack and hurt other children without experiencing compassion or regret; they may destroy inanimate objects; be egotistic and irresponsible; or appropriate what does not belong to them, etc.; worst of all, educational influence usually proves helpless with regard to them. Their regressed drives have come to terms with their regressed ego, and in the absence of conflict between the two there is no sufficient incentive for them to behave otherwise. They are incapacitated by a mental state which has to be understood as the result of "total regression" (or rather partial id plus partial ego regression). Not to be "age adequate" characterizes the essential nature of their disturbance.

The alternative reaction of a child whose drives have regressed is the following: his ego remains firm and refuses to give in to the demand for primitive satisfactions, however great the pressure toward them may be. He keeps up his former reasonable functioning, the height of his achievements, and the moral and ethical demands made on his behavior by his conscience (superego). But this attitude, although more ambitious and in the developmental sense more appropriate than the former one, leads as inevitably to pathology, though of a different kind. The child becomes a prey to severe anxieties and to internal conflicts in which his ego and superego engage in battle with the drives. The result is an infantile neurosis built on the pattern of adult neuroses, with symptom formation set up as a compromise between the conflicting inner agencies.[5]

From the foregoing it is obvious that it is the more highly developed child with the better organized personality who tends to produce not infantilisms but neurotic symptoms. To appreciate this last fact may serve to make pediatricians more tolerant and more understanding toward the neurotic psychopathology of their child patients with which, not without reason, they often feel out of sympathy.

SUMMARY

Mutual interests of pediatricians and child analysts are described and obstacles to mutual understanding are indicated. *Regression*, a mental process, is described with the aim of extending the application of psychoanalytic concepts to pediatrics. Regression in drive and libido development and in ego development are discussed in order to illuminate the psychic states of health and illness in child development. Although temporary regressions are characteristic of healthy development, permanent regressions are associated with deviant development.

[5] It may be confusing to the pediatrician that in these neurotic cases, too, apparently simple psychosomatic manifestations exist side by side with the complex psychological symptoms; further, that some of this symptomatology scarcely differs from the infantilisms mentioned above (for example, enuresis, incontinence). The child analyst's answer to this is that the difference lies not in the outward appearance of the pathological manifestations but in their inner structures. The infantilisms are returns to forms of behavior which have been age adequate for an earlier stage of development; the neurotic symptoms are rooted in two sides of the personality and constitute an attempt to combine opposing tendencies: they express in one and the same action the primitive drive with its urge for satisfaction and the ego's fight against this satisfaction taking place.

25

Children in the Hospital

(1965)

I

FOREWORD

By now, the insights contained in psychoanalytic child psychology have been used for the handling of children in many areas, for their upbringing in home and school, their management in health and sickness, for child law and adoptive procedures. The opening up of every additional

First published as "Foreword" and Chapter 15, "Conclusion," in *Children in the Hospital,* by Thesi Bergmann in collaboration with Anna Freud. New York: International Universities Press, 1965, pp. 9-10 and pp. 135-151.

The book is based on observations collected by Thesi Bergmann in her capacity as hospital therapist in a receiving hospital for children with chronic diseases. The case histories of the children referred to are all described in this book.

field always has been due to the efforts of some interested individual who applied himself to it singlehandedly, devotedly, and without much recognition until others followed suit. This, exactly, is the manner in which Thesi Bergmann took up work with chronically ill children, to pursue it quietly and unobtrusively, over almost twenty years, collecting data concerning their behavior, increasing understanding of their plight, and helping them to improve their fate.

It is my respect and appreciation for labors of this kind which have prompted me to join forces with her in shaping her findings for publication. While the material in this book and many of the conclusions drawn from it are wholly hers, the formulation of the text, the responsibility for the final selection from her examples, and the concluding chapter are wholly mine. I have done this work in the hope that the reader will enjoy the excellence of her observations, follow her argumentation, and profit in his own work from her experiences.

II

CONCLUDING REMARKS

When assessing the practical value of the material presented in the preceding pages, a number of considerations have to be taken into account, such as the following:

Severe, Chronic versus Minor, Acute Illness

It is a characteristic of this book that Thesi Bergmann's observations are derived from work with children whose lives were disrupted by the most dangerous and crippling bodily afflictions. Nevertheless it seems to me erroneous to conclude that this diminishes its relevance for those parents, nurses or physicians who deal habitually with the more benign and transitory forms of children's diseases. The differences to be noted in the patients' reactions to the two types of illness are matters of degree and quantity rather than basic differences in quality; more important still, they concern external physical realities rather than the internal psychic realities of the child, with all the discrepancies which exist between the former and the latter.

SURGERY

Any interference with the child's body, whether major or minor, is likely to arouse his fantasies and fears with regard to being attacked, mutilated, deprived of a valuable part of his own self. It makes surprisingly little difference whether the intervention is as serious as in the cases of Linda or Jackie, or as insignificant as with Marion.[1] Whatever has been seen in one of the children described above is also present in the usual cases of tonsillectomy, adenoidectomy or hernia repair, occasions which are regarded by many of the children concerned with no less dread than Carl regarded being placed in the respirator or with which Henry and Larry met their dangerous operations.[2]

On the other hand, the differences between major and minor, serious and negligible, which are insufficiently re-

---

[1] [Linda was a spastic diplegic, Jackie needed a spinal operation; while Marion, an asthmatic child, dreaded to have a blood sample taken.]

[2] [Carl was completely paralyzed following polio, Henry was a paraplegic, and Larry had tuberculosis of the hip.]

acted to by the child patient himself, loom very large in the minds of the medical and nursing staff, who are used to an objective and wholly realistic appraisal of events. Our attempts to reveal the children's intimate reactions may be met with incredulity by the adults in question so long as they concern procedures which are harmless and insignificant to their eyes, as are impending visits to the dentist, injections, inoculations, or completely noninjurious events such as sun-ray treatments. What blocks understanding here is the normal adult's unfamiliarity with the child's subjective, irrational, emotional approach. Adult understanding comes more readily where psychic reality and external reality coincide and the child's fears are concerned with unquestionably serious situations which cannot fail to evoke anybody's concern and sympathy; on the other hand, once the child's helpless terror has been brought home to the environment on these occasions, it is easier to establish the fact that, so far as fantasies, anxieties, and affects are concerned, the piercing of a boil, the taking of a blood sample, or the extraction of a tooth may loom as large as the actual removal of an eye or the amputation of a limb. What needs to be understood is the fact that in both instances, whether objectively justified or not, the patient's emotions are very real and the child is in need of help. That in this book's exposition the reader is invited to follow a path of understanding which leads from the major to the minor events may well have its advantages over the usual course which goes in the opposite direction.

ILLNESS AS PUNISHMENT

In the child's conception there is a similar lack of difference between severe illness and its lighter forms. Any intercurrent infection, caught inadvertently, is understood by many children as the consequence of naughtiness and revives the memory of things eaten, warm clothing and rubbers discarded or fought against, puddles walked into, etc., in the face of parental prohibition. What weighs heavily on the child in these instances is neither the actual act of disobedience, nor its alleged bodily consequence as such, but their symbolic value, namely, what appears to the child as a confirmation of the belief that wrongdoing, however secretly performed, is open to punishment, and that other, still undetected misdeeds, whether actually carried out or merely contemplated in fantasy, will likewise be followed by retribution of some kind. This idea intensifies all the fears which in any case accompany childhood development, and it arouses intolerable pangs of conscience irrespective of whether fate metes out the supposed "punishment" in the form of rheumatic illnesses (as with Ernest or Ruth), or in the milder form of common colds, sore throats, upsets of the stomach and digestive tract.

DURATION OF ILLNESS

The enormous difference between the chronic and acute states is significant for the adult environment rather than for the children themselves, especially for the younger ones. This of course does not mean that a year (or more) of hospitalization or bodily incapacity seems short to any child; even the shortest terms of being confined, of being in the hospital, on a diet, under motor restriction, seem intolerably long or even eternal to all children, whether they last twenty-four hours, three days, a week or a fortnight. The operative factor here is that the sense of time functions differently in earlier than in later ages. Adults behave objectively about time; i.e., they measure it with the help of clock and calendar, and this reality-adapted attitude gives way only occasionally, when time "passes incredibly quickly" with some pleasurable occupation; or when it "drags on," "hangs heavy on their hands," appears "interminable" when they are bored, or in pain, or anxiously awaiting some event. In the very young, however, these latter subjective appraisals of time are the order of the day—in fact are the only attitude to time of which they are capable. Not only are calendar and clock still beyond their intellectual grasp; it is of greater importance that their measuring of time is carried out not by their ego, i.e., the sensible and rational part of their personalities, but by the strength and urgency of their wishes which turn all periods of time into waiting times, namely, waiting for gratification of their impulses. What young children, especially those of the toddler age, accomplish least of all is postponement of wish fulfillment, whether the wish is a crudely instinctual one or merely a wish for comfort, company, entertainment, activity, motor outlet, relief from discomfort, pain or anxiety. Consequently, all periods of illness are painfully long for the child, whatever their objective length. Here too, understanding is easier for the adults if they acquire their insights from contact with the chronic rather than the acute illnesses. In cases of the first kind of the child's despair about the duration of his incapacity is readily grasped and shared by parents and hospital staff, whereas his fretting and impatience in the case of short, acute spells is dismissed more easily as "unreasonable" and, consequently, met with little sympathy or with facile promises that discomfort or deprivation will "soon be over," "not last long," "only take a minute," i.e., with reassurances which are out of harmony with the child's inner experience and therefore fail to be effective in allaying his anxieties.

When looking after chronically ill children, however, one particular point should not be overlooked. As it happens when people, children or adults, have come to live under traumatic conditions for extended periods of time (see ch. 14 in this volume), the human organism as a whole adapts to the existing state of affairs, whether this is one of increased danger, heightened pain, discomfort or unpleasure. Where we would expect the young child to be adversely affected, angry or up in arms fighting against the pain inflicted upon him, we may find to our surprise that this negative experience has become for him part of "normal life" and is expected and coped with as such. It is, as Thesi Bergmann remarks in her observations, only the unexpected addition to the usual quota of discomfort or restriction which arouses the young patient's indignation.

THE STUDY OF CHILDREN'S REACTIONS TO ILLNESS

There are obvious advantages offered by a hospital setting such as Rainbow's. In the usual quick turnover of a general pediatric ward, there is little for the observer to see apart from the immediate impact on the children of separation from home, admission to unfamiliar surroundings, with the consequent reactions of shock, or anxiety, or protest, or withdrawal, often intermixed and overlaid with attitudes of apparent indifference, compliance, and acceptance. The acutely ill patient, in contrast to the chronic one, has no time to proceed beyond the distress of the unrelated newcomer, to transfer confidence and dependence onto the hospital staff, and to change thereby from a shadowy figure to a distinct individual, revealing the doubts, conflicts, difficulties, and fantasies about his illness which we have described above. On the other hand, it is precisely this intimate, personal knowledge of the child on which help, support, and reassurance for him can be based; and it is easier to apply to the acutely ill patients what has been learned in the orthopedic, tuberculosis or poliomyelitis hospitals than to gather the necessary insights during the hurried contacts with the shifting population of an ear, nose, and throat ward.

Interaction between Mind and Body

If the descriptions given in this book are accepted as valid —and we hope they are—it may be appropriate to extract from them some conclusions as to the normal interactions between mind and body in the early ages.

In our time, when the *psychosomatic* basis of many illnesses is in the process of being accepted by the medical profession, it seems hardly necessary to present additional examples of "mind over matter" or to stress the importance of emotional factors in such illnesses as asthma, certain heart conditions, etc. It is also a well-known fact that the younger the child, the closer is normally the connection between mind and body, because, in the relative absence of mental outlets through thinking, reasoning, and speech, the emotions are discharged through physical channels via skin eruptions, upsets in the feeding and sleeping rhythm, the digestice tract. Therefore, what we tried to illustrate in the preceding chapters is no more than the experience that, even in the severe illnesses of our organic patients, attitudes and emotions such as hope, despair, compliance, fear, and guilt played a part, precipitating the onset of the disease or contributing to it, delaying recovery or speeding it up, and occasionally even determining the final outcome in a positive or negative direction.

THE IMPACT OF PHYSICAL HAPPENINGS ON THE MIND

Compared with the attention paid to psychosomatic factors, the impact of physical happenings on the mind and on personality formation constitutes a neglected chapter; we have tried, accordingly, to document it amply in the preceding pages.

The medical and nursing personnel must inevitably be guided in their actions by the needs which arise during the various physical crises or the exigencies of pre- and post-operative situations. This, nevertheless, does not alter the fact that every single happening during illness, as well as every single action performed during its course and for its sake, beneficial as it may be in the physical sense, also has its potential adverse repercussions on the child's mind. The following are merely some representative examples of these:

1. The mere incidence of pain and discomfort, especially in early infancy, upsets the delicate *balance between pleasure and unpleasure,* which lies at the basis of mental development and determines the infant's positive or negative attitude to life. We know now that the newborn's earliest concept of himself is located in the kernel of pleasurable sensations connected with the physical experiences of feeding, satiation, body comfort, etc. The infant "loves" all these pleasures and shrinks from all experiences of pain and discomfort, which have a retarding and disrupting effect on his ego growth. For this reason, painful illnesses at the beginning of life, as well as painful medical procedures, are

justifiably dreaded in the interest of mental development.

2. Another potential interference with the progressive personality development of the older child is the situation of *"being nursed,"* and this quite apart from and often in striking contrast to his physical need for the nurse's help. Adult patients who, while healthy, feel certain of their independence in body matters can during physical illness permit themselves to return temporarily to the state of a helpless infant whose body is under other people's care and jurisdiction. It is impossible for children to accept nursing in the same spirit. For them, to have attained a measure of physical independence from the adult world and to have personal control over their own bodies are great developmental achievements which they prize highly and are reluctant to renounce. They may show this by obstructive and uncooperative behavior as a defense against the regressive move which the situation demands from them; or they may feel unable to keep up their more mature status and slip back entirely into passive compliance, allowing themselves to be handled without resistance. Both reactions are unwelcome and unhelpful, from the practical point of view of dealing with the ill body as well as from the aspect of smooth, progressive mental development.[3]

3. It is not difficult to understand that nursing and medical staff feel reluctant if they are asked to take into account the meaning which their handling has for the child, i.e., of the fantastic interpretations and transformations which their practical actions undergo in the child's mind.

---

[3] Adult men who ward off latent passive-feminine tendencies in their personality structure are often notoriously bad patients. Like the children, they put up a fight against the passive experience of being nursed.

Not every child is objective enough to praise the nurse as a "corker," because she pursues her course of action dutifully, regardless of his protests (as nine-year-old Dave, a child afflicted with polio, did). Most children are, instead, in the grip of the fears and fantasies which are touched on and reinforced by the physical experience. Thus, the taking of a blood sample is translated into an attack by hostile forces. Operations are registered in the mind as interference with the intactness of the body and experienced according to age and level of development as annihilation, mutilation, or castration.

Hospitalization or isolation because of infection gives substance to ever-present fears of being rejected and of being unworthy. Diets are reacted to as deprivations and are experienced as especially intolerable when there is a strong fixation to the oral infantile phase, during which food and love are equated by the child. Medical investigations are feared by many children because they are "examinations" in the true sense of the word, i.e., inspections of the body which may reveal damage self-inflicted through masturbation. Circumcision, if performed after infancy, is invariably interpreted as punishment. Medical interferences with the body openings (such as enemas, ear sprays) are reacted to as if they were acts of seduction. Painful procedures of all kinds are apt to arouse and make manifest in many children their latent masochistic tendencies.

The point is frequently made that it would add to the heavy burden carried by the hospital staff if emotional implications were taken seriously by them, alongside the physical ones with which they are concerned. Whether this would in fact be the case is still an open question. As matters stand at present, no greater gulf can be imagined than that existing between the practical, factual, and realistic approach of most medical and nursing personnel on the pediatric wards and the unrealistic, affective response of their patients—a gulf which in many instances precludes cooperation and the building up of positive relationships, and causes as much exasperation on one side as it causes distress and unhappiness on the other. As was pointed out in the introduction [to the book], it is as much the task of the "hospital therapist" to introduce the staff to the intricacies of the child patient's mental and emotional functioning as it is her task to guide the children toward a clearer grasp of the physical and medical necessities. In my opinion, such advances toward mutual understanding do not add complications to the situation. On the contrary, they can serve only to ease the present strain on both parties, to clear the atmosphere, and thereby to improve the conditions which are favorable for the process of recovery.

The Technique of "Mental First Aid" in Children's Hospitals

After reading what we have to offer, people may complain that our book contains no clear-cut guidance on two important topics: (1) how to gain access to those intimacies of the child patient on the knowledge of which help for him has to be based; (2) and how to determine what form of help should be offered in the various instances. Although procedures are described with regard to many individual cases, no clues are given why they were selected; whether it is reasoning or intuition by which the hospital therapist was prompted to spin out preparation for surgery with one girl while hastening it with another; to respect one child's defensive denial while working to replace it in another child by a more realistic attitude; to reassure some children while in another case simply allowing the child's grief to run its course.

All we can offer in our defense is that the omission of such answers is neither accidental nor unintentional. In spite of the urgent need for an acceptable and accepted technique of "mental first aid" in the hospital, so far no such technique is in existence. Even though attempts in this direction are being undertaken in various places,[4] none of them have gone far enough, or been proved valid enough, to be published, taught, and generally recommended. Up to now, this type of work is in the experimental stage, and it is left to the discretion of each pioneering worker to open up the path of communication with the child patients and to choose appropriate remedies for the internal difficulties and complexities which are encountered. That such a method is one of trial and error is unavoidable; on the whole this seems preferable to me than to advocate readymade solutions before their validity has been tested sufficiently and their worth been proved.

With regard to the actual procedures adopted for the cases described above, all that can be said of them is that, according to the need of the moment, they were borrowed from a number of other fields and adapted *ad hoc* to the given conditions of the hospital environment, the fields being those of child rearing, education, play therapy, child guidance, and child analysis. As mentioned before, the understanding of the facts observed was based throughout on the psychoanalytic theory of child development which im-

[4] Among others, in the Kinderkliniek Academisch Ziekenhuis in Leyden, Holland under Prof. N. G. M. Veeneklaas.

plies that children, while emotionally dependent on their parents, are personalities in their own right with their own underworld of instincts and desires; their own consciences and demands on themselves; and their own rational ego trying to keep the balance between impulse and ideals and with it between the pressures from the inner and the outer world. While this task of achieving a relative inner balance is not an easy one for any child, it is taken for granted here that it becomes immeasurably more difficult when anxieties, frustrations, and deprivations due to illness are added to it.

So far as establishing actual contact with the child's inner world is concerned, this does not seem to us to present insuperable difficulties. This type of communication is based on the fact that children have a natural need and wish to confide and share their feelings. In the absence of the parents they transfer this wish to a substitute figure if given the time, the opportunity, and the privacy to do so, the last named probably being the most difficult to achieve under conditions of the ward. In the presence of the parents, it is the latter's positive relations to the hospital which enable the child to displace his confidence and communicate freely without experiencing a conflict of loyalty. Only where the child himself is oblivious of the true cause of his distress does this natural approach need reinforcement from the recognized techniques of how to undo inner defenses and unravel the processes of the unconscious mind.

To apply these remarks in greater detail to our cases:

There are simple, human situations where the hospital therapist is called upon merely to assume the mother's basic role of *giving comfort*. This usually happens when the mother herself is too distressed and shaken by the event to perform her task.

Likewise, in some cases, the hospital therapist usurped a task which normally falls within the province of an understanding mother. In fact, no young child is able to weather the ups and downs of external reality without being swamped by fear, guilt, and anxiety-arousing fantasies. To keep up a reality-adapted attitude he has to lean heavily on the mature reason of the mother, whose role it is to clarify the issues and to remove over and over again the misunderstandings derived from his emotional irrationality and his primitive defensive ways of coping with events, reversing affects to the contrary ones, denying facts and necessities. Where, for some reason such as absence, lack of understanding, lack of sympathy, the mother herself fails the child in this respect, the role of "*auxiliary ego*" can be taken over profitably by the hospital therapist.

In another case, the hospital therapist acted as *educators* do, namely, on the intuition that an authoritative decision by the adult can be helpful in putting an end to situations where the child's complaints and hesitations serve ulterior motives such as attention seeking, provocation, masochism. When intuition is right, the intervention acts as a relief for the child, as it did in this case. On the other hand, there are no real safeguards against guessing wrong or against basing the decision not on the child's need but on the adult's exasperation with the child's unreasonable attitude.

With May's food refusal and Jane's preparation for surgery the method used was that of *play therapy*, i.e., inducing the child to displace the area of anxiety or conflict to the dolls and using the dolls to play out solutions which are then secondarily applied to the child herself.

In the cases of Ronnie and Larry success was achieved by

means of *"corrective experience,"* a method of therapy which usually is effective only with the very young. To make up for the mother's strict handling or the mother's neglect, the therapist, and the nurses under her direction, assumed the role of permissive and caring mother figures in relation to whom the child was able to lessen conflicts and take forward steps in development—an achievement which the child had been unable to accomplish in relation to the real mother.

With Ernest, Cindy, and Ruth the procedure resembled that in the usual child *guidance treatment* where, after the child's confidence has been won, guilt feelings and masturbation conflicts are verbalized, discussed, and relieved. While these conflicts lay near the surface of the mind, with no real obstacle blocking these children's awareness of the problem, the situation was different in the case of Elizabeth. With her, the connections had to be pursued patiently from the subject of the bad, seducing companions, to her own badness, until at last the core of her worry, namely, the image of her "bad father," could be reached.

Finally, real *analytic interpretation* was carried out on Betty's nightmares to unearth their repressed content of mourning and anxiety.

A Future Technique of "Mental First Aid"

From the experiences collected in this book, we can perhaps extract some hints permitting us to envisage a future organized technique of "mental first aid" in the hospital, its prerequisites, its scope, its nature, and its limitations.

In view of the wide divergence in the case material and the physical afflictions of the children, such a technique will have to be flexible, i.e., applicable to disturbances which range from the surface to the depth. Since therapy is carried out within the hospital setting, it has to involve not only the parents of the patient, as in child guidance work, but equally the nursing and medical staffs. Since the approach ranges from the human to the scientific and covers every aspect of the child's life, such as physical health, illness, normal and abnormal mental life, an orientation in these various fields will be essential for the worker; so will observational skill and a thorough grounding in the essentials of a developmental child psychology.

There will always be children who can cope with traumatic happenings without therapeutic help (such as Dave), as well as those whose disturbance is too severe to be influenced by a first aid scheme (such as Stephen). Also beyond the scope of such a scheme will be those children who refuse to transfer allegiance from their parents (such as Ann and Judy). Nevertheless, the majority of child patients in the hospital, whether acutely or chronically ill, will benefit greatly from any plan under which the needs of their minds are considered to be as important as the needs of their bodies.

26

Three Contributions to a Seminar on Family Law
(1965 [1963–1964])

I

ON THE DIFFICULTIES OF
COMMUNICATING WITH CHILDREN

THE LESSER CHILDREN IN CHAMBERS[1]

When Mr. Justice Streit summons Larry, Benjamin, and Dee Lesser to his chambers to inform himself about their preferences regarding future custody, he is lucky to be spared almost all the major difficulties which usually arise

---

[1] For the case of the Lesser family, see Goldstein and Katz (1965, Chapter I). The children were seen in chambers when both parents, in the course of separation and divorce proceedings, claimed custody of the children.

when adults in authority try to communicate with children. None of the three meet his questions with the blank wall of silence or the contradictory statements which are often the child's automatic defense when a delicate or dangerous situation is investigated. None of them intentionally hides his thoughts, opinions, and feelings, as children do whenever they suspect possible criticism, reproach, or ridicule. They make no attempt to confuse or distort the truth, since he succeeds in being neither feared nor distrusted by them. If nevertheless their statements, especially Larry's, are not as informative as the Judge might wish, this is not due to lack of frankness or cooperation on their part.

What each has to contribute to the picture is inevitably limited to what they know about themselves. To face up to one's real emotions and to probe into one's real motives is not a capacity which we expect to find in children. On the contrary, children of all ages have a natural tendency to deceive themselves about their motivations, to rationalize their actions, and to shy back from full awareness of their feelings, especially where conflicts of loyalty come into question. To pierce through these defenses demands more than usual skill from the investigator. Verbal and non-verbal communications (attitudes, behavior) have to be scrutinized, assessed, and translated into their underlying meaning; openings offered by the child, all unknowingly,

During the springs of 1963 and 1964, when the author was a member of the Yale Law School faculty, these papers were prepared for and presented to a seminar on The Family and the Law, which, under the direction of Professor Joseph Goldstein and Dr. Jay Katz, examined problems concerned with the disposition of children in a variety of legal settings.

First published in *The Family and the Law* by Joseph Goldstein and Jay Katz. New York: The Free Press, 1965, pp. 261-264, 960-962, 1051-1053.

have to be pursued and utilized. In short, an entry has to be found into the child's inner world of emotions, fantasies, and judgments, irrespective of the fact whether this is hidden only from the interviewer or from the child himself as well. The ability to make such contacts is demanded from psychiatric diagnosticians or child analysts as part of their professional equipment. In a legal investigation such as in the Lesser case, it also becomes the Judge's task.

Where Larry is concerned, it is of course true that no six-year-old can feel at ease when he is interviewed by a stranger and that such a situation invariably produces a wary and respectful blandness which proves rather unrevealing. Nevertheless, Larry as informant is not completely unproductive, even when questioned by an adult in authority. Almost immediately, even if involuntarily, he reveals the main measure which he has adopted to defend himself against the pressures and upsets of his broken family life. He does not attempt to master what happens by understanding it, as his six-year-old intellect might well be able to do, but on the contrary proclaims an attitude of "not knowing," a turn of speech which is repeated over and over in his conversations with the Judge. Spontaneously and immediately he begins by informing the Judge that he "does not know" what his middle initial stands for and proceeds from there to all the other things he "does not know," such as the purpose of the building he is in; the person and the function of the Judge; the type of visits by brother and father which he "does not get"; his place of living; the type of school he attends; the time when school breaks up; the days in the week or the months in the year; the number of words he can read, etc. Expressions such as "I should know, but I don't," return repeatedly.

Obviously, he behaves like somebody who complains that "no one tells me anything," and this plea for knowledge is the opening offered to the adult interviewer. If the examination had been a clinical-diagnostic and not a judicial one, the psychiatrist would have been blamed at this point for not recognizing and making better use of the offered opportunity. There is little doubt that a frank explanation and discussion of the family situation not only would have gratified and relieved this bewildered child, but also would have opened up a path to his confidences and, probably, brought forth a flood of further complaints and information. The psychiatrist needs to say no more to the child on such an occasion than a sympathetic: "Isn't it awful how they never explain things to you, as if you were a stupid little boy," thereby firmly establishing himself as an ally of the child against the nonunderstanding and enigmatic adult world.

In clinical experience, Larry's attitude of "not knowing anything" is not infrequently found in children who live in an atmosphere of parental quarrel or who try to close their eyes and ears to the recognition of sexual irregularities in father or mother. Even though this defense protects the child from insights which he is not ready to digest, it can become a serious handicap if it spreads from the home situation to the world at large, to school, and to the learning process in general. There already is a hint in this direction in Larry's diffidence about his reading ability, although in his case the unsatisfied wish to know is still more obvious than the determined fight against knowledge which may take its place later with many other children.

For whatever they may be worth to the Court as relevant information, there are also some hints given by Larry how much he misses his father. Although they are veiled and indirect, as information given by children often is, they are probably more reliable than the perfunctory, "Yes, Sir," to the Judge's standard question. "Do you love your father?" or, "Do you do what your father tells you?" One is that the father is the powerful dispenser of electric trains, an item which Larry brings in spontaneously, not in answer to a question; obviously according to the child's mind, he can give what the mother cannot give. Secondly, he can do things which have to be left undone in his absence, such as taking the extra wheels off the bicycle, a statement which betrays some of the helplessness felt by the fatherless child. The third indication is contained in the boy's behavior at the end of the interview when he is reluctant to leave the judge's presence. In analytic language we would call this a piece of "transference" and understand it as a quick attachment of a "fatherless" boy to the big man who has given him some time and shown some interest in him, and whom the child does not want to give up again, even though his questions have remained unanswered and his curiosity is unsatisfied. If it is our intention to learn more about Larry's conflicting loyalties to mother or father, here is again an opening offered which would make it possible to verbalize and ventilate the question.

Finally, Larry's "all right," as he leaves the Judge against his inclination, can be taken as an instructive demonstration of the boy's habitual, rather passive acquiescence and compliance when he is faced with unsatisfied wishes and with frustrating situations not under his control.

The transition from six-year-old Larry to fourteen-year-old Benjamin demands a complete readjustment in the questioner's approach. Where Larry is diffident, befogged, and betrays his attitudes involuntarily rather than revealing them intentionally, Benjamin makes the Judge's task easy by being highly verbal and open in his communications. He does not lose any time in setting the tone of the interview himself by stating that he was hoping he "would get the chance to talk to someone in that particular field" (of law). Although overtly the remark refers to his own position as "Chairman of the Law and Political Science Conference" in school, it also contains the hidden hint to the Judge that he cannot be talked down to, that no opening gambit of routine questions is necessary for him, and that, so far as he is concerned, the problem of his parents should be approached in a man-to-man atmosphere of intelligent detachment, tolerance, and understanding for the weaknesses of human nature. Altogether, he does not hesitate to provide the information which is sought as a guide for the Court's decision, namely, that his preference is for living with his father, that this is his own "decision," influenced by neither parent, and that he is quite ready to pursue what he takes as his rights even if it had to be through "some sort of appeal from that decision by the Judge."

It is interesting to note that in spite of their frank interchange of opinion, Benjamin and the Judge also occasionally block each other's lines of approach. The boy ignores the offering to talk about basketball and the Judge's role in it and insists on keeping the interview on more adult ground. The Judge on his side does not enter into Benjamin's interest in the law and his school functions with regard to it, trying to keep the interview to the personal matters in hand. Momentarily they tangle both on the power question, each affirming their right to decide the final issue.

Although Benjamin's preferences are not in doubt and this is all the information needed by the Court, it may also be instructive to pursue the matter further and to get a glimpse of the happenings in Benjamin's mind behind the outward veneer of intellectual mastery. Obviously, there is more feeling here than the boy likes and cares to admit to himself. He denies in so many words that there is "bitterness" in him, he praises his father for doing "a good job" in providing a home for him, while he is "surely" on very good terms with his mother and "naturally" still loves her. But he also reveals how this apparent impartiality is achieved, namely, by becoming "somewhat aloof" from both so that it is "not so hard when the final break comes." We see here an adolescent who has escaped from his feelings to his intellect because, in reality, he has lived with the parents' quarreling "a good many years"—"so many" that he cannot "enumerate" them; that he feels "that in a sense they are both wrong," and that the only way to manage is to live on compromise. That, behind this open disillusionment, there is even deeper distaste and even fear of the task of judging them is borne out by his double attitude to the legal profession. In spite of his marked interest in the law, there is an equally marked disinclination to become a judge or lawyer. Attraction to and turning away from the necessity of designating father or mother as the guilty party here fight openly against each other. Perhaps the Judge is right here if he remains cautiously on the outward fringe of this hidden conflict of loyalties and avoids opening up a depth of feeling with which the boy manages to cope with his own efforts, by means of an intelligence which is admittedly beyond his years.

There is less information about the nature of the interviews with Dee, aged seventeen, but still sufficient evidence to show how she has tried to cope with the situation. Unlike Benjamin, who "tosses it up and comes up with his own conclusions," she much prefers to leave the decision of this most private concern to an impartial Judge, thereby escaping the responsibility of hurting either her father's or her mother's feelings. One wonders whether Mr. Justice Streit guesses what device has enabled her to take this attitude. In her testimony she reveals unmistakably that she has managed to transfer the meaning of "home" from the disturbed image of the person of the parents to the safe picture of the "house" itself, with the result that she holds on to living in the house as other girls would hold on to either father or mother. For Dee, the house has become a symbol of the home base to which one belongs (probably a symbol of the parents when they were still united), and in a way it has ceased to matter which one of the two quarreling parents is in actual occupancy.

Whether the Judge has understood Dee's not quite usual way of solving her problem or not seems immaterial here. He has a right to expect that she will settle down to any decision so long as she did not have to inflict it on her parents by herself.

In this manner each of them finds his own escape from judging the parents harshly: Larry by confusion, Benjamin by intellectualization, Dee by displacement of her feelings.

II

A NEGLECTED CHILD IN LAW

JEAN DREW[2]

There are some lessons to be learned from Jean Drew's case, for the complexity of human development as well as for family law in various of its aspects.

The Psychotic Parent

Jean's mother is not a neglecting indifferent, immoral, i.e., a "bad," parent in the ordinary sense of the word. On the contrary, her "moral" standards seem to be high and she verbalizes excellent attitudes toward bringing up children. Her close tie to Jean is expressed in her wish for the girl's companionship; her bitter complaints that "Jean never wanted to go any place with her or do anything with her"; the fact that "she was almost out of her mind to realize Jean did not want to return home"; her threats to kill herself if Jean does not return home; the terrible scene at the bus stop when she prostrates herself on the floor of the depot begging Jean not to go to school; and finally her commitment of herself to a mental hospital after she has lost Jean's support. It belongs to the reverse side of this parental dependence and solicitude for the child that Mrs. Pulaski also nags Jean constantly, deprives her of the normal pleas-

[2] For the case of Jean Drew, see Goldstein and Katz (1965, Chapter III, Part Two). Jean Drew, at the age of fifteen, was charged with delinquency, though she had previously been referred to court, always because of an inability to get along with her divorced psychotic mother.

ures of life, accuses her of imagined acts of misbehavior, and punishes her unreasonably and unmercifully.

Jean responds to this incomprehensible mixture of demandingness, love, hate, and overwhelming injustice with an ambivalence in her own feelings. She is sorry for her mother, pities her, feels needed by her, is protective of and responsible for her, reveals guilt, remorse, concern, and loyalty. At the same time she also hurls invectives at her such as "I hate her," "I never want to see her again," "She is a pig and she doesn't love me and I hate her." While her repeated running away reflects the negative side, her equally frequent willingness to return home expresses the positive side of her relationship to her mother.

For Jean, as for many other children who grow up with a parent diagnosed as paranoid schizophrenic, the bond of affection which ties them to the ill father or mother exerts an unholy influence on their development. They are frequently "the more tolerant and understanding" in the partnership, as Jean is described to be, thereby reversing the normal roles of parent and child. The ill parents whom they cannot help loving, nevertheless cannot be respected by them, nor can they wish to grow up like them as children do normally. The abnormality of the parent's behavior is perceived by them, first dimly, in time sharply. In either case they are frightened by it, as Jean admits to be when "her mother sticks her tongue out, starts scratching her head," and has a strange look in her eyes. Like Jean, such children also are invariably at odds with the neighbors against whom the parent raves and rants in the child's hearing, as Mrs. Pulaski does, and who retaliate as openly by branding her as crazy. Faced by a mother of whose bizarre behavior Jean is deeply ashamed, and by a community with which she cannot identify in loyalty to her mother, Jean and others like her are pushed into an unhealthy social isolation. This state of affairs is summed up expressively in a sentence contained in the Intake Sheet of the Juvenile Court at the preliminary hearing after Jean's first runaway escapade: "This mother is impossible to live with and Referee has never seen an unhappier child."

The Timing of State Intervention before or after the Delinquent Act

Under these external and internal circumstances Jean spends her early years with the results showing in feelings of self-denigration, self-consciousness, uncertain tempers, and difficult relationships to contemporaries and adults expressed by coarse language, rude, noisy, "sassy" manners and argumentativeness. On the bodily side there are weak eyes, scars remaining after childhood accidents, and a one-sided facial paralysis.

What has been submitted to within the home in childhood becomes a matter for police attention with the approach of adolescence. At this time Jean first runs away from her mother, a reaction which is repeated on three other occasions in the same and following year. It is significant for her social orientation at this time that Jean runs for help to neighbors, even turns herself in to the police voluntarily. These escapades are no more than open bids for removal from a home which has become intolerable and from a tie which she cannot break by herself in spite of everything. When these appeals fail, then—and only then—follow a police complaint about deportment, an incident of breaking and entering, and an attempt at suicide. By then, Jean has collected a police record of impressive length with five charges listed; her attitude is described as worse than when the Sheriff's office first had contact with her; and the finding of delinquency is reaffirmed in Court.

What can be traced in the story without difficulty is the "unhappy" child's further growth into an unstable dissocial adolescent. The intervention, which was asked for by her at age thirteen as a protective and preventive measure, is finally granted by the Court two years later but as the result of trial for a delinquent act which, without the delay, need never have occurred.

Problems in Assessment and Prediction

There are two reports before the Court, each giving a completely different assessment of the subject under examination. The probation counselor, who has probed extensively into Jean's past and present, and describes her many internal and external difficulties, sees her nevertheless as a "very nice personality in a great many ways," with "many good qualities," "high moral standards," "certain ambitions for herself," i.e., somebody who "with the proper help could become a rather fine girl." The psychologist, on the other hand, who approaches her with a battery of tests has little or nothing good to say about her functioning intelligence, her social adaptation or her emotional relationships, and gives a glowing outlook on probably increasing crudity and sensuous development. Luckily, the recommendations made by both agree on removal from home and placement in a good training school, although many schools might well have been discouraged in the efforts from the outset by the findings of the tests.

In the further course of events Jean Drew's reports from school do not confirm the current belief that standardized psychological tests provide more objective personality assessments of children and allow for more accurate predictions of their future development than ordinary unaided contacts with them. On the contrary, while Jean fulfills all the expectations of her counselor, the unfolding of her personality in school runs counter to almost the whole range of test results. According to reports from the school, within eighteen months, the girl of dull-normal intelligence (IQ 83, Wechsler) becomes "a very bright girl," "the best geometry student." Her "poor community relationships" and "antisocial tendencies" (California Test of Personality) do not prevent her from becoming within the same time one of the leaders on campus, captain of her cottage baseball team, and elected president of student government. Findings on the same test (C.T.P.) that she feels "just barely capable of standing on her own two feet" and her "poor common-sense reasoning ability" (Wechsler) contrast sharply with the reported "high degree of insight into herself, a realistic evaluation of her home and of her past," which her letters to her mother reveal a year later. The "ambitious goals beyond her capacity" (Rorschach) are actually nearing fulfillment in her school performance. Granted that the tests gave an accurate assessment of Jean's "maladjustment in most areas" (C.T.P.) at the time of trial, what testing obviously was not able to convey for the purpose of prediction was the degree to which her inner potentialities were held in check by external pressure.

That there is in Jean an almost automatic correspondence

between intellectual performance and emotional upset is borne out by the events in her second school year, when her mother's placement in a state hospital arouses her worries and guilt feelings and consequently her excellent grades of all A's except one C drop to all B's with the exception of one C.

The Role of Internal and External Factors in the Production of Abnormality

There are many children in whom the influences and conflicts of their childhood produce either early pathology or a more or less complete blocking of healthy progressive development. By the time they have reached adolescence, the interactions between internal givens and environmental influences have become so entangled and ingrained in them that we meet them as confirmed neurotics, or delinquents, or as individuals who function intellectually, emotionally, or morally on a substandard. In these instances, no change of environmental circumstances by itself will bring about internal improvements, and rehabilitation can be expected only from the patient, long-term analytic disentangling of the dynamic conflicts, compromises, and inhibitions within the personality.

For the purpose of understanding Jean Drew's case, it is important to note that she does not belong in this category. In spite of the severity and potential harmfulness of her environmental conditions, her inner potentialities for warm emotionality, for intellectual achievements, and for moral and social adaptation have remained latent but unharmed and were ready to unfold as soon as external pressure was removed. We may take it as a sign of the present-day insufficiency of available social services that the removal of pressure happened so late in Jean's life and that she was allowed to go as far as she did on the road toward dissociality. If the delinquent escapade of Jean's had not occurred to alert the Court, there is little doubt that one more individual would have taken the path toward suicide, promiscuity, and intellectual malfunction without any inherent necessity to end up this way.

III

GUIDES TO ADOPTION AND FOSTER CARE

CINDY[3]

There are several respects in which the story of Cindy differs from that of other children who are given up by their parents at birth or soon thereafter. There is no time in Cindy's life when her basic material needs are not fulfilled, that is, when she is lacking for proper nourishment, appropriate clothing, hygienic housing, or when she is treated harshly. She does not suffer the fate of institutionalized children whose individuality is submerged in enforced community life at an age when the normal infant yearns for personal relationships. Her placements are not made according to the rules of expediency and practical necessity but with reference to her own "best interests" so far as these are conceived and formulated. In short, a great deal of agency time and thought is spent on her as on an important single individual. That nevertheless some tragic mistakes are made

[3]For the case of Cindy Brown, see Goldstein and Katz (1965, pp. 1034-1051).

in handling her case and that unnecessary suffering is caused to the child cannot be attributed to the usual scarcity of facilities, or to anybody's bad faith or shirking of effort, but merely to an insufficient knowledge of some of the complexities which govern mental growth.

The First Stage

No fault can be found with the agency worker's criticism of Cindy's first placement or with the Court's decision to remove her from Mrs. Andrew's care. On the contrary, whoever is fully aware of an infant's needs in the first year of life will agree that this home was unsuitable since it offered her no more than an incomplete family, a working mother, the haphazard handling by a series of makeshift baby-sitters. One can only subscribe to the Court's opinion "that such conditions might and do exist in numerous cases of natural parenthood" but that there is every reason against selecting them deliberately when better opportunities can be given to a child for starting her life.

It is in accordance with the Court's findings that Cindy, at the age of ten months, presented the typical picture of an infant who has been born normal, but who has been allowed to remain insufficiently stimulated and underdeveloped so far as emotional attachment and sensory and motor potentialities are concerned. As such infants do—unless they are grossly neglected or unduly frightened—Cindy smiled indiscriminately at everybody, but her expression remained bland and blank and nothing in the environment aroused sufficient interest in her to protest against it or to induce her to reach out for it.

The Second Stage

Again, I can only subscribe to the agency's opinion that Cindy, in this state, needed more than average maternal care. What she had missed and what was sorely needed for her development was a stable central figure whom she could recognize as the invariable dispenser of food, comfort, and affection and to whom, in return, her own awakening emotions could attach themselves firmly. Such a tie is necessary for the infant's learning to discriminate between the familiar and unfamiliar, the known and unknown in the environment. It is only in the interaction with such a loved figure that the infant develops intelligent interest and directs attention to the material objects and happenings in his surroundings. The mother's pleasure in his successes in reaching, touching, grasping, recognizing, and moving stimulates his own satisfaction and spurs him on to make new efforts and advances. Where this exchange is missing, the child remains dull, uninterested, and lacking in responses, as Cindy did.

At the time when Mrs. Johnson took over, more was expected of her than the usual developmental stimulation, which is the duty of the ordinary mother; the task before her was more of a remedial, therapeutic nature. Responses had to be elicited belatedly since much valuable time had remained unused in the first year of life. Luckily, Cindy was still young enough to have them elicited, and thereby to escape the fate of many other children about whom less trouble is taken with the result that they are branded as dull, retarded, of substandard mentality at some later date in their lives, usually at school entry.

However this may be, it needed all of Mrs. Johnson's resources of maternal affection, ambition, understanding, perseverance, time, bodily and mental effort to effect changes, and it is greatly to her and the agency's credit that these were brought about. Within eleven months, Mrs. Johnson and Cindy had grown together into a devoted mother-child couple, and on the basis of this growth, the child had caught up practically on all the deficiencies of her development for the whole range of feelings, speech, intelligence, interest, motor skills, and bodily controls.

The Third Stage

Any child of two and a half years who loses his mother through death can be certain of the automatic sympathy accorded to him by all the adults near enough to watch his fate. Even where the father remains as an active figure in a child's life, he cannot make up for the interruption in the bond forged between infant and mother by the day-to-day and minute-to-minute care. Deprived of the basic relationship on which his wider affections and attitudes to the environment have been built, the child is left in the unhappy state of a bewildered and disoriented little orphan.

Owing to the very urgency of their needs, their dependent helplessness, and their complete inability to look after themselves, young children cannot spend much time on mourning and are forced instead to accept substitute care and to all external intents and purposes to adapt to altered circumstances. This does not mean that their unhappinesses are less severe than they will be in later life. But it obscures the recognition by the adult world that a serious blow has been dealt to their sense of security, to the smooth progress of their forward development as well as to their very ability to form deep and lasting attachments, the so-called "capacity for object relationship" which is one of the most valuable attributes acquired by an individual in his first human love relationship. Separated by fate from their first love object, most children establish their further emotional attachments on a more tentative, less satisfying or trusting, and—as future life will show—on a more shallow basis.

Seen against the background of experience with individuals who have undergone such and similar fates, the agency's action to seek further placement for Cindy seems to me an unenlightened, dangerous, and unwarranted step. For the child, the consequences are not mitigated by the fact that the new placement is made for the purpose of adoption, i.e., for the sake of future permanency. Nor does all the careful work which is spent on preparation help since you cannot prevent emotional upset in a two-and-a-half-year-old by approaching him through intellect and reason. So far as Cindy and her own understanding of the event are concerned, she loses the only effective mother whom she ever had in her life and, moreover, one whom she had acquired after delay, hardship, and emotional neglect. It is difficult to conceive how she can weather the experience without being harmed, even if harm remains under the surface for the present, and becomes visible only at a later date.

Since the agency recognized Cindy's needs at the end of Stage One, would it not have been possible for more knowledgeable planning to omit Stage Two altogether and to carry Cindy directly to an adoptive mother willing and able to do Mrs. Johnson's job?

Conclusion

According to the psychoanalyst's experience, the best interests of an infant are safeguarded under the condition that three needs are fulfilled: the need for *affection* (for the unfolding and centering of the infant's own feelings); the need for *stimulation* (to elicit inherent functions and potentialities); and the need for *unbroken continuity* (to prevent damage done to the personality by the loss of function and destruction of capacities which invariably follow on the emotional upheavals brought about by separation from, death or disappearance of the child's first love objects). The authorities who decided Cindy's fate showed themselves well aware of the first two items in the prescription, while they disregarded the third. At the least they seem to have clung to the belief that an individual's capacity to love remains unchanged irrespective of the presence or absence of the loved person. This may be true in later life for most normal adults, but it becomes what I called before a tragic error when applied to the emotional life of a two-year-old. In the young child, the capacity for outgoing love is still bound up inextricably with the reliable presence of the person who has been instrumental in calling forth this emotion and in interchange with whom it has developed.

APPENDIX

RESPONSE OF THE STAFF OF THE DOBUCE
COUNTY WELFARE DEPARTMENT TO
DR. ANNA FREUD'S CRITIQUE OF THE
"CINDY" CASE[4]

It is a great privilege to have Dr. Freud's comments to
study. They are being distributed to our total child welfare
staff, and we hope to see further use of them made throughout the State. They have serious implications for any
adoption program that undertakes placement of children
beyond early infancy.

One can hardly look at the case of Cindy without questioning whether it was "right" to put her through the
tremendous upheaval that was involved in her moving
from the foster mother who had established with her the
saving relationship. People in the field of child placement
have had to face such qualms in thousands of cases and in
many have decided against placement.

Dr. Freud attributes our adoptive placement of Cindy to
insufficient knowledge about mental growth. She could not
have known from the case material that the particular
knowledge to which she refers was painstakingly considered in reaching our decision. We are much aware of the
emphasis psychoanalysis has placed on ego psychology and
of the continuously expanding and changing concept of
ego development. This knowledge is invaluable in our
work, especially as it pertains to the ego vulnerability of
small children, a field of knowledge to which Dr. Anna
Freud has made pioneering and monumental contributions.
To the best of our awareness, however, the development of
this knowledge did not include the study of adopted chil-

[4] This response is here included in its entirety. It was first published in Goldstein and Katz (1965, pp. 1053-1054).

dren whose adoption had been planned and arranged as thoughtfully and carefully as we think Cindy's was. From cumulative experience in child placement, the knowledge of our profession is that a child can transfer his love to a new maternal person, given certain essential conditions. These are that the child is known to have a strong, deep and mutually satisfying love relationship with a mother person, and that the substitute chosen is both aware of the meaning to the child of his loss, and capable of loving deeply. In any placement, both bodies of knowledge must be weighed. Admittedly, prejudicial emphasis of one over the other leads to error.

That we lean toward taking the step of placement in many cases despite the anticipated hurt is attributable to many factors, among them the weight we place upon permanency. Adoptive parents are asked to make a broad and permanent commitment to the child. Foster boarding parents are not offering this. While foster boarding parents do, in some instances, continue with the child throughout his minority, they are not obliged to. We must also live with, but try to prevent, the many occasions on which foster parents request the removal of the child in terms of their own needs and obligations.

If a child is permanently losing his parents, our first approach is to explore the possibility of adoption. When adoption is not possible, the child is often subjected to frequent moves and may never have the opportunity to form a deep attachment. We find this result often potentially more damaging than the loss of a loved parent at a vulnerable age.

In this case we worked with the "Johnsons" in relation to whether they would want to adopt "Cindy." They ultimately reached the very painful decision that they would not. Unfortunately this was not in our case material and could not have been taken into consideration by Dr. Freud.

However, Dr. Freud is not proposing that Cindy should have remained with the Johnsons. Her suggestion is that

Cindy should have gone to an adoptive home upon removal from the first adoptive home.

When Cindy was in the Andrews home, we were very much concerned about her potential for normal emotional and mental development. It seemed possible that she was severely damaged for life. Furthermore, and this is an extremely vital point, she was not legally free for adoption. We saw it as our responsibility (1) to determine whether the natural parents were a resource to her and (2) to give her the best and earliest possible chance for developing the closeness to a mother that we saw as essential. If she could not do the latter, we could not see her as "adoptable" and could not have responsibly suggested to any family that they adopt her.

Perhaps under optimal conditions an adoptive family could have been ready (at the time of the court order removing Cindy from the Andrews home) to take Cindy for better or for worse, on the chance that she would become legally free. But where is that family to be found? If people as deep in their devotion as the Johnsons proved to be could not make the permanent commitment after Cindy had been freed by the court and had made great strides toward normal development, could anyone have made it at the height of her disturbance?

Dr. Freud comments that preparation of Cindy for her critical move was approached through intellect and reason. We are quite taken aback by this interpretation of the preparation. Our objective, accomplished to a significant degree, we think, was to involve Cindy emotionally in working through the awesome task she faced. Methods of enlisting her participation at a feeling level included development of reliance on and trust in the worker who could then support her through the separation trauma, as well as utilization of what intellectual and reasoning capacity she possessed at this time. Also included was repetition "dosage." We did not attempt to prevent emotional upset, but rather to prevent regressive withdrawal and repression of her grief and anger. Perhaps Dr. Freud is implying that the ego of a two-year-old child is insufficiently developed to permit this kind of participation. If so, we would qualify our disagreement, by a readiness for more complete existing knowledge or further research.

Sometimes we are struck with the extent to which American society has accepted, in fact, embraced, adoption as a solution. We appreciate being reminded of the pitfalls for us as practitioners in this society.

In summary, we did weigh the knowledge that Dr. Freud refers to, as we made our decision. Our resources were, indeed, limited in terms of both human potentials and legal, societal, institutional structures. We do need more knowledge testing the weight of various factors in producing emotional health or illness.

It has been tantalizing to have Dr. Freud's comments and no opportunity to discuss them with her. We appreciate the chance to weigh her views and to reply. We value her experience, the range of her thought and the depth of her concern very highly.

27

Psychoanalytic Knowledge and Its Application to Children's Services

(1964)

As child analysts, we occasionally turn away from our specific concern with therapy to take a more general interest in the various services for children. We are then invariably struck by a number of impressions, some of which are not easy to reconcile with each other. We realize that the need for a better understanding of the child's personality is felt keenly by the workers in the other fields and, further, that this is unquestionably on objective grounds. We feel that,

Based on an address entitled "Psychoanalytic Knowledge of the Child and Its Application to Children's Services," given at the 20th Anniversary membership meeting of the Citizen's Committee for Children of New York, at the Cosmopolitan Club, April, 1964. It is here published for the first time.

due to our own investigations, we are in possession of the very facts which are capable of being applied to the problems in these disciplines. Nevertheless, more often than not, our efforts are met by an unwillingness, or inability to understand, to accept, or to integrate the information about child development which we have to offer.

DIFFICULTIES OF COMMUNICATION

Usually, it is the analysts themselves who are blamed for this failure of success in interaction. There is, for one, a language barrier between psychoanalysis and other fields. In the course of time, psychoanalysts have developed not only their own new concepts but also their own new terms, and this terminology, which is strange to outsiders, has to be retranslated into ordinary language for them to be acceptable. This is a task which, though not difficult in itself, is often neglected to the detriment of communication. Further, such teaching has to be done not from the theoretical angle but by utilizing the practical problems in the field to which psychoanalysis is to be applied. Here, analysts often fail due to lack of adequate preparation for the task. No child therapist who has not gone through an apprenticeship of work with normal children has much chance to grasp and elucidate the problems of a teacher in an ordinary classroom. To understand fully the problems of a children's sick nurse, some familiarity is needed with the sickroom, with night duty, with the general fractiousness and uncooperativeness of children during illness. Pediatricians who deal with the severest physical handicaps and abnormalities are, on the whole, far removed from a concern with normal developmental progress on the psychological side. So are lawyers, who have little contact with children except under extreme conditions of hardship, abandonment, need of care and protection, etc. On the other hand, teaching on the other worker's case material, useful as it is as a device, carries with it its own disadvantages. To shed light on individual cases, pieces of information have to be drawn in, torn out of the theoretical setting in which they belong and within the framework of which they are logical and often self-explanatory. It is inevitable in such discussions that certain sides of the child's nature will be overemphasized to the detriment of others. Inevitably, the information which is imparted will have to remain sketchy, incomplete, and, what is worse, often abstruse sounding under such conditions.

These handicaps which we meet when we try to apply psychoanalytic knowledge to the services for children are important. Nevertheless, they are not the only, and not even the most important.

In spite of our various efforts to spread knowledge about child development, and in spite of advances made in the course of the last thirty or forty years, some basic difficulties of communication have remained. In what follows I select from them for discussion the problems of communication in three areas: education, medicine, and law.

It may be asked what prevents teachers, doctors, and lawyers from accepting freely the data which the child analyst can offer, and from making full use of them. The answer is surprisingly simple: because historically, as social institutions, schools, hospitals, and law courts came into being long before psychoanalysis and are organized according to principles which are alien to analytic findings and, in many instances, threatened and opposed by them. *Schools* were originally built on the concept that a child's intellect and his emotions are two separate parts of his personality which do not interact with each other, i.e., that the teacher could safely disregard his pupils' fantasies, fears, emotions while developing his powers of concentration and reasoning, and while filling up his mind with objective knowledge. *Hospitals* were organized similarly according to the idea that body and mind, although belonging to one and the same individual, are divorced from each other sufficiently to allow the treatment of illness and the handling of the child patient to proceed without taking into account his panics, his loyalties, and above all his frightening fantasies of damage to his body. *Family law*, so far as it deals with the provision made for minors in divorce, adoption, custody proceedings, has always been oriented with regard to the best interests of the child which to the Court seemed safeguarded if the child's religion, morality, and financial security were protected.

In all three instances, psychoanalytic teaching runs counter to the former beliefs: emotion and intellect can now be shown to interact in many ways, to the detriment as well as to the advantage of school performance; body and mind can be shown to influence each other and to be inseparable in the production of psychosomatic illness, in the child's reaction to operations, hospitalization, convalescence, etc. The "best interests" of the child are served best, according to analytic experience, if his emotional needs rather than his religious and moral concerns are taken into account.

It is these basic differences of outlook which inhibit and limit the scope and pace of the inroads which the psychoanalyst can make in his dealings with the children's services. To assess his successes and failures in the three areas is a worthwhile task but a lengthy one, far beyond the possibilities of this paper where it can merely be touched on in approximation.

SCHOOLS, AND THEIR RELATION TO PSYCHOANALYTIC FINDINGS

There is one particular finding which the progressive schools have seized on with enthusiasm, namely, that interest can be transferred from the child's most private concerns and fantasies to the material taught in lessons. If not blocked, the child's natural curiosity about sexual matters can be led over to curiosity as such, and this again into the wish to learn. In that manner, exploration of the body and its parts becomes a wish to explore the world and leads to proficiency in geography. Admiration and awe of the father's strength lead, as shown in the fairy tales, to fascination with the powerful animals and an interest in zoology, provided that teaching begins with the lions, tigers, and elephants instead of with the tame and less impressive domesticated creatures. Kings, queens, princes, and heroes figure largely in the children's own fantasies, partly as representatives of the parents, partly fulfilling secret wishes about their own aggrandizement. Preoccupation with them leads easily to a passion for historical tales, provided that history is taught from this aspect and does not confine itself to a memorizing of cold facts and dates. By making use of those innumerable facets of the child's own interests, and of the manner in which they can be "sublimated," the progressive school has succeeded in turning many of the chores of learning into a pleasurable continuation of spontaneous play.

On the other hand, analysts have made other findings which are no less important and which the schools ignore; for example, the difference between play and work. To become a successful scholar, the child needs to do more than merely transfer his energy and interest from his passions to his tasks. He also needs to complete the line of development which leads from play to work, and this implies the ability to pursue an activity, regardless of the pleasure gain of the moment, until a final result has been achieved. Without teaching this "application to the task," or this step toward sustained effort and delay of satisfaction, the results of the progressive school remain incomplete and unsatisfactory.

There are other findings from which the school system has failed to benefit so far. As analysts, we believe firmly that what happens in a child's early years is more decisive for his development than what happens later. This applies to schooling no less than to the events concerning the emotions. Teaching the youngest has more impact on the children's future knowledge and ability to learn than teaching adolescents.

In striking contrast to this, in nearly every school system provisions go in the opposite direction. Elementary school teachers are paid less and held in lower esteem than high school teachers; school buildings and equipment are improved for older rather than for younger children. Worst of all, there are plans for raising the school-leaving age before the age for school entry is lowered. It appears to me, many of the present urgent problems of schooling, especially for the underprivileged child, could be solved or ameliorated if all of them were given the beneficial opportunity of early nursery school education.

Another important piece of knowledge, so far ignored by the school system, is the fact that in the early years the intake of knowledge is closely connected with the relationship to the teacher and this relationship does not develop, or does not survive, if there are too many children in one class. Twenty children can relate to one teacher and vice versa. Where the numbers reach thirty or forty, personal relations go by the board, and much of the effectiveness of teaching is lost.

Thus, in spite of the present-day worry about the unruly adolescents, analytic findings point in the opposite direction concerning public education: that schooling should begin early, in the form of nursery schools; that all classes for the young should be kept small; and that whatever money may be spent on training teachers for the young is well spent in view of their impact on development.

MEDICINE AND ITS RELATION TO PSYCHOANALYTIC FINDINGS

In addition to the many things written recently about children in hospitals, their reaction to separation from home under the conditions of pain, illness, etc., there is one main point which child analysts who have worked with pediatricians here or elsewhere have found worth stressing.

Many physicians who deal with children find themselves highly interested in what the child's mind can do to his body, i.e., in psychosomatic illness. They feel fairly convinced by now that many of the common illnesses of childhood are produced by the emotional side of the child's personality, such as, for example, many of the feeding disturbances, the disturbances of elimination, the headaches, the stomach troubles, even a heightened vulnerability to infection. In short, the concept of psychosomatic illness has found comparatively easy acceptance by the pediatricians.

On the other hand, we find it very difficult indeed to awaken the pediatrician's interest to the same degree in the repercussions of the bodily happenings on the child's mind. As analysts, we find that the child's mental development is influenced by the pain and discomfort which accompany illness; by medical and surgical interventions; by restrictions of motility and diet imposed by medical necessity. These are measures which strike the medical practitioner or pediatrician as so essential that somehow their effects are not pursued beyond the realm of the body into the child's mind, where they cause a multitude of upsets, give rise to long-lasting anxieties, undo recent achievements in independence, set up regression to more infantile states, etc. To fill in that gap in knowledge and produce a better equilibrium between the appreciation of psychosomatic illness and of the impact of bodily disturbance on mental development seems to be the next task in hand when dealing with the medical profession.

FAMILY LAW AND ITS RELATION TO PSYCHOANALYTIC FINDINGS

As regards family law, a closer interrelation between the legal profession and psychoanalysis is of fairly recent origin. It is true that some Juvenile Courts on the European continent were in tentative contact with workers in the psychoanalytic field,[1] as long as thirty or forty years ago, but no

[1] See August Aichhorn (1925) and other publications in prewar Vienna, Austria.

permanent cooperation was built on these beginnings. This had to wait for the constructive interest which arose in one of the oldest and most renowned legal centers of the United States, the Yale Law School.

There, at the present moment, the psychoanalytic teachings are scrutinized systematically for the possibility of applying their data to the various eventualities when children come within the scope of court proceedings. So far, it seems that psychoanalytic findings are able to throw light on the following subjects which fall under the category of family law:

Where *custody* of a child has to be determined, valuable guides are offered by the analyst's knowledge concerning the harmful effects of separating a child from either mother or father, and the variation of these effects according to the child's age.

Where *visiting rights* have to be granted (or withheld), analysis offers information concerning the importance of loyalty conflicts and the child's ability or inability to tolerate them without being harmed.

Where parents are *mentally ill*, clinical data elicited in child analysis show up the links between parental disturbance and the appearance of neurotic, psychotic or delinquent pathology in the child. These can act as guides to determine when and how far *state intervention* is warranted as a preventive measure in such cases.

Where children have to be placed in foster care, there are ample analytic data to demonstrate the psychological harm done by *multiple placement*.

Where *adoption* proceedings are concerned, knowledge is available with regard to the child's specific problems in relation to his adoptive and natural parents, with special reference to typical distresses, danger moments, and critical chronological ages.

Where *corporal punishment* comes into question, analysis has much to add to its discussion from studies of the various types of discipline and their differing effect on the social adaptation of the child.

Where *criminal* events happen in a family (murder, assault), the traumatic impact on the children has been studied and assessed.

In short, there is no doubt that psychoanalytic study of child development in its normal and abnormal aspects can prove useful to the family courts in many minor and major ways. It seems to me that its biggest contribution may consist in constructing a revised definition of what is in the "best interests" of a child.

The best interests of a child are served, according to our point of view, by all measures which promote his smooth progression toward normal maturity. The latter, in its turn, depends above all on the coincidence of three factors: on the free interchange of affection between child and adult; on ample external stimulation of the child's inborn, internal potentialities; and on unbroken continuity of care.

Part IV

This section, which corresponds to Part III in Volume IV, consists of brief writings. It readily falls into two groups:

(1) introductions and comments to research work carried out at the Hampstead Child-Therapy Clinic,
(2) introductions to the work of colleagues outside the Clinic.

The items are presented in chronological order in each group. The first group, chs. 28-32, dealing with work at the Hampstead Child-Therapy Clinic, is of course closely related to Part I of this volume.

Editor's note

28

Introduction to Gabriel Casuso's "Anxiety Related to the 'Discovery' of the Penis" (1957)

Analysts who have followed the publications in our psychoanalytic journals from their beginnings may remember a column in the original German issue which was reserved for observations made on children. The communications selected for it were written by parents or teachers who had undergone analysis themselves, and thereby had their eyes opened for signs of happenings in the child's mind which escaped the notice of unanalyzed observers. They recorded sayings and forms of behavior which showed the child under the impact of his sexual strivings. These descriptions

---

First published in *The Psychoanalytic Study of the Child*, 12:169-170, 1957.

473

ceased to be published later on when the existence of infantile sexuality had been established beyond doubt, and no further evidence from direct observation seemed necessary to validate the analytic findings in this particular respect.

After reading Casuso's description of certain events in the life of his infant son, readers may feel that the publication of communications of this kind should be begun again in our days and that the observing and recording activity of analyzed parents might help toward filling an important gap in our analytic knowledge. Although in recent years the interest of many analysts and child analysts has been concentrated on the first year of the child's life, there is still much uncertainty concerning the ways and means which should be employed to unearth suitable material. Reconstruction from the analyses of later stages of development has provided us with all we know about the libidinal phases, the oedipus and the castration complexes; but reconstruction becomes less certain, and less fruitful, where the preverbal period is concerned. Even though analysis may expect the complications of the early mother relationship to be repeated in the transference, they will be less confident concerning the reappearance of past happenings where, for example, the intricacies of building up the body ego are in question.

Direct observation of developmental steps may, therefore, prove invaluable and indispensable. But to take cognizance of an infant's changing mood swings, of his fleeting moments of anxiety or pleasure, interest, or need for comfort, is no easy matter. It is done best on the basis of the type of twenty-four-hour contact which is denied to the objective, academic, scientific observer. Motherless children who are cared for by objective strangers labor, as we know, under disadvantages which confuse the issues. This points to the parents as the only people who are sufficiently in contact with the infant and knowledgeable about him to observe minutely. The recording of their observations will be all the more valuable, the more their attention is alerted and any inevitable subjectivity corrected by their analytic experience.

Casuso's short paper may convince readers that this can be done.

29

Introduction to "Inconsistency in the Mother as a Factor in Character Development: A Comparative Study of Three Cases" by Anne-Marie Sandler, Elizabeth Daunton, and Anneliese Schnurmann (1957)

There is a variety of ways in which a mother's neurosis or personality disturbance can act unfavorably on a child's development; and there is a variety of ways in which the interaction of the partners in the preoedipal mother rela-

First published in *The Psychoanalytic Study of the Child,* 12:209-210, 1957.

tionship can be explored. In our Hampstead Child-Therapy Clinic the method of choice is the procedure outlined by Dorothy Burlingham et al. in "Simultaneous Analysis of Mother and Child" (1955). This implies that mother and child are analyzed independently of each other, by two different workers; that the analysts do not communicate with each other so as not to exert any influence on the treatment of the other partner; and that they report to a third analyst who coordinates the material and scrutinizes it for whatever types of interaction may emerge.

The following "Comparative Study of Three Cases" of the Hampstead Child-Therapy Clinic, on the other hand, has not been carried out on the basis of this exacting method, nor is it equally ambitious in its aims. It represents the independent effort of three analytic child therapists who were struck by marked similarities in the manifest behavior and symptomatology of their patients and entered into discussion with each other, wondering whether similar environmental factors in the children's backgrounds might be held responsible for the result. Their exploration convinced them that the harmful factor at work in all three cases was to be found neither in a similarity of the mothers' personalities (of whom only one was in analysis), nor in the family circumstances or historical events which differed with each child. The point of identity lay in a particular type of fear of the mother which was present in all three cases and reinforced in the children the same archaic and fantastic anxieties. The similarity between the mothers, summed up by the authors under the term of "inconsistency," went no further than the fact that they aroused this fear.

The three authors of this paper are aware of the limitations of a comparative study of this nature; it cannot elicit all the details of interchange between the id content of two personalities by way of following the processes of identification, internalization, or positive and negative response to subtle provocation. On the other hand, they are confident that their paper may be useful in trying to trace the ways in which external environmental influences are translated into internal pathogenic agents. In their cases the path led from the threatening quality of the first love object to an increase of id anxieties. This, in its turn, produced an overstressing of defenses, alternating with complete breakdowns in defense activity; and furthered the inhibitions, the lack of control, and with them the inconsistencies of personality development by which the three children are characterized.

30

Introduction to Kata Levy's "Simultaneous Analysis of a Mother and Her Adolescent Daughter: The Mother's Contribution to the Loosening of the Infantile Object Tie"
(1960)

Up to the present date, nine mother-child couples have been in simultaneous analysis in our Hampstead Child-Therapy Clinic, or are in such analyses at present. The material gained from these studies is useful for a number of purposes.

First published in *The Psychoanalytic Study of the Child,* 15:378-380, 1960.

Above all, it is invaluable for highlighting the points of interaction between the abnormalities of mother and child, as Dorothy Burlingham et al. have shown in an earlier paper (1955). In that paper which deals with the treatments of a highly disturbed woman and her young child (who entered analysis before the age of four), the authors maintain that "the influence of the mother's actions, her manifest attitude, her conscious and above all her unconscious fantasies, is neither straightforward nor uniform." Ilse Hellman et al., in a recent study of the treatments of a mother and her schoolboy son (1960), confirmed this assertion in all respects. The detailed clinical demonstrations of these authors represent a welcome step forward from the indications derived from child guidance work to the effect that "most mental disturbances of children can be traced back to the disturbances of their parents"; that a particular mother does "not want" her child to grow up, to become clean, to lose his symptoms, etc., precise information backed up by analytic findings taking the place in this manner of the former rather vague generalizations.

Secondly, our material suggests that not all the children studied in this project show direct reactions to their mothers' symptoms, but that some of them are affected only indirectly, so far as their mothers' illness interferes, or has interfered, with the latter's capacity for effective mothering. In these cases, the resultant disturbances of the children can be of a completely different nature from those of their mothers and show none of the characteristic consequences of identification, of the overlapping of fantasy activity, and of the *folie-à-deux* phenomena described by the authors mentioned above.

Thirdly, our study throws light on some important facts

which govern the therapeutic possibilities in child analysis and limit them in certain cases. Where the neurotic symptom, the conflict, or the regression of a child not only is anchored in the young patient's own personality but is further held in place by powerful emotional forces in the parent to whom the child, in his turn, is tied, the therapeutic action of analysis may well be slowed up or, in extreme cases, made impossible. Our material shows instances in which interpretations to the child have become effective, or regressive libidinal positions have been given up, in direct relation to the mother's relinquishing either a fixed pathological position of her own or, in other cases, relinquishing her pathological hold on the child.

Finally, I should like to maintain that the tool of simultaneous analysis can also be used profitably to throw light on other developmental problems. To understand the interaction between parents and their children is of the highest importance not only where the first foundations of the personality or the roots of mental illness are concerned. As a child moves forward on the developmental scale, each step demands the giving up of former positions and gains, not only from the child himself but also from the parents. It is only in the most healthy and normal cases that both sides—parents and child—wholly welcome the progressive move and enjoy the child's increasing maturity and gradually increasing libidinal and moral independence. More often it is one or the other partner who lags behind, the child being unable to free himself from fixations, or the parent clinging to attitudes of protectiveness and mothering which have become unjustified. In the worst cases, mother and child may join forces in a regressive move. Such interlocking then becomes particularly fateful with the onset of puberty.

In a research project on "Adolescence," undertaken in the Hampstead Child-Therapy Clinic (and directed by L. Frankl and Ilse Hellman), the analytic study of the various manners in which individual adolescents strive to free themselves from the infantile object ties to their parents plays a prominent part. Here, again, the simultaneous analyses of mothers and their children have proved helpful. Whereas we receive no more than a dim impression of the parent's responses in those cases where the adolescent alone is in treatment, simultaneous analysis enables us to trace the contributions made by both sides to the success or failure of this particular developmental task.

I have mentioned this fourth use of simultaneous analysis in detail to introduce the paper by Kata Levy on the "Simultaneous Analysis of a Mother and Her Adolescent Daughter" (1960). I hope that it may serve to illustrate that this particular mother-child couple entered treatment for the usual therapeutic reasons and for the elucidation of the links between their respective disturbances. But in the course of the work, their analyses became significant for the exploration of the struggle of a neurotic adolescent to free herself from her preoedipal and oedipal attachments, and of her mother's part in this. Kata Levy describes the story from the mother's side only, and shows her own battle. The story of the daughter's analysis, with all its implications for the mother-child as well as for the adolescent problem is presented in a separate paper by Marjorie Sprince (1962).

31

Preface to *The Hampstead
Psychoanalytic Index*
by John Bolland and
Joseph Sandler et al.
(1965)

_____

As a sample of work done in the Hampstead Child-Therapy
Clinic, the case of Andy has a variety of purposes.

As a clinical example it illustrates successful analytic
treatment carried out in the case of a very young boy who
suffered from developmental upsets and made his environment suffer through his aggressive outbursts, his disturbances of sleep, and his difficult behavior. Analysis in his

First published in *The Monograph Series of The Psychoanalytic
Study of the Child*, No. 1. New York: International Universities
Press, 1965.

case is shown to have proved therapeutic with regard to early symptom formation and truly preventive so far as the threat of a later full-blown infantile neurosis was concerned.

There are various ways in which the mother of a two-and-a-half-year-old participates in plans for his treatment: it can take the form of simultaneous analysis of mother and child; or of treatment of the child through the mother (guided by the analyst); or of straightforward child analysis with added guidance of the mother. What was chosen in Andy's case was the third possibility, but with "mother guidance" given in a special form. Without undergoing analysis or any form of psychotherapy herself, Andy's mother was included in the analytic process, shared in her son's involvement with transference and resistance, as well as in his receiving and working through of interpretation and enlightenment. At the end of treatment, both mother and child could be seen to emerge together on a new level of understanding, liberation, and development. The consecutive steps of this satisfying venture are illustrated in detail by the weekly reports which form Chapter 5 of the Monograph.

For the rest, Andy's case is used to demonstrate the "indexing" of analytic material, which is one of the ways in which analysts may learn to lay down their personal clinical impressions to be shared with others. How this is being done in the Hampstead Clinic is explained at length in Chapter 1. What we hope to construct by this laborious method is something of a "collective analytic memory," i.e., a storehouse of analytic material which places at the disposal of the single thinker and author an abundance of facts gathered by many, thereby transcending the narrow confines of individual experience and extending the possibilities for insightful study for constructive comparisons between cases, for deductions and generalizations, and finally for extrapolations of theory from clinical therapeutic work.

32

Foreword to Humberto
Nagera's *Early Childhood
Disturbances, the Infantile
Neurosis, and the Adulthood
Disturbances*
(1966 [1965])

Nagera's monograph bears witness to the child analyst's
dissatisfaction with the present mode of diagnostic thinking. As stated by him, we are not content any longer to sub-
sume all childhood disorders under the all-embracing title
of an "infantile neurosis," as analysts tended to do in former eras of psychoanalysis. Nor do we consider it an ade-

First published in *The Monograph Series of The Psychoanalytic
Study of the Child*, No. 2. New York: International Universities
Press, 1966.

quate solution to search for our answer to all diagnostic questions in any one period of childhood, whether late, in the oedipal phase, as the classical view sets out, or early in the first year of life, as more recent views assert. Nor are we ready to accept the exclusive indictment of either faulty object relationships or faulty ego development, which many modern authors treat as the only potential sources of trouble.

What the author of this monograph does to remedy the position is a careful apportioning of pathogenic impact to external and internal interferences at any time of the child's life; the location of the internal influences in any part of the psychic structure or in the interaction between any of the inner agencies; and the building up, step by step, of an orderly sequence of childhood disorders, of which the infantile neurosis is not the base, but the final, complex apex.

What satisfies the student of analysis in an exposition of this nature is the fact that on the one hand it is rooted in the notion of a hypothetical norm of childhood development, while on the other hand it establishes a hierarchy of disturbances which is valid for the period of immaturity and meaningful as a forerunner of adult psychopathology.

33

Foreword to Marion Milner's
On Not Being Able to Paint
(1957)

Marion Milner's treatment of psychic creativity differs in several respects from those well-established approaches to art to which psychoanalytic readers owe whatever familiarity with the subject they possess. She chooses as the object of her scrutiny not the professional and recognized artist but herself as a "Sunday painter"; not the finished masterpiece but her own fumbling and amateurish beginner's efforts to draw and paint. In short, she analyzes not the mysterious and elusive ability of the genius who achieves self-expression through the medium of painting, but—as the title of

First published in the second revised edition of *On Not Being Able to Paint* by Marion Milner. London: Heinemann; New York: International Universities Press, 1957.

the book suggests—the all too common and distressing restrictions by which the creativity of the average adult individual is held in check.

It is fascinating for the reader to follow the author's attempts to rid herself of the obstacles which prevent her painting, and to compare this fight for freedom of artistic expression with the battle for free association and the uncovering of the unconscious mind which make up the core of an analyst's therapeutic work. The amateur painter, who first puts pencil or brush to paper, seems to be in much the same mood as the patient during his initial period on the analytic couch. Both ventures, the analytic as well as the creative one, seem to demand similar external and internal conditions. There is the same need for "circumstances in which it is safe to be absent-minded" (i.e., for conscious logic and reason to be absent from one's mind). There is the same unwillingness to transgress beyond the reassuring limits of the secondary process and "to accept chaos as a temporary stage." There is the same fear of the "plunge into no-differentiation" and the disbelief in the "spontaneous ordering forces," which emerge once the plunge is taken. There is, above all, the same terror of the unknown. Evidently, it demands as much courage from the beginning painter to look at objects in the external world and see them without clear and compact outlines as it demands courage from the beginning analysand to look at his own inner world and suspend secondary elaboration. There are even the same faults committed. The painter interferes with the process of creation when, in the author's words, he cannot bear the "uncertainty about what is emerging long enough, as if one had to turn the scribble into some recognisable whole when, in fact, the thought or mood seeking expression had not yet reached that stage." Nothing can resemble more closely than this the attitude of haste and anxiety on the analyst's or patient's part which leads to premature interpretation, closes the road to the unconscious, and puts a temporary stop to the spontaneous upsurge of the id material. On the other hand, when anxieties and the resistances resulting from them are overcome, and the "surrender of the planning conscious intention has been achieved," both—painter and analysand—are rewarded by "a surprise, both in form and content." It is only at this juncture that we meet the essential difference between the analytic process and the process of creation. The legitimate result of analysis is the inner experience of formerly unknown affects and impulses which find their final outlet in the ego processes of verbalization and deliberate action. The creative process in art, on the other hand, "remains within the realm in which unknown affects and impulses find their outlet, through the way in which the artist arranges his medium to form harmonies of shapes, colours or sounds"; whether deliberate action is affected or not in the last issue, the main achievement is, according to the author, "a joining of that split between mind and body that can so easily result from thinking in words."

Marion Milner's book is written throughout from the eminently practical aspect of self-observation and self-expression. Abstraction is relegated to an Appendix in which her theoretical opinions on creativity find expression.

Readers who have personal experience with any form of creative work, whether literary or artistic, will welcome the enlightening description of "emptiness as a beneficent state before creation," and will acknowledge willingly, although shame-facedly, the truth of her brilliant explanation of the confusion in the creator's (especially an author's) mind between the orgastic feelings during creation and the value of the created. Her treatment of this particular aspect of artistic productivity seems to me one of the most rewarding chapters of the book.

With regard to the analytic controversy whether psychic creativity seeks, above all, "to preserve, re-create the lost object," the author takes the stand that this function of art, although present, is a secondary one. According to her, the artist's fundamental activity goes beyond the re-creation of the lost object to the primary aim of "creating what has never been" by means of a newly acquired power of perception. There is, here, another correspondence with the results of analytic therapy. For the patient, too, we aim at more than mere recovery of lost feelings and abilities. What we wish him to achieve is the creation of new attitudes and relationships on the basis of the newly created powers of insight into his inner world.

There is, lastly, a highly interesting treatise on negativistic attitudes toward psychic creativity in which certain inhibitions to create are ascribed to a fear of regression to an undifferentiated state in which the boundaries between id and ego, self and object become blurred. Owing to this anxiety, no "language of love," i.e., no medium, can be found in which to "symbolise the individual's pregenital and genital orgiastic experiences." These views coincide in a welcome manner with certain clinical observations of my own concerning states of affective negativism, in which the patient's ability to express object love is blocked by the fear of an all too complete emotional surrender.[1] Future studies of this kind will owe much to Marion Milner's lucid explanation of this "unconscious hankering to return to the blissful surrender, this all-out body giving of infancy."

[1] See Volume IV, ch. 10.

34

Preface to *Chronic Schizophrenia* by Thomas Freeman, John L. Cameron, and Andrew McGhie (1958)

It is a special merit of this book that it offers more than the sober title leads us to expect. The authors themselves describe their efforts as a "clinical, interpretative and therapeutic study of schizophrenia." They address themselves primarily to those who—like themselves—work with chronic, hospitalized, severely deteriorated schizophrenic patients, and they make no claim for wider application of their findings. This modesty on their part, on the other hand, should

First published in London: Tavistock Publications, and New York: International Universities Press, 1958.

not obscure the fact that readers from many other fields of work can derive profit and stimulation from the careful clinical descriptions and challenging theoretical considerations of this monograph.

In Chapter II, for example, the theory of mental functioning ostensibly serves the purpose only of providing a theoretical framework—taken from psychoanalysis—against which the authors wish their clinical observations to be viewed. But, beyond accomplishing this task, the chapter also provides valuable instruction for all psychiatrists who are interested in the analytic approach to mental illness, whatever their specific range of case or treatment. It will be welcomed as well by students of psychoanalysis proper as an exceptionally clear and succinct summary of certain basic principles of psychoanalytic thinking.

Chapters VI to IX are relevant for all workers in the field of analytic psychology. Here, the authors use the severe deteriorations of personality structure as they occur in the chronic schizophrenic to discuss in detail those primitive levels of mental life where the distinction between the self and the environment is lacking, with disastrous results for such important functions as perception, thinking, memory, etc. Here, students of ego psychology are presented with vivid clinical pictures of the disturbance of the normal, conscious thought processes and of their lowering to the level of the "primary process," i.e., to that form of mental functioning which normally reveals itself in dream activity only. Further, the authors show in detail how the "confusion of identity," which results from this state of mind, destroys the individual's attachment to his environment and substitutes the most primitive processes of "merging with the object" for the normal, adult forms of emotional relationships.

In Chapter X, finally, readers are introduced to the painstaking methods by which the patients are induced —wherever possible—to re-establish contact with the environment. Child analysts, and other workers with young children, will note with interest that the therapeutic tools used and recommended by the authors are in many respects identical with the methods used in the upbringing of infants. In the young infant—as in the schizophrenic patient —we find egocentric, autistic behavior, together with confusion between himself and the environment, both corresponding to a state "before the boundaries between the self and not-self are adequately formed." The infant acquires this distinction through his attachment to stable, need-satisfying, reliable figures in the outside world. It is the identification with and introjection of such figures which enables him to build up his ego and sets him on the path to normal functioning.

The authors show convincingly that the formation of such stable relationships is indispensable in the therapy of chronic, institutionalized schizophrenic patients and they describe in which ways they themselves and, above all, the members of the nursing staff were able to serve as figures of this kind.

35

Foreword to Margarete
Ruben's *Parent Guidance
in the Nursery School*
(1960 [1959])

Margarete Ruben's small handbook on parent guidance does not really stand in need of special recommendation. It is as serious in purpose as it is modest in appearance and, as it seems to me, it cannot fail to satisfy a demand and fill a gap, while simultaneously conveying an accurate picture of the carefulness which the author and her co-workers exercise when meeting the individual mother's need.

The professional readers of this publication, whether workers or authors in the same field, will have no difficulty in recognizing the basic analytic tenets which form the

First published by International Universities Press, New York, 1960.

background of the counseling: the role of the body needs for food and sleep; the infant's attachment to the mother; the emotional importance of intake and elimination; the sequences in the development of sex and aggression; the conflicts and complexes arising from the child's ties to his objects, etc. The author shows convincingly that, to her, parent guidance means to draw on this fund of knowledge, without ever dispensing more than the mother in question can assimilate at the given moment.

Many years ago, when some analytic colleagues and I made our first contacts with the field of education, we frequently found ourselves unable to prescribe the proper course of action for parents, owing to the scanty and tentative nature of the knowledge which we possessed. Today, when many more relevant data are at our disposal, there are other considerations which make us cautious. The most significant of these is an objection which is itself derived from analytic experience. The successful upbringing of a young child, as we know, depends not on his mother's objective knowledge but on her subjective emotional attitudes; and difficulties of handling the child arise, above all, wherever the mother's unconscious fantasies and leanings, her defenses, conflicts, symptoms, in short, her psychopathology, block the way to understanding and appropriate management.

I have no doubt about the truth of this statement. A woman's capacity for mothering is subject to a multitude of complex disturbances, no less so—or even more—than all other human capacities and relationships. On the other hand, I see mothering not only as an instinctive attitude but also as a skilled task, and an increasingly difficult one under present conditions when the actions of mothers are no longer guided by tradition. Intelligent observation, information about basic facts of human development, and understanding of an individual child's behavior, as they are offered in this book, will strengthen the mothers' own goodwill, even in those cases where they have to struggle with their own emotions.

Margarete Ruben herself stresses in her Introduction that the limits for all counseling are set by the parents' personalities.

36

Heinz Hartmann: A Tribute
(1965 [1964])

The pioneers of psychoanalysis, among whom Heinz Hartmann is an outstanding figure, have been known at all times to wage war on more than one front. As uncompromising representatives of a new discipline, they inevitably find themselves in opposition to the academic and clinical departments in which they have grown up. As innovators and explorers in their chosen field, they cannot help incurring the distrust and misgivings of their new colleagues. If, like Hartmann, they simultaneously stand firm on all the valued and tested acquisitions of psychoanalysis, they expose themselves also to the reproach of "orthodoxy" from the side of

Based on introductory remarks made at a special meeting of the New York Psychoanalytic Society in honor of Heinz Hartmann's seventieth birthday, at the New York Academy of Medicine, November 4, 1964. First published in the *Journal of the American Psychoanalytic Association*, 13:195-196, 1965.

the more extreme of the analytic revolutionaries. It is only on rare occasions, such as anniversary celebrations, that the dissenting voices recede into the background and make room for universal acclaim and an adequate evaluation of their role within the fabric of the analytic movement and the growth and development of analytic theory.

In spite of this precarious position at the top of a profession, Heinz Hartmann, in his teaching activities and publications, seems to have completely disregarded or even remained oblivious to the battle which was staged around him. In the place of polemics, criticism of fellow workers, or bids to win approval, there is only the author's deep immersion in the problems which engage his own interest and for which he tries to gain the students', the readers', or the audiences' attention.

The range and sequence of these topics and their bearing on the structure of psychoanalysis as a whole are well known by now. From the narrower conception of the ego as the seat of anxiety, conflict, and defense, Hartmann moved to the ego's conflict-free sphere, that is, from what had been taken so far as the only truly analytic field of study to an area which until then had remained the preserve of academic psychology. To the intersystemic approach to the pathogenic disharmonies between id, ego, and superego and to the more global ideas of precocious or retarded ego development, he added the painstaking intrasystemic approach to the ego as such, the attempts to specify when and where its functions undergo acceleration or the opposite in relation to the drives or to one another, and where ego functions of one kind are interfered with by ego functions of another kind. He enriched not only theoretical but clinical psychoanalysis by his distinction between a primary and secondary ego autonomy and the important bearing this difference has on the resistance of ego functions to regressive pulls. Never satisfied with a one-sided scrutiny of the instinctual forces only, he did not share the analyst's usual hesitation to turn also to the superficial layers of the mind and to find significant clues in what he called "the sign and signal function" of the behavior of the individual. With regard to the ontogenetic origins of the ego, Hartmann's explorations went backward in time from a structural division of the personality to the undifferentiated id-ego sphere, testing and searching in the earliest constellations to find evidence for the existence of primary ego energies and innate directives for the unfolding of the ego's varied potentialities. His work on sublimation and neutralization of sex and aggression added the dimension of qualitative energy change to that of displacement of aim. His treatises on morality and the concept of health are instructive patterns of objectivity and restraint when applying psychoanalytic thinking to the fields of moral, aesthetic, and social values.

In this variety of studies, Heinz Hartmann's main aim seems to have remained an unswerving one: to raise the status of psychoanalysis from that of a depth psychology to that of a general theory of the mind which impartially embraces depth and surface; id, ego, and superego; in short, the total of the human personality. That he was unusually successful in his endeavors is borne out by "the remarkable degree to which his ideas have shaped and become assimilated into current psychoanalytic thinking," as the editors of the English edition of his *Ego Psychology and the Problem of Adaptation* aptly and with justification point out.

37

Foreword to Jeanne Lampl-de
Groot's *The Development
of the Mind*
(1965)

The author of this book belongs to a small but prominent
group of psychoanalysts who served their apprenticeship in
Vienna in the '20s of the century and who are now, one
after the other, approaching, celebrating, or looking back
on their 70th birthday.

The members of this group were fortunate in their professional career in several respects. They entered the analytic field late enough to be spared many of the setbacks,
hardships, and attacks by a hostile world to which the
pioneering generation had been subjected. They were early
enough, on the other hand, to be taught by the originator

First published by New York: International Universities Press,
1965.

of psychoanalysis himself, and to develop their ideas in lively interchange with him. They entered the Vienna Society when scientific life there was at its height. And, when this Society broke up, they dispersed all over the world, to become the mainstay of analytic branches elsewhere, valued teachers in new analytic Institutes, editors of or contributors to analytic journals, and guiding figures in the International Psycho-analytical Association.

Jeanne Lampl-de Groot is conducting her life as an analyst in conformity with this exacting tradition. In practical terms, this implies that she does a great deal of hard work with minimal interruptions; that she carries out as many analytic treatments herself as she supervises therapy done by others; that by means of training analyses, seminar and lecture work, she cooperates in producing succeeding generations of well-informed and capable representatives and teachers of psychoanalysis. It implies above all that she extracts from her activities the insights needed to break new ground and increase the volume of psychoanalytic knowledge, a task to which she brings considerable acumen, conscientiousness, prudence, and complete scientific integrity. That her interest embraces a wide range of psychoanalytic problems and that, with her, theoretical deduction never appears divorced from clinical experience, is borne out by the scope, the quality, and the variety of papers presented in this book.

Part V

38

Doctoral Award Address
(1967 [1964])

Whenever dinner guests are presented to an assembled company, whatever they have to say for themselves can only be an anticlimax compared with the high expectations that have been raised about them. That is a risk which I take knowingly tonight after Dr. Waelder's introduction, since I do not want to bypass the opportunity to express my gratitude for the honor and the many signs of goodwill which I have received.

Although I have been given the choice of talking on any subject of my liking, there is no other on my mind at present, except the very impressive events of this memorable day. Concerning them, I am intrigued by two questions for

Afterdinner Speech delivered on June 12, 1964 at Jefferson Medical College on the occasion of receiving an honorary degree of Doctor of Science. First published in the *Journal of the American Psychoanalytic Association*, 15:833-840, 1967.

which, before coming here, I had not found an answer. There must be many sciences competing for the honor of being publicly recognized on the occasion of the Commencement Exercises here; why has the choice fallen on the science of psychoanalysis? And further, there are many worthy representatives of psychoanalysis; for what reason have I been singled out among them? It is to these two topics that I want to speak tonight.

The first, obviously, is easier to tackle. Events such as the honoring of psychoanalysis never occur without preparation. What I had not known before coming here was that Jefferson Medical College had given previous signs that this was going to happen. It is never an easy step for a medical school to introduce psychoanalysis into the curriculum, but Jefferson made this move several years ago. The students of the School have been introduced to psychoanalysis for a considerable time by analysts such as Drs. Robert Bookhammer, Paul Poinsard, Abraham Freedman, John A. Koltes. More recently, the residents have been drawn into the orbit of psychoanalytic thinking by Drs. Guttman and Waelder. That one of these analysts, appointed to the staff, is not even a medical man, nor a psychiatrist, seems to me to signify Jefferson's recognition that psychoanalysis, far from being only a subspecialty of psychiatry, represents a body of knowledge in its own right, a theory of mental functioning, normal and abnormal, the true substratum and cornerstone of psychology. If these signs are read correctly, the honor accorded to psychoanalysis today appears no longer as sudden or as surprising.

The second, personal question is more difficult to approach. All I can do at present is to review for you, and me, a number of possible solutions.

During the ceremonies today, I could not help looking at all those who graduated together with me, and to place my own status in relation to theirs. I did not wish to rank myself with the eminent scientists who received honorary degrees, like myself, since this seemed presumptuous. Instead I viewed myself in comparison with the large group of young medical men, and outlined in my mind the main points of contrast between us.

One basic difference, of course, springs to the eye: what I received as a gift, they have worked hard for. With each young man who came up the steps as a student, and went down as a graduate, I could imagine the years of intensive work which culminated in that particular moment. Also, I was certain that not one of them asked himself the question which was on my mind: "Why me?" They had selected themselves for the fate of graduation, and their own efforts, bent in that direction, had brought about the desired result.

Another difference between the recipients of ordinary and honorary degrees is no less obvious. What is commencement for the former, i.e., beginning of a professional life, is not the same for the latter. No honors come to a beginner. Honorary degrees are received at best at the climax of a career, more frequently at the very end of it. They represent somehow a finalizing, not a commencement ceremony.

I am sure, further, that before any degree is conferred on a student by a reputable medical school, much examination and appraisal of the individual goes beforehand. If I remember correctly how the relevant phrase runs: "that the student in question has been examined in detail by all the people concerned in his training and that he has satisfied all requirements." I expect that the Honoraries also have to satisfy requirements, but what I miss is the awareness of ever having been examined. With the students, no personal considerations are allowed to play a part and, to assure the scrupulous honesty of the whole process, all personal favors are excluded which might be instrumental in pushing their claim to graduation. Can I really rest assured that the same scrupulous honesty and impartiality were exercised regarding my selection; that there were no personal friends and colleagues who spoke up in my favor?

The situation seems even more ominous if my thoughts move from the decision about graduation in the direction of the selection procedures which assure admission to a medical school to the original applicants. I have been told that usually not more than 10 to 15 percent of the applicants are permitted entrance to a medical school of the rank of Jefferson's. Their curriculum vitae is gone through carefully and, if the facts are satisfactory, the applicant is summoned for a personal interview. What about me, then, in comparison with this? It is true that I have been summoned here for personal viewing and that I have duly appeared today. But was that not unduly late in the whole process? And did it not follow acceptance to the School instead of preceding it?

Worse still about the curriculum vitae: I was never asked for it. Not that I minded that particular omission. On the contrary, I had to regard the fact as fortuitous, since it is an unconventional one, of the kind at which no decent university looks twice. On the other hand, I feel it remains an obligation to lay it before the College which admitted me to its ranks, and I decided to do it now, where, *post factum*, no further risk is attached to its presentation.

CURRICULUM VITAE OF A LAY ANALYST

I share, in fact, with all other lay analysts the lack of a medical education. I also have in common with a few remaining analysts of my generation the circumstance that our analytic training took place at a period before the official psychoanalytic training institutes came into being. We were trained by our personal analysts, by extensive reading, by our own, unsupervised efforts with our first patients, and by lively interchange of ideas and discussion of problems with our elders and contemporaries. At the time, my own analytic apprenticeship seemed a haphazard affair to me, following no clear line. The rationale underlying it did not dawn on me until several years later when I read what my father wrote concerning the training of analysts: "A scheme of training for analysts has still to be created. It must include elements from the mental sciences, from psychology, the history of civilization and sociology, as well as from anatomy, biology and the study of evolution . . . an ideal which can and must be realized" (1926b, p. 252). And further, in the same connection: "Analytic training, it is true, cuts across the field of medical education, but neither includes the other. If—which may sound phantastic to-day— one had to found a college of psycho-analysis, much would have to be taught in it which is also taught by the medical faculty: alongside of depth-psychology, which would always remain the principal subject, there would be an introduction to biology, as much as possible of the science of sexual life, and familiarity with the symptomatology of psychiatry. On the other hand, analytic instruction would include branches of knowledge which are remote from medicine and which the doctor does not come across in his practice: the history of civilization, mythology, the psychology of religion and the science of literature. Until he is well at home in these subjects, an analyst can make nothing of a large amount of his material" (p. 246).

This ambitious scheme, as you know, has not been realized up to date, but it must have been the basis of the guidance which I was given at the time. "Familiarity with the symptomatology of psychiatry" was offered to me thanks to the permission to attend the rounds in the psychiatric teaching hospital of Vienna, then under Professor Wagner-Jauregg. This was an exciting time in the particular department where I was a guest, with Paul Schilder as first, and Heinz Hartmann as second clinical assistant. The ward rounds, especially when led by Schilder, were highly instructive, and what they taught was never forgotten by me. We all listened spellbound to the revelations made by the patients, their dreams, delusions, fantastic systems, which the analytically knowledgeable among us fitted into a scheme. We also had the chance to witness the first results of fever therapy, initiated then by Wagner-Jauregg.

Clinical experience—practical contact with human beings, as it was called at the time—which was demanded from every analyst, was supplied for me by teaching school, a five-year contact with young children. This proved important for me, as my curriculum will show, since in later life analysts usually return to, and single out for application, the very fields in which they had their first, preanalytic, practical experience.

The main part of the study, of course, as outlined in the programmatic quotation given above, was depth psychology, this always remaining the principal subject. Depth psychology, for the analyst in training, meant psychoanalytic work itself. I quote here from the address given by Maxwell Gitelson, as president of the International Psycho-Analytical Association at the recent Annual Meeting of the American Psychoanalytic Association in Los Angeles (1964). He said: "the integrity of the classical model of the psychoanalytic situation [is] the only available condition for the controlled study of human individual psychology in its deepest sense" (p. 472). The psychoanalytic work with patients, carried on over years, remained the main source of learning. In pre-Institute times, there were differences also in this respect from the usual practice of today. American candidates nowadays treat three cases before qualification, European candidates in many Institutes only two. In our Hampstead Clinic, our students analyze three children, in exceptional instances sometimes four. But this does not compare with what happened in my past. We had five, six, seven, or eight patients at a time and continued in this manner not for two or three years, but for five or ten before our older colleagues considered us full-grown members. I realize now, looking back, that it was much more difficult to qualify without an established training program and an objectively fixed training period. For many years, the analytic beginner in the Society was looked down on as "inexperienced." I remember that even the discussion group which we initiated among ourselves for the exchange of opinions was officially called the "Children's Seminar," not because child cases were discussed there, but because the discussants themselves were considered to be in analytic infancy.

What, then, was the order of cases we were given to treat? We were lucky in that respect since all the classical forms of neurosis were still available for study. I remember well that my first case was a globus hystericus; my second case a full-blown obsessional neurosis in an adolescent girl who almost killed her mother in her compulsive oversolicitude for her health by wrapping her up in warm shawls and nearly strangling her, so that the police had to be called in to save the helpless woman from the girl's clutches. Working inhibitions and a phobia concluded this first group of patients, from whom I gradually passed on to traumatized cases, cases of seduction, perverts, near delinquents, a delusional and a paranoid woman, both sent to me with the diagnosis of neurosis. From there, the way led to the addicts and the homosexuals, and, in good time, to candidates in training, where I made my first acquaintance with the character neuroses. When this happened, the first learning period seemed to be completed.

To be trained in this unorthodox way had its advantages. One was that one was supposed to be completely familiar with the classical technique before there was any thought of introducing modifications of it, or adaptations; my first independent move here was to adapt the technique for adults to fit the treatment of children. Another advantage was that no one was expected to produce theoretical papers at the beginning of his career, as many young analysts feel urged to do now. On the contrary, where theory was concerned, to sit and listen and not say anything was considered an asset, not a failing in a young analyst. I remember that I adhered religiously to this pattern, although I made up for lost speaking opportunities at later dates.

My first excursion from the clinic to theory led me to the study of the defense mechanisms of the ego. In contrast to many colleagues, I was never concerned one-sidedly with either id, ego, or superego, but always with the interactions between them. The dynamics of mental life which fascinated me, to my mind, found their clearest expression in the defense organization of the ego, with the attempts of the rational personality to deal with the irrational. After extending my interest from adult analysis to child analysis and from clinical to theoretical problems, I also turned to the various applications of analysis. Beginning in Vienna, and continuing in England and the United States, I tried to select from analytic knowledge what can be useful for education, for teaching, for pediatrics, for the law. That, in short, is my curriculum vitae. Measured in time, it comprises a working period of approximately forty-five years.

One more personal addition: When I was a young girl and dissatisfied with my appearance—as girls often are—I felt comforted by a saying then popular in Vienna: "After a certain age every woman gets the face that she deserves," i.e., the face she creates for herself. Today, I want to apply this assertion to the work of every psychoanalyst: I think it is true that after a certain age and point of his career, every psychoanalyst creates for himself the type of work that he deserves. In Professor Castle's Commencement Speech this morning, we heard how wide a choice there is for the medical man, how many fields to select from, and how difficult it is in the beginning to predict whether the individual persons will turn into clinicians or theoreticians, or administrators, i.e., which fate they will carve out for themselves in medicine. What is true for the medical graduate is applicable to the analytic graduate. Some become analytic practitioners; some apply psychoanalysis only to psychiatry; some even restrict themselves to psychotherapy; some enter a field of application and remain there; some turn to theory, etc. So far as I am concerned, I feel I have been well treated by fate and have been given more than I deserved. At present, I am lucky enough to be organizer of an institution which combines in itself almost all the aspects of psychoanalysis: teaching, therapy, techniques, theory, research, application to prevention, education, pediatrics, etc. There is no better life for the analyst than to be able to be in constant contact with all the facets of human behavior, from childhood to adulthood and from normality to the severest forms of pathology.

And one final remark. When I return home tomorrow, as a new Sc.D., people not familiar with university usage may ask in which of the sciences I received my doctorate. I hope I have your agreement if I answer: "The science of psychoanalysis, of course."

Bibliography

ADATTO, C. P. (1958), Ego Reintegration Observed in Analysis of Late Adolescents. *Int. J. Psycho-Anal.*, 39:172-177.

AICHHORN, A. (1923-1948), *Delinquency and Child Guidance: Selected Papers*, ed. O. Fleischmann, P. Kramer, & H. Ross. New York: International Universities Press, 1964.

——— (1925), *Wayward Youth.* New York: Viking Press, 1935.

——— (1932), Erziehungsberatung. *Z. psychoanal. Päd.*, 6:445-488.

——— (1948), Delinquency in a New Light. *Delinquency and Child Guidance*, ed. O. Fleischmann, P. Kramer, & H. Ross. New York: International Universities Press, 1964, pp. 218-235.

ALPERT, A. (1959), Reversibility of Pathological Fixations Associated with Maternal Deprivation in Infancy. *The Psychoanalytic Study of the Child*, 14:169-185.*

APLEY, J. (1962), The Role of the Paediatrician. In: *Clinical Problems of Young Children: The Proceedings of the 18th Child Guidance Inter-Clinic Conference.* London: National Association for Mental Health, pp. 30-35.

* *The Psychoanalytic Study of the Child*, currently 24 Volumes, edited by Ruth S. Eissler, Anna Freud, Heinz Hartmann, Marianne Kris. New York: International Universities Press; London: Hogarth Press, 1945-1969.

BALINT, M. (1934), Der Onanieabgewöhnungskampf in der Pubertät. Z. *psychoanal. Päd.*, 8:374-391.

—— (1962), The Theory of the Parent-Infant Relationship (ix). *Int. J. Psycho-Anal.*, 43:251-252.

BARNES, M. J. (1964), Reactions to the Death of a Mother. *The Psychoanalytic Study of the Child*, 19:334-357.

BARRON, A. T., see BURLINGHAM, D.

BERGEN, M. E. (1958), The Effect of Severe Trauma on a Four-Year-Old Child. *The Psychoanalytic Study of the Child*, 13:407-429.

BERGMANN, T. (1960), Application of Analytic Knowledge to Children with Organic Illness. In: *Recent Developments in Psychoanalytic Child Therapy*, ed. J. Weinreb. New York: International Universities Press, pp. 139-148.

—— & FREUD, A. (1965), *Children in the Hospital*. New York: International Universities Press.

BERNFELD, S. (1923), Über eine typische Form der männlichen Pubertät. *Imago*, 9:169-188.

—— (1924), *Vom dichterischen Schaffen der Jugend*. Vienna: Psychoanalytischer Verlag.

—— (1935), Über eine einfache männliche Pubertät. Z. *psychoanal. Päd.*, 9:360-379.

—— (1938), Types of Adolescence. *Psychoanal. Quart.*, 7:243-253.

BIBRING, G. L. (1959), Some Considerations of the Psychological Processes in Pregnancy. *The Psychoanalytic Study of the Child*, 14:113-121.

—— (1960), Work with Physicians. In: *Recent Developments in Psychoanalytic Child Therapy*, ed. J. Weinreb. New York: International Universities Press, pp. 39-52.

——(1966), Old Age: Its Liabilities and Its Assets. In: *Psychoanalysis—A General Psychology*, ed. R. M. Loewenstein, L. M. Newman, M. Schur, & A. J. Solnit. New York: International Universities Press, pp. 253-271.

BLOS, P. (1962), *On Adolescence: A Psychoanalytic Interpretation*. Glencoe, Ill.: Free Press.

BOLLAND, J., SANDLER, J., ET AL. (1965), *The Hampstead Psy-*

choanalytic Index: A Study of the Psychoanalytic Case Material of a Two-and-a-Half-Year-Old Child [Monograph Series of the Psychoanalytic Study of the Child, No. 1]. New York: International Universities Press.

BONNARD, A. (1958), Pre-Body-Ego Types of (Pathological) Mental Functioning. *J. Amer. Psychoanal. Assn.*, 6:581-611.

——— (1961), Truancy and Pilfering Associated with Bereavement. In: *Adolescents*, ed. S. Lorand & H. I. Schneer. New York: Hoeber, pp. 152-179.

——— (1967), Primary Process Phenomena in the Case of a Borderline Psychotic Child. *Int. J. Psycho-Anal.*, 48:221-236.

BORNSTEIN, B. (1949a), The Analysis of a Phobic Child: Some Problems of Theory and Technique in Child Analysis. *The Psychoanalytic Study of the Child*, 3/4:181-226.

——— (1949b), Discussion following the presentation of Phyllis Greenacre's paper [see Greenacre (1950)] at the New York Psychoanalytic Society. Abstr. in: *Psychoanal. Quart.*, 18:277.

BOWLBY, J. (1951), *Maternal Care and Mental Health*. Geneva: World Health Organization.

——— (1958), The Nature of the Child's Tie to His Mother. *Int. J. Psycho-Anal.*, 39:350-373.

——— (1960a [1958]), Separation Anxiety. *Int. J. Psycho-Anal.*, 41:89-113.

——— (1960b), Grief and Mourning in Infancy and Early Childhood. *The Psychoanalytic Study of the Child*, 15:9-52.

——— (1961a), Processes of Mourning. *Int. J. Psycho-Anal.*, 42:317-340.

——— (1961b), Note on Dr. Max Schur's Comments on Grief and Mourning in Infancy and Early Childhood. *The Psychoanalytic Study of the Child*, 16:206-208.

——— ROBERTSON, JAMES, & ROSENBLUTH, D. (1952), A Two-Year-Old Goes to Hospital. *The Psychoanalytic Study of the Child*, 7:82-94.

BREUER, J. & FREUD, S. (1893-1895), Studies on Hysteria. *Standard Edition*, 2.†

† See footnote ∫.

BÜHLER, C. (1935), *From Birth to Maturity*. London: Routledge & Kegan Paul.

BURLINGHAM, D. (1932), Child Analysis and the Mother. *Psychoanal. Quart.*, 4:69-92, 1935.

―――― (1935), Empathy between Infant and Mother. *J. Amer. Psychoanal. Assn.*, 15:764-780, 1967.

―――― (1951), *Twins: A Study of Three Pairs of Identical Twins*. New York: International Universities Press.

―――― (1958), Identical-Twin Studies Based on the Integration of Observational and Analytical Data. *Proc. Roy. Soc. Med.*, 51:943-945.

―――― (1961), Some Notes on the Development of the Blind. *The Psychoanalytic Study of the Child*, 16:121-145.

―――― (1964), Hearing and Its Role in the Development of the Blind. *The Psychoanalytic Study of the Child*, 19:95-112.

―――― (1965), Some Problems of Ego Development in Blind Children. *The Psychoanalytic Study of the Child*, 20:194-208.

―――― (1967), Developmental Considerations in Occupations of the Blind. *The Psychoanalytic Study of the Child*, 22:187-198.

―――― & BARRON, A. T. (1963), A Study of Identical Twins: Their Analytic Material Compared with Existing Observation Data of Their Early Childhood. *The Psychoanalytic Study of the Child*, 18:367-423.

―――― & GOLDBERGER, A. (1968), The Re-education of a Retarded Blind Child. *The Psychoanalytic Study of the Child*, 23:369-390.

―――― ―――― & LUSSIER, A. (1955), Simultaneous Analysis of Mother and Child. *The Psychoanalytic Study of the Child*, 10:165-186.

―――― see also FREUD, A.

BUXBAUM, E. (1933), Angstäusserungen von Schulmädchen im Pubertätsalter. *Z. psychoanal. Päd.*, 7:401-409.

―――― (1945), Transference and Group Formation in Children and Adolescents. *The Psychoanalytic Study of the Child*, 1:351-365.

CAMERON, J. L., see FREEMAN, T.

CASUSO, G. (1957), Anxiety Related to the "Discovery" of the Penis: An Observation. *The Psychoanalytic Study of the Child*, 12:169-174.

COLEMAN, R. W., KRIS, E., & PROVENCE, S. (1953), The Study of Variations of Early Parental Attitudes. *The Psychoanalytic Study of the Child*, 8:20-47.

―――― see also PROVENCE, S.

COLONNA, A. B. (1968), A Blind Child Goes to the Hospital. *The Psychoanalytic Study of the Child*, 23:391-422.

―――― see also NAGERA, H.

DAUNTON, E., see SANDLER, A.-M.

DERSHOWITZ, A. M., see KATZ, J.

DEUTSCH, H. (1944), *The Psychology of Women*, Vol. I. New York: Grune & Stratton.

―――― (1967), *Selected Problems of Adolescence*. New York: International Universities Press.

EISSLER, K. R. (1950), Ego-Psychological Implications of the Psychoanalytic Treatment of Delinquents. *The Psychoanalytic Study of the Child*, 5:97-121.

―――― (1953), Notes upon the Emotionality of a Schizophrenic Patient and Its Relation to Problems of Technique. *The Psychoanalytic Study of the Child*, 8:199-251.

―――― (1955), An Unusual Function of an Amnesia. *The Psychoanalytic Study of the Child*, 10:75-82.

―――― (1958), Notes on Problems of Technique in the Psychoanalytic Treatment of Adolescents. *The Psychoanalytic Study of the Child*, 13:223-254.

―――― (1959), On Isolation. *The Psychoanalytic Study of the Child*, 14:29-60.

ERIKSON, E. H. (1946), Ego Development and Historical Change. *The Psychoanalytic Study of the Child*, 2:359-396.

―――― (1950), *Childhood and Society*. New York: Norton.

―――― (1959), *Identity and the Life Cycle* [*Psychological Issues*, Monogr. 1]. New York: International Universities Press.

FEDERN, P. (1912), [Contribution to:] *Die Onanie: 14 Beiträge zu einer Diskussion der Wiener Psychoanalytischen Vereinigung*. Wiesbaden: Bergmann, pp. 68-82.

────── (1952), *Ego Psychology and the Psychoses.* New York: Basic Books.

FENICHEL, O. (1938), Review of *The Ego and the Mechanisms of Defence. Int. J. Psycho-Anal.,* 19:116-136.

────── (1945), *The Psychoanalytic Theory of Neurosis.* New York: Norton.

FERENCZI, S. (1912), On Onanism. *Sex in Psychoanalysis.* New York: Basic Books, 1950, pp. 185-192.

FOLKART, L., *see* THOMAS, R.

FRAIBERG, S. (1955), Some Considerations in the Introduction to Therapy in Puberty. *The Psychoanalytic Study of the Child,* 10:264-286.

FRANKL, L. (1958), Enquiry into the Difficulty of Diagnosis by Comparing the Impressions in the Diagnostic Interviews with the Material Elicited in the Course of the Child's Analysis. *Proc. Roy. Soc. Med.,* 51:945-946.

────── (1961a), Some Observations on the Development and Disturbances of Integration in Childhood. *The Psychoanalytic Study of the Child,* 16:146-163.

────── (1961b), The Child and His Symptoms. In: *Psychosomatic Aspects of Paediatrics,* ed. R. MacKeith & J. Sandler. New York & London: Pergamon Press, pp. 114-118.

────── (1963), Self-Preservation and the Development of Accident Proneness in Children and Adolescents. *The Psychoanalytic Study of the Child,* 18:464-483.

────── & HELLMAN, I. (1963), A Specific Problem in Adolescent Boys. *Bull. Phila. Assn. Psychoanal.,* 13:120-129.

────── ────── (1964), The Ego's Participation in the Therapeutic Alliance. In: *Child Psychotherapy,* ed. M. W. Haworth. New York: Basic Books, pp. 229-236.

FREEMAN, T., CAMERON, J. L., & McGHIE, A. (1958), *Chronic Schizophrenia.* London: Tavistock Publications; New York: International Universities Press.

FREUD, ANNA (1926-1927), *Introduction to the Technique of Child Analysis.* New York & Washington: Nervous & Mental Disease Publ. Co., 1929; also in: *The Psycho-Analytical Treat-*

ment of Children. New York: International Universities Press, 1959 [see Volume I‡].

—— (1936), *The Ego and the Mechanisms of Defense.* New York: International Universities Press, rev. ed. 1966 [Volume II].

—— (1957), Die Kinderneurose. In: *Das psychoanalytische Volksbuch,* ed. P. Federn & H. Meng. Bern & Stuttgart: Hans Huber, pp. 203-214.

—— (1961 [1959]), Defense Mechanisms. *Encyclopaedia Britannica.* Chicago, London, Toronto: William Benton.

—— (1962), Assessment of Childhood Disturbances. *The Psychoanalytic Study of the Child,* 17:149-158 [see Volume VI, pp. 138-147].

—— (1963a), The Concept of Developmental Lines. *The Psychoanalytic Study of the Child,* 18:245-265 [see Volume VI, pp. 62-92].

—— (1963b), Regression as a Principle in Mental Development. *Bull. Menninger Clin.,* 27:126-139; also in: *Normality and Pathology in Childhood: Assessments of Development.* New York: International Universities Press [see Volume VI, pp. 93-107].

—— (1965a), *Normality and Pathology in Childhood: Assessments of Development.* New York: International Universities Press [Volume VI].

—— (1965b [1964]), Some Recent Developments in Child Analysis. In: *Psychotherapy and Psychosomatics,* 13:36-46. Basel & New York: Karger.

—— (1965c), Diagnostic Skills and Their Growth in Psycho-Analysis. *Int. J. Psycho-Anal.,* 46:31-38 [see Volume VI, pp. 10-24].

—— (1966), Adolescence As a Developmental Disturbance. Presented at the 6th International Congress for Child Psychiatry [see Volume VII].

—— (1968), *Indications for Child Analysis and Other Papers.* New York: International Universities Press [Volume IV].

‡ The Volume numbers in brackets refer to *The Writings of Anna Freud.* New York: International Universities Press, 1966-

—— & Burlingham, D. (1942), *War and Children.* New York: International Universities Press, 1943 [see Volume III].

—— —— (1943), *Infants Without Families.* New York: International Universities Press, 1944 [see Volume III].

—— *see also* Bergmann, T.

Freud, Sigmund (1894), The Neuro-Psychoses of Defence. *Standard Edition*, 3:43-68.§

—— (1896a), Further Remarks on the Neuro-Psychoses of Defence. *Standard Edition*, 3:159-184.

—— (1896b), The Aetiology of Hysteria. *Standard Edition*, 3:189-221.

——(1900), The Interpretation of Dreams. *Standard Edition*, 4 & 5.

—— (1901), The Psychopathology of Everyday Life. *Standard Edition*, 6.

—— (1905), Three Essays on the Theory of Sexuality. *Standard Edition*, 7:125-245.

—— (1908), Character and Anal Erotism. *Standard Edition*, 9:167-175.

—— (1909a), Analysis of a Phobia in a Five-Year-Old Boy. *Standard Edition*, 10:5-149.

—— (1909b), Notes upon a Case of Obsessional Neurosis. *Standard Edition*, 10:153-318.

—— (1911), Psycho-analytic Notes on an Autobiographical Account of a Case of Paranoia (Dementia Paranoides). *Standard Edition*, 12:3-82.

—— (1912), Contribution to a Discussion on Masturbation. *Standard Edition*, 12:239-254.

—— (1915), Instincts and Their Vicissitudes. *Standard Edition*, 14:109-140.

—— (1916-1917 [1915-1917]), Introductory Lectures on Psycho-Analysis. *Standard Edition*, 15 & 16.

§ *The Standard Edition of the Complete Psychological Works of Sigmund Freud*, 24 Volumes, translated and edited by James Strachey. London: Hogarth Press and the Institute of Psycho-Analysis, 1953-

———— (1917 [1915]), Mourning and Melancholia. *Standard Edition*, 14:237-260.

———— (1918 [1914]), From the History of an Infantile Neurosis. *Standard Edition*, 17:3-123.

———— (1919), Preface to Reik's *Ritual: Psycho-Analytic Studies*. *Standard Edition*, 17:257-263.

———— (1922), Some Neurotic Mechanisms in Jealousy, Paranoia and Homosexuality. *Standard Edition*, 18:221-232.

———— (1924 [1923]), A Short Account of Psycho-Analysis. *Standard Edition*, 19:191-209.

———— (1926a [1925]), Inhibitions, Symptoms and Anxiety. *Standard Edition*, 20:77-174.

———— (1926b), The Question of Lay Analysis. *Standard Edition*, 20:179-258.

———— (1927), The Future of an Illusion. *Standard Edition*, 21:64-145.

———— (1930 [1929]), Civilization and Its Discontents. *Standard Edition*, 21:59-149.

———— (1931), The Expert Opinion in the Halsmann Case. *Standard Edition*, 21:251-253.

———— (1933 [1932]), New Introductory Lectures on Psycho-Analysis. *Standard Edition*, 22:3-182.

———— (1940 [1938]), An Outline of Psycho-Analysis. *Standard Edition*, 23:141-207.

———— see also BREUER, J.

FREUD, W. E. (1967), Assessment of Early Infancy: Problems and Considerations. *The Psychoanalytic Study of the Child*, 22:216-238.

———— (1968), Some General Reflections on the Metapsychological Profile. *Int. J. Psycho-Anal.*, 49:498-501.

FRIEDLANDER, K. (1941), Children's Books and Their Function in Latency and Pre-puberty. *Amer. Imago*, 3:129-150, 1942.

FRIEDMANN, O., see HELLMAN, I.

FRIES, M. E. (1946), The Child's Ego Development and the Training of Adults in His Environment. *The Psychoanalytic Study of the Child*, 2:85-112.

FURMAN, E. (1956), An Ego Disturbance in a Young Child. *The Psychoanalytic Study of the Child*, 11:312-335.

———— (1957), Treatment of Under-Fives by Way of Their Parents. *The Psychoanalytic Study of the Child*, 12:250-262.

FURMAN, R. A. (1964a), Death and the Young Child: Some Preliminary Considerations. *The Psychoanalytic Study of the Child*, 19:321-333.

———— (1964b), Death of a Six-Year-Old's Mother during His Analysis. *The Psychoanalytic Study of the Child*, 19:377-397.

———— & KATAN, A., EDS. (1969), *The Therapeutic Nursery School*. New York: International Universities Press.

FURST, S. S., ed. (1967), *Psychic Trauma*. New York: Basic Books.

GAUTHIER, Y. (1965), The Mourning Reaction of a Ten-and-a-Half-Year-Old Boy. *The Psychoanalytic Study of the Child*, 20:481-494.

GELEERD, E. R. (1957), Some Aspects of Psychoanalytic Technique in Adolescents. *The Psychoanalytic Study of the Child*, 12:263-283.

———— (1958), Borderline States in Childhood and Adolescence. *The Psychoanalytic Study of the Child*, 13:279-295.

GILLESPIE, W. H. (1963), Some Regressive Phenomena in Old Age. *Brit. J. Med. Psychol.*, 36:203-209.

GITELSON, M. (1948), Character Synthesis: The Psychotherapeutic Problem in Adolescence. *Amer. J. Orthopsychiat.*, 18:422-431.

———— (1962), The Curative Factors in Psycho-Analysis. *Int. J. Psycho-Anal.*, 43:194-205.

———— (1964), On the Identity Crisis in American Psychoanalysis. *J. Amer. Psychoanal. Assn.*, 12:451-476.

GOLDBERGER, A., *see* BURLINGHAM, D.

GOLDSTEIN, J. & KATZ, J. (1965), *The Family and the Law: Problems for Decision in the Family Law Process*. New York: Free Press.

———— *see also* KATZ, J.

GREENACRE, P. (1950), The Prepuberty Trauma in Girls. *Psychoanal. Quart.*, 19:298-317.

———— (1960), Considerations Regarding the Parent-Infant Relationship. *Int. J. Psycho-Anal.*, 41:571-584.

———— (1962), The Theory of the Parent-Infant Relationship: Further Remarks. *Int. J. Psycho-Anal.*, 43:235-237.

———— (1967), The Influence of Infantile Trauma on Genetic Patterns. In: *Psychic Trauma*, ed. S. S. Furst. New York: Basic Books, pp. 108-153.

GROUP FOR THE ADVANCEMENT OF PSYCHIATRY (1957), *The Diagnostic Process in Child Psychiatry.* Report No. 38, formulated by The Committee on Child Psychiatry.

GYOMROI, E. L. (1963), The Analysis of a Young Concentration Camp Victim. *The Psychoanalytic Study of the Child*, 18:-484-510.

HALL, J. WAELDER (1946), The Analysis of a Case of Night Terror. *The Psychoanalytic Study of the Child*, 2:189-228.

HARNIK, J. (1923), Various Developments Undergone by Narcissism in Men and Women. *Int. J. Psycho-Anal.*, 5:66-83, 1924.

HARTMANN, H. (1939a), *Ego Psychology and the Problem of Adaptation.* New York: International Universities Press, 1958.

———— (1939b), Psychoanalysis and the Concept of Health. *Essays on Ego Psychology.* New York: International Universities Press, 1964, pp. 1-18.

———— (1950a), Psychoanalysis and Developmental Psychology. *Essays on Ego Psychology.* New York: International Universities Press, 1964, pp. 99-112.

———— (1950b), Comments on the Psychoanalytic Theory of the Ego. *Essays on Ego Psychology.* New York: International Universities Press, 1964, pp. 113-141.

————(1951), Technical Implications of Ego Psychology. *Essays on Ego Psychology.* New York: International Universities Press, 1964, pp. 142-154.

———— (1952), The Mutual Influences in the Development of Ego and Id. *Essays on Ego Psychology.* New York: International Universities Press, 1964, pp. 155-181.

———— (1954), Problems of Infantile Neurosis. *Essays on Ego*

Psychology. New York: International Universities Press, 1964, pp. 207-217.

———— (1955), Notes on the Theory of Sublimation. *Essays on Ego Psychology*. New York: International Universities Press, 1964, pp. 215-240.

———— (1960), *Psychoanalysis and Moral Values*. New York: International Universities Press.

———— (1964), *Essays on Ego Psychology: Selected Problems in Psychoanalytic Theory*. New York: International Universities Press.

———— KRIS, E., & LOEWENSTEIN, R. M. (1946), Comments on the Formation of Psychic Structure. *The Psychoanalytic Study of the Child*, 2:11-38.

———— ———— ———— (1964), *Papers on Psychoanalytic Psychology* [*Psychological Issues*, Monogr. 14]. New York: International Universities Press.

HEINICKE, C. M. & WESTHEIMER, I. (1965), *Brief Separations*. New York: International Universities Press.

HELLMAN, I. (1958), Research on Adolescents in Treatment. *Proc. Roy. Soc. Med.*, 51:942-943.

———— (1962), Hampstead Nursery Follow-up Studies: I. Sudden Separation and Its Effect Followed Over Twenty Years. *The Psychoanalytic Study of the Child*, 17:159-174.

———— (1964), Observations on Adolescents in Psycho-Analytic Treatment. *Brit. J. Psychiat.*, 110:406-410.

———— FRIEDMANN, O., & SHEPHEARD, E. (1960), Simultaneous Analysis of Mother and Child. *The Psychoanalytic Study of the Child*, 15:359-377.

———— see also FRANKL, L.

HILL, J. C. (1926), *Dreams and Education*. London: Methuen.

HOFFER, W. (1946), Diaries of Adolescent Schizophrenics. *The Psychoanalytic Study of the Child*, 2:293-312.

———— (1950), Development of the Body Ego. *The Psychoanalytic Study of the Child*, 5:18-24.

———— (1952), The Mutual Influences in the Development of Ego and Id: Earliest Stages. *The Psychoanalytic Study of the Child*, 7:31-41.

BIBLIOGRAPHY 529

—— (1954), Defensive Process and Defensive Organization. *Int. J. Psycho-Anal.*, 35:194-198.

HOLDER, A. (1968), Theoretical and Clinical Notes on the Interaction of Some Relevant Variables in the Production of Neurotic Disturbances. *The Psychoanalytic Study of the Child*, 23:63-113.

—— see also SANDLER, J.

ISAACS, S. (1935), *The Psychological Aspects of Child Development.* London: Evans.

JACKSON, E. B. (1947), Rooming-in Plan for Mothers and Newborn Infants. *Conn. Med. J.*, 2:175-176.

—— (1948), A Hospital Rooming-in Unit for Four Newborn Infants and Their Mothers. *Pediatrics*, 1:28-43.

—— & KLATSKIN, E. H. (1950), Rooming-in Research Project: Development of a Methodology of Parent-Child Relationship Study in a Clinical Setting. *The Psychoanalytic Study of the Child*, 5:236-274.

JACOBSON, E. (1961), Adolescent Moods and the Remodeling of Psychic Structures in Adolescence. *The Psychoanalytic Study of the Child*, 16:164-183.

—— (1964), *The Self and the Object World.* New York: International Universities Press.

—— (1965), The Return of the Lost Parent. In: *Drives, Affects, Behavior*, Vol. 2, ed. M. Schur. New York: International Universities Press, pp. 193-211.

JAMES, M. (1960), Premature Ego Development: Some Observations upon Disturbances in the First Three Years of Life. *Int. J. Psycho-Anal.*, 41:288-294.

—— (1962), The Theory of the Parent-Infant Relationship (iv). *Int. J. Psycho-Anal.*, 43:247-248.

JOFFE, W. G. & SANDLER, J. (1965), Notes on Pain, Depression, and Individuation. *The Psychoanalytic Study of the Child*, 20:394-424.

—— see also SANDLER, J.

JONES, E. (1922), Some Problems of Adolescence. *Papers on Psycho-Analysis.* London: Baillière, Tindall & Cox, 5th ed., 1948, pp. 389-406.

KATAN, A. (1937), The Role of Displacement in Agoraphobia. *Int. J. Psycho-Anal.*, 32:41-50, 1951.

—— (1960), The Nursery School as a Diagnostic Help to the Child Guidance Clinic. In: *Recent Developments in Psychoanalytic Child Therapy*, ed. J. Weinreb. New York: International Universities Press, pp. 93-107.

—— see also FURMAN, R. A.

KATAN, M. (1950), Structural Aspects of a Case of Schizophrenia. *The Psychoanalytic Study of the Child*, 5:175-211.

KATZ, J., GOLDSTEIN, J., & DERSHOWITZ, A. M. (1967), *Psychoanalysis, Psychiatry and Law*. New York: Free Press.

—— see also GOLDSTEIN, J.

KESTENBERG, J. S. (1967-1968), Phases of Adolescence: Parts I, II, & III. *J. Amer. Acad. Child Psychiat.*, 6:426-463; 6:577-614; 7:108-151.

KHAN, M. M. R. (1963), The Concept of Cumulative Trauma. *The Psychoanalytic Study of the Child*, 18:286-306.

KING, T. (no date), *From the Pen of F. Truby King* [Chapters Compiled from the Writings and Lectures of the Late Truby King, by R. F. Snowden & H. Deem]. Auckland: Whitcombe & Tombs.

KLATSKIN, E. H., see JACKSON, E. B.

KLEIN, M. (1932), *The Psycho-Analysis of Children*. London: Hogarth Press.

KOCH, E. & SANDLER, J. (1966), The Psychopathology of Rages and Temper Tantrums: A Study of Four Cases Recorded in the Hampstead Psychoanalytic Index. Mimeographed.

KRIS, E. (1938), Review of *The Ego and the Mechanisms of Defence. Int. J. Psycho-Anal.*, 19:136-146.

—— (1950a), Notes on the Development and on Some Current Problems of Psychoanalytic Child Psychology. *The Psychoanalytic Study of the Child*, 5:24-46.

—— (1950b), Introduction to *The Origins of Psychoanalysis*, by S. Freud. New York: Basic Books, 1954.

—— (1951), Opening Remarks on Psychoanalytic Child Psychology. *The Psychoanalytic Study of the Child*, 6:9-17.

—— (1952), *Psychoanalytic Explorations in Art*. New York: International Universities Press.

—— (1955), Neutralization and Sublimation: Observations on Young Children. *The Psychoanalytic Study of the Child*, 10:30-46.

—— (1956), The Recovery of Childhood Memories in Psychoanalysis. *The Psychoanalytic Study of the Child*, 11:54-88.

—— (1957), A Longitudinal Study in Child Development. Paper originally prepared in 1952 as a report to the Commonwealth Fund, New York. Read in revised form (by S. Provence) at the International Psycho-Analytical Congress, Paris, 1957.

—— see also COLEMAN, R. W.; HARTMANN, H.

KRIS, M. (1957), The Use of Prediction in a Longitudinal Study. *The Psychoanalytic Study of the Child*, 12:174-189.

—— see also SOLNIT, A. J.

KUT ROSENFELD, S. (1958), The Study of a Wasp Fantasy. Unpublished.

—— & SPRINCE, M. P. (1963), An Attempt to Formulate the Meaning of the Concept "Borderline." *The Psychoanalytic Study of the Child*, 18:603-635.

—— —— (1965), Some Thoughts on the Technical Handling of Borderline Children. *The Psychoanalytic Study of the Child*, 20:495-517.

LAMPL-DE GROOT, J. (1950), On Masturbation and Its Influence on General Development. *The Psychoanalytic Study of the Child*, 5:153-174.

—— (1960), On Adolescence. *The Psychoanalytic Study of the Child*, 15:95-103.

—— (1965), *The Development of the Mind: Psychoanalytic Papers on Clinical and Theoretical Problems*. New York: International Universities Press.

LANDAUER, K. (1935), Die Ich-Organisation in der Pubertät. *Z. psychoanal. Päd.*, 9:380-420.

LANDER, J. (1942), The Pubertal Struggle Against the Instincts. *Amer. J. Orthopsychiat.*, 12:456-462.

LAUFER, M. (1964), Ego Ideal and Pseudo Ego Ideal in Adolescence. *The Psychoanalytic Study of the Child*, 19:196-221.

────── (1965), Assessment of Adolescent Disturbances: The Application of Anna Freud's Diagnostic Profile. *The Psychoanalytic Study of the Child*, 20:99-123.

────── (1966), Object Loss and Mourning during Adolescence. *The Psychoanalytic Study of the Child*, 21:269-293.

────── (1968), The Body Image, the Function of Masturbation, and Adolescence: Problems of the Ownership of the Body. *The Psychoanalytic Study of the Child*, 23:114-137.

LEVY, K. (1960), Simultaneous Analysis of a Mother and Her Adolescent Daughter: The Mother's Contribution to the Loosening of the Infantile Object Tie. *The Psychoanalytic Study of the Child*, 15:378-391.

LEWIN, B. D. (1961), Reflections on Depression. *The Psychoanalytic Study of the Child*, 16:321-331.

LIPTON, R. C., see COLEMAN, R. W.

LOEWENSTEIN, R. M. (1956), Some Remarks on the Rôle of Speech in Psycho-Analytic Technique. *Int. J. Psycho-Anal.*, 37:460-468.

────── see also HARTMANN, H.

LORAND, S. & SCHNEER, H. I., Eds. (1962), *Adolescents: Psychoanalytic Approach to Problems and Therapy*. New York: Hoeber.

LUDOWYK GYOMROI, E., see GYOMROI, L. E.

LUSSIER, A. (1960), The Analysis of a Boy with a Congenital Deformity. *The Psychoanalytic Study of the Child*, 15:430-453.

────── see also BURLINGHAM, D.

McGHIE, A., see FREEMAN, T.

McCOLLUM, A. T., see RITVO, S.

McDONALD, M. (1964), A Study of the Reactions of Nursery School Children to the Death of a Child's Mother. *The Psychoanalytic Study of the Child*, 19:358-376.

MAENCHEN, A. (1946), A Case of Superego Disintegration. *The Psychoanalytic Study of the Child*, 2:257-262.

MAHLER, M. S. (1952), On Child Psychosis and Schizophrenia: Autistic and Symbiotic Infantile Psychoses. *The Psychoanalytic Study of the Child*, 7:286-305.

——— (1961), On Sadness and Grief in Infancy and Childhood: Loss and Restoration of the Symbiotic Love Object. *The Psychoanalytic Study of the Child*, 16:332-351.

MASSERMAN, J. H. (1943), *Behavior and Neurosis: An Experimental Psychoanalytic Approach to Psychobiologic Principles*. Chicago: Chicago University Press.

MEERS, D. R. (1966), A Diagnostic Profile of Psychopathology in a Latency Child. *The Psychoanalytic Study of the Child*, 21:483-526.

——— see also SANDLER, J.

MENNINGER, K. A. (1954), Regulatory Devices of the Ego Under Major Stress. *Int. J. Psycho-Anal.*, 35:412-420.

MICHAELS, J. J. & STIVER, I. P. (1965), The Impulsive Psychopathic Character according to the Diagnostic Profile. *The Psychoanalytic Study of the Child*, 20:124-141.

MILNER, M. (1952), Aspects of Symbolism in Comprehension of the Not-Self. *Int. J. Psycho-Anal.*, 33:181-195.

——— (1957), *On Not Being Able to Paint*. London: Heinemann; New York: International Universities Press.

MODEL, E., see THOMAS, R.

MONCHAUX, C. DE (1958), Pooling of Case Material: A Methodological Project. *Proc. Roy. Soc. Med.*, 51:946-947.

NAGERA, H. (1963), The Developmental Profile: Notes on Some Practical Considerations Regarding Its Use. *The Psychoanalytic Study of the Child*, 18:511-540.

——— (1964a), On Arrest in Development, Fixation, and Regression. *The Psychoanalytic Study of the Child*, 19:222-239.

——— (1964b), Autoerotism, Autoerotic Activities, and Ego Development. *The Psychoanalytic Study of the Child*, 19:-240-255.

——— (1966a), Sleep and Its Disturbances Approached Developmentally. *The Psychoanalytic Study of the Child*, 21:-393-447.

―――― (1966b), *Early Childhood Disturbances, the Infantile Neurosis, and the Adulthood Disturbances* [*Monograph Series of the Psychoanalytic Study of the Child*, No. 2]. New York: International Universities Press.

―――― (1969), Children's Reactions to the Death of Important Objects. *The Psychoanalytic Study of the Child*, 24 (in press).

―――― & COLONNA, A. B. (1965), Aspects of the Contribution of Sight to Ego and Drive Development: A Comparison of the Development of Some Blind and Sighted Children. *The Psychoanalytic Study of the Child*, 20:267-287.

―――― see also SANDLER, J.

NEUBAUER, P. B. (1960), The One-Parent Child and His Oedipal Development. *The Psychoanalytic Study of the Child*, 15:286-309.

―――― (1967), Trauma and Psychopathology. In: *Psychic Trauma*, ed. S. S. Furst. New York: Basic Books, pp. 85-107.

NOSHPITZ, J. D. (1957), Opening Phase in the Psychotherapy of Adolescents with Character Disorders. *Bull. Menninger Clin.*, 21:153-164.

NUNBERG, H. (1910), On the Physical Accompaniments of Association Processes. In: *Studies on Word Association: Experiments in the Diagnosis of Psychopathological Conditions*, by C. G. Jung. London: Heinemann, 1918.

―――― (1913), The Unfulfilled Wishes According to Freud's Teaching [*Neurol. Polska*, 3]. *Practice and Theory of Psychoanalysis*, Vol. II. New York: International Universities Press, 1965, pp. 1-12.

―――― (1917), [A Case of Hypochondriasis]. Abstr. in: *Int. Z. Psychoanal.*

―――― (1920), On the Catatonic Attack. *Practice and Theory of Psychoanalysis*. New York: International Universities Press, 2nd ed., 1961, pp. 3-23.

―――― (1921), The Course of the Libidinal Conflict in a Case of Schizophrenia. *Practice and Theory of Psychoanalysis*. New York: International Universities Press, 2nd ed., 1961, pp. 24-59.

―――― (1924), States of Depersonalization in the Light of the

Libido Theory. *Practice and Theory of Psychoanalysis*. New York: International Universities Press, 2nd ed., 1961, pp. 60-74.

——— (1925), The Will to Recovery. *Practice and Theory of Psychoanalysis*. New York: International Universities Press, 2nd ed., 1961, pp. 75-88.

——— (1926), The Sense of Guilt and the Need for Punishment. *Practice and Theory of Psychoanalysis*. New York: International Universities Press, 2nd ed., 1961, pp. 89-101.

——— (1928), Problems of Therapy. *Practice and Theory of Psychoanalysis*. New York: International Universities Press, 2nd. ed., 1961, pp. 105-119.

——— (1930), The Synthetic Function of the Ego. *Practice and Theory of Psychoanalysis*. New York: International Universities Press, 2nd ed., 1961, pp. 120-136.

——— (1932), *Principles of Psychoanalysis*. New York: International Universities Press, 1955.

——— (1934), The Feeling of Guilt. *Practice and Theory of Psychoanalysis*. New York: International Universities Press, 2nd ed., 1961, pp. 137-149.

——— (1937), Theory of the Therapeutic Results of Psychoanalysis. *Practice and Theory of Psychoanalysis*. New York: International Universities Press, 2nd ed., 1961, pp. 165-173.

——— (1938), Psychological Interrelations between Physician and Patient. *Practice and Theory of Psychoanalysis*. New York: International Universities Press, 2nd ed., 1961, pp. 174-184.

——— (1939), Ego Strength and Ego Weakness. *Practice and Theory of Psychoanalysis*. New York: International Universities Press, 2nd ed., 1961, pp. 185-198.

——— (1943), Limitations of Psychoanalytic Treatment. *Practice and Theory of Psychoanalysis*. New York: International Universities Press, 2nd ed., 1961, pp. 199-208.

——— (1947), Problems of Bisexuality as Reflected in Circumcision. *Practice and Theory of Psychoanalysis*, Vol. II. New York: International Universities Press, 1965, pp. 13-93.

——— (1961), *Curiosity*. New York: International Universities Press.

—— & FEDERN, E., EDS. (1962, 1967), *Minutes of the Vienna Psychoanalytic Society*, Vol. I: 1906-1908; Vol. II: 1908-1910. New York: International Universities Press.

OMWAKE, E., *see* RITVO, S.

PROVENCE, S. & LIPTON, R. [COLEMAN] (1962), *Infants in Institutions*. New York: International Universities Press.

—— *see also* COLEMAN, R. W.; RITVO, S.

RANGELL, L. (1967), The Metapsychology of Psychic Trauma. In: *Psychic Trauma*, ed. S. S. Furst. New York: Basic Books, pp. 51-84.

REICH, A. (1950), On the Termination of Analysis. *Int. J. Psycho-Anal.*, 31:179-183.

REIK, T. (1919), *Ritual: Psychoanalytic Studies*. New York: International Universities Press, 1958.

REXFORD, E. N., ED. (1966), *A Developmental Approach to Problems of Acting Out*. New York: International Universities Press.

RIBBLE, M. A. (1943), *The Rights of Infants*. New York: Columbia University Press.

RITVO, S. (1966), Correlation of a Childhood and Adult Neurosis (Summary). *Int. J. Psycho-Anal.*, 47:130-131.

—— & SOLNIT, A. J. (1958), Influences of Early Mother-Child Interaction on Identification Processes. *The Psychoanalytic Study of the Child*, 13:64-85.

—— —— (1960), The Relationship of Early Ego Identifications to Superego Formation. *Int. J. Psycho-Anal.*, 41:295-300.

—— McCOLLUM, A. T., OMWAKE, E., PROVENCE, S., & SOLNIT, A. J. (1963), Some Relations of Constitution, Environment, and Personality as Observed in a Longitudinal Study of Child Development: A Case Report. In: *Modern Perspectives in Child Development*, ed. A. J. Solnit & S. Provence. New York: International Universities Press, pp. 107-143.

ROBERTSON, JAMES (1958), *Young Children in Hospital*. London: Tavistock Publications; New York: Basic Books.

—— *see also* BOWLBY, J.

ROBERTSON, JOYCE (1962), Mothering as an Influence on Early Development: A Study of Well-Baby Clinic Records. *The Psychoanalytic Study of the Child*, 17:245-264.

———— (1965a), Mother-Infant Interaction from Birth to Twelve Months: Two Case Studies. In: *Determinants of Infant Behaviour*, ed. B. M. Foss. London: Methuen, pp. 111-124.

———— (1965b), Three Devoted Mothers. *Samiksa*, 18:10-26.

ROCHLIN, G. (1961), The Dread of Abandonment: A Contribution to the Etiology of the Loss Complex and Depression. *The Psychoanalytic Study of the Child*, 16:451-470.

———— (1965), *Griefs and Discontents: The Forces of Change*. Boston: Little, Brown.

ROOT, N. N. (1957), A Neurosis in Adolescence. *The Psychoanalytic Study of the Child*, 12:320-334.

ROSENBLATT, B. (1963), A Severe Neurosis in an Adolescent Boy. *The Psychoanalytic Study of the Child*, 18:561-602.

———— see also SANDLER, J.

ROSENBLUTH, D., see BOWLBY, J.

RYCROFT, C. (1956), Symbolism and Its Relationship to the Primary and Secondary Processes. *Int. J. Psycho-Anal.*, 37:137-146.

RUBEN, M. (1960), *Parent Guidance in the Nursery School*. New York: International Universities Press.

SANDLER, A.-M. (1963), Aspects of Passivity and Ego Development in the Blind Infant. *The Psychoanalytic Study of the Child*, 18:343-360.

———— DAUNTON, E., & SCHNURMANN, A. (1957), Inconsistency in the Mother as a Factor in Character Development: A Comparative Study of Three Cases. *The Psychoanalytic Study of the Child*, 12:209-225.

———— & WILLS, D. M. (1965), Preliminary Notes on Play and Mastery in the Blind Child. *J. Child Psychother.*, 1:7-19.

SANDLER, J. (1960), On the Concept of Superego. *The Psychoanalytic Study of the Child*, 15:128-162.

———— (1962), The Hampstead Index as an Instrument of Psycho-Analytical Research. *Int. J. Psycho-Anal.*, 43:287-291.

———— (1965), The Hampstead Child-Therapy Clinic. In: *As-*

pects of Family Mental Health in Europe. Geneva: World Health Organization, pp. 109-123.

—— (1966), Disorders of Narcissism (in preparation).

—— (1967), Trauma, Strain, and Development. In: *Psychic Trauma,* ed. S. S. Furst. New York: Basic Books, pp. 154-174.

—— HOLDER, A., & MEERS, D. (1963), The Ego Ideal and the Ideal Self. *The Psychoanalytic Study of the Child,* 18:139-158.

—— & JOFFE, W. G. (1965a), Notes on Childhood Depression. *Int. J. Psycho-Anal.,* 46:88-96.

—— —— (1965b), Notes on Obsessional Manifestations in Children. *The Psychoanalytic Study of the Child,* 20:425-438.

—— & NAGERA, H. (1963), Aspects of the Metapsychology of Fantasy. *The Psychoanalytic Study of the Child,* 18:159-194.

—— & ROSENBLATT, B. (1962), The Concept of the Representational World. *The Psychoanalytic Study of the Child,* 17:128-145.

—— ET AL. (1962), The Classification of Superego Material in the Hampstead Index. *The Psychoanalytic Study of the Child,* 17:107-127.

SANDLER, J., *see also* BOLLAND, J.; JOFFE, W. G.; KOCH, E.

SCHARL, A. E. (1961), Regression and Restitution in Object Loss: Clinical Observations. *The Psychoanalytic Study of the Child,* 16:471-480.

SCHMIDEBERG, M. (1931), Psychoanalytisches zur Menstruation. *Z. psychoanal. Päd.,* 5:190-202.

SCHNURMANN, A., *see* SANDLER, A.-M.

SCHUR, M. (1960), Discussion of Dr. John Bowlby's Paper [Grief and Mourning in Infancy and Early Childhood]. *The Psychoanalytic Study of the Child,* 15:63-84.

SHAMBAUGH, B. (1961), A Study of Loss Reactions in a Seven-Year-Old. *The Psychoanalytic Study of the Child,* 16:510-522.

SHEPHEARD, E., *see* HELLMAN, I.

SINGER, M. B. (1960), Fantasies of a Borderline Patient. *The Psychoanalytic Study of the Child,* 15:310-356.

SOLNIT, A. J. (1959), Panel Report: The Vicissitudes of Ego Development in Adolescence. *J. Amer. Psychoanal. Assn.*, 7:523-536.

——— (1960), Hospitalization: An Aid to Physical and Psychological Health in Childhood. A.M.A. *J. Dis. Child.*, 99:155-163.

——— & KRIS, M. (1967), Trauma and Infantile Experiences: A Longitudinal Perspective. In: *Psychic Trauma*, ed. S. S. Furst. New York: Basic Books, pp. 175-220.

——— see also RITVO, S.

SPIEGEL, L. A. (1951), A Review of Contributions to a Psychoanalytic Theory of Adolescence. *The Psychoanalytic Study of the Child*, 6:375-393.

SPITZ, R. A. (1945), Hospitalism: An Inquiry into the Genesis of Psychiatric Conditions in Early Childhood. *The Psychoanalytic Study of the Child*, 1:53-74.

——— (1957), *The First Year of Life*. New York: International Universities Press, rev. ed. 1965.

——— (1959), *A Genetic Field Theory of Ego Formation*. New York: International Universities Press.

——— (1960), Discussion of Dr. John Bowlby's Paper [Grief and Mourning in Infancy and Early Childhood]. *The Psychoanalytic Study of the Child*, 15:85-94.

——— & WOLF, K. M. (1946), Anaclitic Depression: An Inquiry into the Genesis of Psychiatric Conditions in Early Childhood, II. *The Psychoanalytic Study of the Child*, 2:313-342.

SPRINCE, M. P. (1962), The Development of a Preoedipal Partnership between an Adolescent Girl and Her Mother. *The Psychoanalytic Study of the Child*, 17:418-450.

——— (1964), A Contribution to the Study of Homosexuality in Adolescence. *J. Child Psychol. Psychiat.*, 5:103-117.

——— see also KUT ROSENFELD, S.

STIVER, I. P., see MICHAELS, J. J.

SYMPOSIUM (1951), Problems of Child Development [Stockbridge, 1950]. *The Psychoanalytic Study of the Child*, 6:9-58.

——— (1962a), The Curative Factors in Psycho-Analysis. *Int. J. Psycho-Anal.*, 43:194-234.

—— (1962b), The Theory of the Parent-Infant Relationship. *Int. J. Psycho-Anal.*, 43:235-257. [*See also* GREENACRE (1960) and WINNICOTT (1960).]

THOMAS, R., FOLKART, L., & MODEL, E. (1963), The Search for a Sexual Identity in a Case of Constitutional Sexual Precocity. *The Psychoanalytic Study of the Child*, 18:636-662.

—— ET AL. (1966), Comments on Some Aspects of Self and Object Representation in a Group of Psychotic Children: An Application of Anna Freud's Diagnostic Profile. *The Psychoanalytic Study of the Child*, 21:527-580.

WAELDER, J., *see* HALL, J. WAELDER.

WAELDER, R. (1967), Trauma and the Variety of Extraordinary Challenges. In: *Psychic Trauma*, ed. S. S. Furst. New York: Basic Books, pp. 221-234.

WEINREB, J. (1960), Problems of Diagnosis and Selection. In: *Recent Developments in Psychoanalytic Child Therapy*, ed. J. Weinreb. New York: International Universities Press, pp. 75-83.

WESTHEIMER, I., *see* HEINICKE, C. M.

WILLS, D. M. (1965), Some Observations on Blind Nursery School Children's Understanding of Their World. *The Psychoanalytic Study of the Child*, 20:344-364.

—— *see also* SANDLER, A.-M.

WINNICOTT, D. W. (1953), Transitional Objects and Transitional Phenomena: A Study of the First Not-Me Possession. *Int. J. Psycho-Anal.*, 34:89-97.

—— (1954), Withdrawal and Regression. *Collected Papers.* New York: Basic Books, 1958, pp. 255-261.

—— (1955), Metapsychological and Clinical Aspects of Regression within the Psycho-Analytical Set-Up. *Int. J. Psycho-Anal.*, 36:16-26.

—— (1960), The Theory of the Parent-Infant Relationship. *Int. J. Psycho-Anal.*, 41:585-595.

—— (1965), A Child Psychiatry Case Illustrating Delayed Reaction to Loss. In: *Drives, Affects, Behavior*, Vol. 2, ed. M. Schur. New York: International Universities Press, pp. 212-242.

WITTELS, F. (1949), The Ego of the Adolescent. In: *Searchlights on Delinquency*, ed. K. R. Eissler. New York: International Universities Press, pp. 256-262.

WOLF, K. M., *see* SPITZ, R. A.

WOLFENSTEIN, M. (1966), How Is Mourning Possible? *The Psychoanalytic Study of the Child*, 21:93-123.

ZETZEL, E. R. (1965), Depression and the Incapacity to Bear It. In: *Drives, Affects, Behavior*, Vol. 2, ed. M. Schur. New York: International Universities Press, pp. 243-276.

──── (1966), 1965: Additional 'Notes upon a Case of Obsessional Neurosis': Freud 1909. *Int. J. Psycho-Anal.*, 47:123-129.

Index

Behavior—*Continued*
regression in, 325, 328, 332-333, 414-416
sign and signal function of, 213-214, 501
social, 217-218
surface manifestations revealing origin of, 100-101, 356-366
translated into unconscious elements, 100-101
Behavior disturbances
in healthy children, 39
initial phases of, 283
see also Childhood disturbances, Developmental disturbances
Bereavement, 179, 186
duration of, in children, 179-182
see also Grief, Mourning
Bergen, M. E., 90, 134, 234, 518
Bergmann, T., 89, 133, 292, 406, 419-420, 425, 518, 524
Bernfeld, S., 138-139, 141, 150-151, 518
Bibring, E., 195
Bibring, G. L., 153, 195, 289, 518
Biology, 511
interest in, 126-127
Bion, W. R., 168
Birth, *see* Fantasies, Sibling
Bisexuality, 65, 199, 246
Bladder control, 269, 413; *see also* Toilet training
Blind children, 8, 16-17, 25, 227, 229, 296, 353
mother of, *see* Mother, Parent guidance
nursery school for, 6-7, 373-374
Profile of, 61
services for mothers of, 6-7; *see also* Mother guidance, Parents
traumatization in, 230
Blos, P., 166, 518
Body
discomfort, 427-430
disturbance of vital functions, 215, 303
illness of, *see* Physical illness
interest in, 129
interferences with: 381, 383-384,

405-406; and fantasies, 428-429; symbolic meaning, 384
needs, fulfillment of, 170-172, 323, 387-389
openings, interference with, 381-384
play with, 329-330
pleasure in, 364
repercussions on mind, 405-406; *see also* Body, interferences with; Development, impact of physical illness
symbolic meaning of interferences with, 384
Body ego, 371, 474
Body image, 311
in borderline cases, 311-312
Body language, 258, 313; *see also* Organ language
Body-mind, 380-381, 463
interaction between, 426-430
lack of differentiation in infant, 370-371
in obsessional neurosis, 259
problem, 243, 251-253, 258, 405
Bolland, J., 88, 483, 518-519, 538
Bonnard, A., 182, 288-289, 519
Bookhammer, R., 508
Borderline cases, 13-14, 39, 44, 109, 125-128, 145-146, 153, 244, 284
assessment of, 301-314
and infantile neurosis, 307-308
Profile of, 61
Boredom, 198-199
Bornstein, B., 249, 519
Bowel control, 413
Bowlby, J., 120, 167-186, 519, 536-538
Boy
aftereffect of suppositories, 384-385
behavior in phallic phase, 308
envy of sister, 57
femininity in, 113-114
heightened castration anxiety in, 308
love for and rivalry with father, 270; *see also* Oedipus complex

Fixation—*Continued*
in blind, 61
gratification and deprivation and, 413-414
incestuous, 151
to mother: 151, 277; lack of, 152
oral, 309, 429
points, 302, 305, 412, 416
pregenital, 48, 129
prephallic, 215
and regression, 108-109; *see also* Regression
Fleischmann, O., 109, 517
Fleming, J., 182
Fliess, W., 105, 202
Folie à deux, 293, 480
Folkart, L., 87, 522, 540
Food
fads, 42, 366
refusals, 48, 397
Foss, B. M., 537
Foster care, 80-83, 356, 450-459, 468
multiple placements, 468
preparation for placement, 454
see also Adoption
Foster parents, 288, 296, 373, 450-459
Fraiberg, S., 144, 522
Frankl, L., 20, 85, 90, 166, 285, 482, 522, 528
Free association, 12-13, 100
and creativity, 489
Freedman, A., 508
Freeman, T., 161, 493-495, 520, 522, 532
Freud, A., v-vii, 24, 32, 34-35, 42, 52, 85-90, 93, 98, 133, 139, 141, 162, 166, 173, 182, 207-209, 211-213, 215, 255, 276-277, 285, 292, 294, 297, 302, 332, 355, 365, 396, 406, 407, 410, 456-459, 492, 517-518, 520, 522-524, 532, 540
Freud, S., 41, 47, 105, 137-138, 141, 169, 171, 188-189, 197, 202, 24-215, 222, 243, 249, 251, 511-512, 519, 524-525, 530, 541
on infantile neurosis, 47

on infant's dependence and helplessness, 188-189
on obsessional character, 214
on psychoanalytic training, 511-512
on symptoms, 41
Freud, W. E., 60-75, 89-90, 525
Friedlander, K., 525
Friedman, M., 5
Friedmann, O., 87, 294, 480, 525, 528
Friendship, 66, 156, 332, 350
Fries, M. E., 120, 525
Frustration, 228, 273, 275, 277, 279-280, 412, 416, 432
acceptance of, 277
and sublimation, 124-125
tolerance: 36, 48, 146, 148, 219, 367; fluctuations in, 225-227
Furman, E., 233-234, 297, 308, 526
Furman, R. A., 182, 297, 526, 530
Furst, S. S., 221, 526-527, 534, 536-538, 540

Gairdner, D., 379
Gangs, 156
Gauthier, Y., 182, 526
Geleerd, E. R., 144, 166, 526
Genetic point of view, 368
Genital zone, primacy of, 137
Genitality, 250
and pregenitality, 151
Gillespie, W. H., 526
Girl
aftereffect of suppositories, 384-385
development of, 277
rejection of femininity, 116
rivalry with mother, 115-116
Gitelson, M., 141, 191, 513, 526
Globus hystericus, 513
Goldberger, A., 87, 294, 477, 480, 520, 526
Goldstein, J., 102, 136, 436-437, 444, 450, 456, 526, 530
Gordon, B., 290
Greed, 327, 411
Greenacre, P., 141, 187-188, 190, 221, 223-225, 228-229, 231, 233, 235, 519, 526-527, 540

Grief
  duration of, in children, 179-182
  in infancy, 173-186
  see also Bereavement, Mourning
Group
  child raised in, 347; see also War
    children, War nursery
  role in adolescence, 138, 156
  tolerance for, and enjoyment of,
    320, 328-335
  see also Child, Residential nursery
Group for the Advancement of Psy-
    chiatry, 409, 527
Guidance
  indications for, 306
  of mother, see Mother guidance,
    Parent guidance
  see also Child guidance, Child
    guidance clinic
Guilt, 157-158, 171, 175, 186, 286,
    426, 434
  and anxiety, 154, 199-200, 272-
    273, 360
  and need for punishment, 199
  and neurosis, 154
  see also Conscience, Superego
Guttman, S. A., 508
Gyomroi, E. L., 86, 182, 527, 532

Hall, J. Waelder, 302, 527
Hampstead Child-Therapy Course
    and Clinic, vi, 1, 3-27, 76-77,
    82, 84, 122, 125, 127, 144,
    152, 189, 208-209, 215, 285,
    290, 294-295, 307, 312-313,
    348, 352, 357, 362, 373-376,
    390, 477, 479-485, 513
  description of activities, 3-8
  Index of, see Psychoanalytic In-
    dex
  research projects of, 4, 7-59
  units of, 4-8
Hampstead War Nurseries, see War
    nurseries
Handicapped child, see Child,
    handicapped
Harnik, J., 141, 527
Hartmann, H., 123, 141, 195, 204-
    220, 499-501, 512, 517, 527-
    528, 531, 532

tribute to, 204-220, 499-501
Haworth, M. W., 522
Head Start, 80
Headache, 409, 466
Health
  concept of, 218-220, 501
  see also Mental health, Normality
Heart conditions, 426
Heinicke, C. M., 180, 528, 540
Hellman, I., 13, 85-87, 90, 166,
    182, 294, 480, 482, 522, 525,
    528, 538
Helplessness, 222-223; see also
    Child, Infant
Heredity, 117; see also Constitu-
    tion, Development, Endow-
    ment
Heroism, 226
Hill, J. C., 128, 528
Hindley, C. B., 379
Hitschmann, E., 195
Hobbies, 214
Hoffer, W., 139, 141, 177, 528-529
Holder, A., 88, 90, 529, 538
Homesickness, 171, 181
Homosexuality, 52, 66, 156, 385,
    514
Honesty, 413
Hospital, 181, 354, 356, 377-378,
    415
  and eating problems, 397
  mental first aid in, 430-435
  not ideal place to study separa-
    tion reactions, 181-182
  therapist: 430-435; as auxiliary
    ego, 433
  visiting rules, 373
Hospitalization, 7, 17, 34, 276, 291-
    292, 322, 338, 361-362, 463
Hypnosis, wish for, 192
Hypochondriasis, 114, 160, 184,
    236
Hysteria, 47-48, 145, 154, 217, 226,
    243, 258; see also Anxiety hys-
    teria

Id, 154
  and analytic technique, 98-99
  in borderline cases, 309
  compulsive manifestations of, 245

Pregnancy, 153
Prepuberty, see Latency, Preado-
    lescence
Prevention, 5, 7-8, 23-25, 59, 295,
    358-361, 408, 447, 516
    of mental illness, 266-267, 271
    and prediction, 135
Preverbal phase, 99, 187-193, 474
Primary deficiencies (organic), 39
Primary process, 494; see also
    Thought processes
Probation officer, 354, 372, 377,
    447
Prognosis, 50, 59, 126, 130; see
    also Prediction
Projection, 119, 126, 145, 159, 161,
    211, 313, 365
Promiscuity, 450
Protective shield, see Stimulus bar-
    rier
"Protest," 169-170, 178, 322, 324
Provence, S., 105-107, 119-120,
    407, 521, 531, 536
Psychiatry, 307, 358, 407, 439, 494,
    511-512, 515
Psychic apparatus, 206, 305
    defective, 304; see also Primary
    deficiencies
    development of, see Development
    immaturity of, 270
    see also Ego, Id, Superego
Psychic energy
    change in, 206
    neutralized, 123
    reservoir and flux, 123
    transformation of, 123-124
    see also Cathexis, Instinctual
    drives, Libido
Psychoanalysis
    absence: of specialization, 12-14;
    of experimentation, 14-17
    applications of, 407-408, 501,
    515-516; of sum total of facts,
    359-361
    and child rearing, 265-280, 286-
    287, 298-300, 355-361, 407-
    408, 460-469
    and children's services, 460-469
    contribution of direct observation
    to, 95-101

a depth psychology, 205, 501,
    511-513
development of, 104-107, 214
difficulties of communicating
    knowledge to other profes-
    sions, 461-464
and family law, 76-78, 436-459,
    461-463, 467-469
a general psychology, 205, 501
history of, 105-106
and pediatrics, see Pediatrics,
    Physical illness
pioneers, of, 499, 502
relationship to child guidance
    clinic, 361-362
research in, see Research, psy-
    choanalytic
teaching of, 460-469, 500, 503,
    516; see also Child psychology,
    psychoanalytic
Psychoanalytic Index, 22-23, 30,
    483-485
    as "collective analytic memory,"
    484-485
Psychoanalytic movement, 195-196
Psychoanalytic theory, 514-516
    introduction of structural point
    of view, 104
    modifications of, 97
    verification, 19-20, 105-106
Psychoanalytic therapy and tech-
    nique
    abrupt termination of, 13, 144,
    161, 192
    adaptations of technique in ado-
    lescent, 144-145
    in adolescence, 13-14, 144-145,
    147-148, 157-164, 482
    adolescent's lack of involvement,
    in, 147-148
    of adults and adolescents, com-
    pared, 145
    adult's life history product of
    own memory, 132
    of child, see Child analysis
    and classical neurosis, 514
    compared with creativity, 489-
    491
    contraindications, 193

Wittels, F., 141, 541
Wolf, K. M., 120, 539, 541
Wolf Man, 216, 302
Wolfenstein, M., 182, 541
Wood, B. S., 379
Word association experiments, 197
Work, 62, 65, 291, 347, 465
    inhibitions, 48, 514

and play, 34, 329-331, 465
    see also Play
Working through, 484

Yale Child Study Center, 19, 79, 105, 107, 118-119

Zetzel, E. R., 182, 541